Surgery of Spinal Cord Tumors Based on Anatomy

Chun Kee Chung
Editor

Surgery of Spinal Cord Tumors Based on Anatomy

An Approach Based on Anatomic Compartmentalization

Springer

Editor
Chun Kee Chung
Department of Neurosurgery
Seoul National University Hospital
Seoul National University
College of Medicine
Seoul, Republic of Korea

Neuroscience Research Institute
Seoul National University
Medical Research Center
Seoul, Republic of Korea

Clinical Research Institute
Seoul National University Hospital
Seoul, Republic of Korea

Department of Brain and Cognitive
Sciences, Seoul National University
College of Natural Sciences
Seoul, Republic of Korea

ISBN 978-981-15-7770-3 ISBN 978-981-15-7771-0 (eBook)
https://doi.org/10.1007/978-981-15-7771-0

This Springer imprint is published by the registered company Springer Nature Singapore Pte Ltd.
The registered company address is: 152 Beach Road, #21-01/04 Gateway East, Singapore 189721, Singapore

Foreword

Surgery for spinal cord tumors was revolutionized after introduction of the magnetic resonance imaging and the operating microscope into the clinical practice. In spite of these advances in diagnostic and surgical equipment, the surgery has been a major challenge for spine surgeons owing to the limited case experience with lack of practical literatures. Since most previous literatures on spinal cord tumors described epidemiology and/or pathologic findings, they have been in short of helping spine surgeons to care of spinal cord tumors. The purpose of this book is to improve the safety and perfectiveness of surgery for spinal cord tumor in a very pragmatic way. Professor Chung emphasizes anatomical layers between the tumor and normal nervous tissue, which would facilitate to remove the tumor safely on the tumor side. This book successfully addresses the unmet need which all the spine surgeons have been felt during their career. Undoubtedly, it would be a book of reference for spinal surgeons who are interested in spinal cord tumor surgery and surely would guide them through the most challenging surgery to the goal of much better outcome. The beauty of this book lies on unleashing shortcomings of the traditional concepts and dogmas and building a general concept of interface between spinal cord tumors and normal nervous tissues, which enables a safer approach to the tumors with anatomical resection of the tumor only.

As a teacher and predecessor of Professor Chung, I am deeply grateful for his endeavor and congratulate Professor Chung and all the contributors for their excellent effort to make a practical book. I expect that this book will be a reference for all spinal surgeons before every surgery for a patient with spinal cord tumors, in order to guarantee better lives of patients they are taking care of.

Hyun-Jib Kim MD, PhD
Professor Emeritus
Department of Neurosurgery
Seoul National University College of Medicine
Seoul, Korea

Preface

My career as a neurosurgeon who has had a rare privilege of performing surgery almost continuously to the patients having spinal cord tumors for almost 30 years leads me to feel obliged to detail my experience as well as the change I made in the planning and doing the surgery, and to let them available to the future generation of neurosurgeons who surely would keep doing surgery to the patients with spinal cord tumors, which is of a potentially devastating impact to the patients themselves as well as the loving persons who shares their lives with the patients. In this regard, I always feel much honor and also pressure since I am not taking care of the particular disease but also the way of life the patient expects to have. When we take the responsibility and honor of providing care to the spinal cord tumor patients, the odds at our hands include the way the patient lives as well as persons who would and should live with their loving one.

Hence during my whole career, I always have tried to overcome my shortcomings and the complications that I had to incur to my respectable patients because of my limited understandings of the disease, in this case spinal cord tumors. In that sense, I owe the overall improvement of surgical planning and surgery summarized here in this book to the patients who embraced complications gracefully and encouraged me. They taught me how to live with those complications. My feeling of indebtedness to the patients is the foremost reason that I decided to write this book on anatomical compartment based spinal cord tumor surgery.

Hence I decided that everything in surgery should be undergone strict scrutiny. There are several things I discarded early in my career. I do not use steroids perioperatively. The evidence favoring the use of steroids was at most marginal or contrary to the belief bringing harms instead of benefit. I encourage patients to walk as early as possible. Hence unless the neurological status does not allow, every patient once they returned to their bed after surgery is urged to walk immediately. Hence in a sense, the patient should walk right from the stretcher car to their bed. I stopped prescribing opioid analgesics around the year 2010, when I began to feel that opioids are not decreasing pain, but leading the patient to the other way that we never expected. Opioids are not relieving pain, but introduce a kind of deviation to turn away from pain. At last, usually the patients were remained with pain with withdrawal symptoms from opioids. Also I encouraged, or coerced in the other way, to stretch their body part if they feel pain in that specific body part. I tried to reduce the analgesia drugs. I am not using the so-called patient controlled analgesia. Also I encouraged the patient to drink as much as possible water daily. In that sense, the patient should be rid of all intravenous lines immediately after they returned to the bed.

I ought to make my patient with my surgery better than or at the least not worse than their preoperative status. With those principles in mind, I let them use their body as much as possible, which make it obvious to me and patients as well what I am wrong at.

I am not immune to the complications, instead my surgical career has been dotted with major complications all the way to the present. What I have tried is that with one complication, I constructed some hypotheses to avoid that complication in the next surgery, although I have to acknowledge that my hypothesis about the incident would not be right. Despite of these limitations I am aware of, I at least changed one thing at a time with a complication that I might prevent.

This book summarizes all my experiences which were acquired from these painful experiences. I have learned much more from my complications than my uneventful surgeries.

Therefore I would like to reiterate my indebtedness to my patients. They could not be too much acclaimed. They taught me, and I have learned from the scratch to what I know at present. I deeply owe them.

To make this book appeared, I owe many people. Firstly I mention one of my patient, Jung Sook Choi, who donated funds to support this project. Then I appreciate Dr. Chang-Hyun Lee, who orchestrated all the projects. Dr. Dong Hwan Kim and Dr. Yong San Ko worked really hard to provide all the data and to edit all the surgical videos. Without them, this book would not be possible. From the contributors, I particularly would like to mention Professor Yong Il Hwang, who contributed an anatomy chapter. He provided the foundation on which all other chapters were based. During my career, I have had an honor of working with the most brilliant persons, who contributed most chapters in this book. They are my colleagues and my former fellows, to whom I would like to use this occasion to expressing my deepest gratitude.

I would like to wrap this preface with appreciating my family. My wife, Professor Hyun Ah Kim should be merited. Without her support and encouragement, I never could stand out with all those life events. I dedicate this book to my loving daughters, Seung Won and Seung Min. I love you.

Seoul, Republic of Korea
October, 2019

Chun Kee Chung

Contents

1 Epidemiology of Spinal Cord Tumors

Seil Sohn and Chun Kee Chung

Abstract

Background. We would like to introduce epidemiology of spinal cord tumors based on academic nationwide studies. Methods. Korean National Health Insurance (NHI) Corporation's database and nationwide cancer registry (KCCR) were used for epidemiology. Newly diagnosed spinal cord tumor was investigated between 2009 and 2012 from NHI data. In KCCR data, primary spinal cord and appendage tumors (PSCATs) were from 2006 to 2010. Results. Of 1600 primary spine tumors diagnosed from 2009 to 2012, 373 (23.3%) were malignant and 1227 (76.7%) were nonmalignant. Differences in primary malignant, primary nonmalignant spine tumor incidence by sex were significant ($P = 0.004, < 0.001$, respectively). The most common histological type was neurilemomas (41.3%), followed by meningiomas (20.1%) and ependymomas (7.6%).

Keywords

Epidemiology · Neoplasm · Population · Spinal cord · Spine

S. Sohn
Department of Neurosurgery, Spine Center, CHA University, CHA Bundang Medical Center, Seongnam-si, Gyeonggi-do, South Korea
e-mail: seilsohn@gmail.com

C. K. Chung (✉)
Department of Neurosurgery, Seoul National University Hospital, Seoul National University College of Medicine, Seoul, Republic of Korea
e-mail: chungc@snu.ac.kr

Neuroscience Research Institute, Seoul National University Medical Research Center, Seoul, Republic of Korea

Clinical Research Institute, Seoul National University Hospital, Seoul, Republic of Korea

Department of Brain and Cognitive Sciences, Seoul National University College of Natural Sciences, Seoul, Republic of Korea

1.1 Introduction

The relative rarity of primary spine tumors limits the level of research, treatment decisions, and health-care planning [1–4]. There have been several reports about population-based incidence rates [3–7]. However, nationwide studies are very rare. In Korea, there have been a few studies about epidemiology of spinal cord tumor [8–11]. In this chapter, we would like to introduce epidemiology of spinal cord tumors based on academic nationwide studies.

C. K. Chung (ed.), *Surgery of Spinal Cord Tumors Based on Anatomy*,
https://doi.org/10.1007/978-981-15-7771-0_1

1.2 Material and Methods

1.2.1 Data Source

In this book, two nationwide databases in Korea were used for epidemiology [8, 11]. First, Korean National Health Insurance (NHI) Corporation's database registered all nationwide inpatient and outpatient data on disease and services (procedures and operations) [9–11]. Disease codes are standardized according to the Korean Classification of Disease, 4th version, which follows the International Classification of Disease, 10th version (ICD-10) [9–11]. In Korea, NHI database is a fee-for-service system. All health-care organizations in Korea use these standardized codes for diseases and procedures.

Second, the Korean Ministry of Health and Welfare initiated the nationwide cancer registry (KCCR) in 1980 [12]. The KCCR expanded cancer registration to cover the entire Korean population since 2003. Data on primary spinal cord and appendage tumors (PSCATs) from 2006 to 2010, including malignant and nonmalignant cases, were identified in the Korea National Cancer Incidence Database (KNCIDB). Primary tumors with the following ICD-O-3 site codes were included in the analysis: C70.1 (spinal meninges), C72.0 (spinal cord), and C72.1 (cauda equina) [8].

1.2.2 Patient Population and Study Design

First, Health Insurance Review and Assessment Service (HIRA) database between January 1, 2008 and December 31, 2012 were used. Every primary tumor occurring within spine is included in this nationwide study. A multidisciplinary panel consisting of spine surgeons, epidemiologists, and a radiation oncologist defined the primary spine tumors. Disagreements were resolved by consensus after discussion.

Primary spine tumor was defined by the following criteria: (1) ICD-10 codes for primary malignant or primary nonmalignant spine tumors, (2) spine magnetic resonance imaging (MRI) within 1 year after initial ICD-10 code assignment, (3) no previous same tumor code history within 1 year, and (4) hospital visit within 3 months after diagnosis. The ICD-10 codes for primary malignant spine tumors were C41.2 (malignant neoplasm of vertebral column), C41.4 (malignant neoplasm of pelvic bones, sacrum, and coccyx), C70.1 (malignant neoplasm of spinal meninges), and C72.0 (malignant neoplasm of spinal cord). The ICD-10 codes for primary nonmalignant spine tumor were D16.6 (benign neoplasm of vertebral column), D16.8 (benign neoplasm of pelvic bones, sacrum, and coccyx), D32.1 (benign neoplasm of spinal meninges), D33.4 (benign neoplasm of spinal cord), and D42.1 (neoplasm of uncertain or unknown behavior of spinal meninges).

Data regarding age, sex, health insurance type, comorbidity were obtained from the NHI database. Comorbidities were classified using the Charlson Comorbidity Index [13, 14].

1.2.3 Statistical Analysis

Frequency of occurrence by demographic characteristics and tumor types for all primary spine tumors were determined. Incidence rates by age at diagnosis, sex, ICD-10 codes, diagnosis year, health insurance type (Medicare or Medicaid), and the number of comorbidities were calculated. All incidence rates were expressed as incidence per 100,000 persons. Age-adjusted rates were standardized to "Age Structure of Population in Korea 2009" as provided by Statistics Korea. Logistic regression analysis was performed to determine the association between age and incidence rate. Rates were compared using the chi-square test or Fisher's exact test. The relationships of incidence rate with diagnosis year and the numbers of comorbidities were compared by using logistic regression analysis. A two-tailed p value of <0.05 was considered indicative of a significant difference. SAS software (version 9.1.3; SAS Institute, Inc., Cary, NC, USA) was used for statistical analysis.

Table 1.1 Description of primary spine tumor incidence by selected characteristics, South Korea, 2009–2012 [1]

Characteristics	Primary malignant spine tumor			Primary nonmalignant spine tumor		
	Count (%)	Rate [95% CI]	*P*	Count (%)	Rate [95% CI]	*P*
Total	373 (100.0)	0 .99[0.89,1.09]		1227 (100.0)	3.24 [3.06,3.43]	
Age at diagnosis, years						
20–29	27 (7.2)	0.38 [0.24,0.52]	**<0.001**†	74 (6.0)	1.04 [0.80,1.27]	**<0.001**†
30–39	46 (12.3)	0.55 [0.39,0.70]		157 (12.8)	1.86 [1.57,2.16]	
40–49	58 (15.5)	0.67 [0.50,0.84]		263 (21.4)	3.02 [2.66,3.39]	
50–59	91 (24.4)	1.44 [1.14,1.73]		325 (26.5)	5.14 [4.58,5.70]	
60–69	64 (17.2)	1.60 [1.21,1.99]		242 (19.7)	6.04 [5.28,6.80]	
70–79	61 (16.4)	2.54 [1.90,3.17]		137 (11.2)	5.70 [4.74,6.65]	
≥ 80	26 (7.0)	3.08 [1.90,4.26]		29 (2.4)	3.43 [2.18,4.68]	
Sex						
Male	212 (56.8)	1.14 [0.98,1.29]	**0.004**†	543 (44.3)	2.91 [2.66,3.15]	**<0.001**†
Female	161 (43.2)	0.84 [0.71,0.97]		684 (55.7)	3.57 [3.30,3.84]	
Categories						
Vertebral column (C41.2, D16.6)	146 (39.1)	0.39 [0.32,0.45]		126 (10.3)	0.33 [0.27,0.39]	
Pelvic bone, sacrum, coccyx (C41.4, D16.8)	25 (6.7)	0.07 [0.04,0.09]		4 (0.3)	0.01 [0.00,0.02]	
Meninges (C70.1, D32.1)	10 (2.7)	0.03 [0.01,0.04]		217 (17.7)	0.57 [0.50,0.65]	
Spinal cord (C72.0, D33.4)	192 (51.5)	0.51 [0.44,0.58]		812 (66.2)	2.15 [2.00,2.29]	
Uncertain (D42.1)				68 (5.5)	0.18 [0.14,0.22]	
Secondary malignancy (C79.5, M4950)						
Diagnosis year						
2009	85 (22.8)	0.17 [0.13,0.21]	0.215*	261 (21.3)	0.53 [0.46,0.59]	**0.005***
2010	81 (21.7)	0.16 [0.13,0.20]		290 (23.6)	0.58 [0.51,0.65]	
2011	100 (26.8)	0.20 [0.16,0.24]		339 (27.6)	0.68 [0.60,0.75]	
2012	107 (28.7)	0.21 [0.17,0.25]		337 (27.5)	0.67 [0.60,0.74]	
Health insurance type						
Medicare	348(93.3)	0.92 [0.82,1.02]	**<0.001**†	1171(95.4)	3.10 [2.92,3.27]	**<0.001**†
Medicaid	25(6.7)	0.07 [0.04,0.09]		56(4.6)	0.15 [0.11,0.19]	
CCI						
0–2	94(25.2)	0.25 [0.20,0.30]	**<0.001***	931(75.9)	2.46 [2.30,2.62]	**<0.001***
3–5	185(49.6)	0.49 [0.42,0.56]		253(20.6)	0.67 [0.59,0.75]	
6–7	56(15.0)	0.15 [0.11,0.19]		31(2.5)	0.08 [0.05,0.11]	
≥ 8	38(10.2)	0.10 [0.07,0.13]		12(1.0)	0.03 [0.01,0.05]	

Bold style indicates statistical significance. Abbreviations: CCI, Charlson Comorbidity Index †Chi-square test, *Logistic regression analysis

1.3 Results

Of 1600 primary spine tumors diagnosed from 2009 to 2012, 373 (23.3%) were malignant and 1227 (76.7%) were nonmalignant. The most frequent tumor type was neoplasm of the spinal cord both in primary malignant (C72.0, 51.5%) and primary nonmalignant (D33.4, 66.2%) spine tumors. Overall incidence rates for C72.0 and D33.4 neoplasms during the study period were 0.99 and 3.24 per 100,000 persons, respectively. The second most common tumor types were neoplasm of the vertebral column (C41.2, 39.1%) in primary malignant spine tumor and neoplasm of meninges (D32.1, 17.7%) in primary nonmalignant spine tumor (Table 1.1).

The incidence rates among our 7 patient age groups ranged from 0.38 to 3.08 per 100,000 persons in primary malignant spine tumor and from 1.04 to 6.04 per 100,000 persons in primary nonmalignant spine tumor. Differences in primary spine tumor incidence by sex were also noted. The overall primary malignant spine tumor incidence rate for males was 1.14 per 100,000 persons, where females had an incidence rate of 0.84 per 100,000 persons ($P=0.004$). In primary nonmalignant spine tumor, the overall incidence rate for males was 2.91 per 100,000 persons, while females had an incidence rate of 3.57 per 100,000 persons ($P=<0.001$, Table 1.2).

Among the types of primary malignant spine tumor, neoplasm of vertebral column (C41.2) and neoplasm of spinal cord (C72.0) were significantly higher in males than in females ($P=0.013$, 0.028, respectively). In primary

Table 1.2 Male–female incidence ratio in South Korea, 2009–2012 [1]

Tumor type (ICD-10 code)	Total		Male		Female		Male–Female Rate Ratio	*P*
	Count	Rate [95% CI]	Count	Rate [95% CI]	Count	Rate [95% CI]		
Primary malignant spine tumor								
Vertebral column (C41.2)	146	0.39 [0.32,0.45]	87	0.47 [0.37,0.56]	59	0.31 [0.23,0.39]	1.51	**0.013**†
Pelvic bones, sacrum and coccyx (C41.4)	25	0.07 [0.04,0.09]	11	0.06 [0.02,0.09]	14	0.07 [0.03,0.11]	0.81	0.592†
Spinal meninges (C70.1)	10	0.03 [0.01,0.04]	4	0.02 [0.00,0.04]	6	0.03 [0.01,0.06]	0.68	0.554*
Spinal cord (C72.0)	192	0.51 [0.44,0.58]	110	0.59 [0.48,0.70]	82	0.43 [0.34,0.52]	1.38	**0.028**†
Primary nonmalignant spine tumor								
Vertebral column (D16.6)	126	0.33 [0.27,0.39]	57	0.31 [0.23,0.38]	69	0.36 [0.28,0.45]	0.85	0.355†
Pelvic bones, sacrum and coccyx (D16.8)	4	0.01 [0.00,0.02]	1	0.01 [−0.01,0.02]	3	0.02 [−0.00,0.03]	0.34	0.330*
Spinal meninges (D32.1)	217	0.57 [0.50,0.65]	73	0.39 [0.30,0.48]	144	0.75 [0.63,0.87]	0.52	**<0.0001**
Spinal cord (D33.4)	812	2.15 [2.00,2.29]	377	2.02 [1.82,2.22]	435	2.27 [2.06,2.48]	0.89	0.095†
Uncertain (D42.1)	68	0.18 [0.14,0.22]	35	0.19 [0.13,0.25]	33	0.17 [0.11,0.23]	1.09	0.728†

Bold style indicates statistical significance. Male to female rate ratio = male rate/female rate. †Chi-square test, *Fisher's exact test

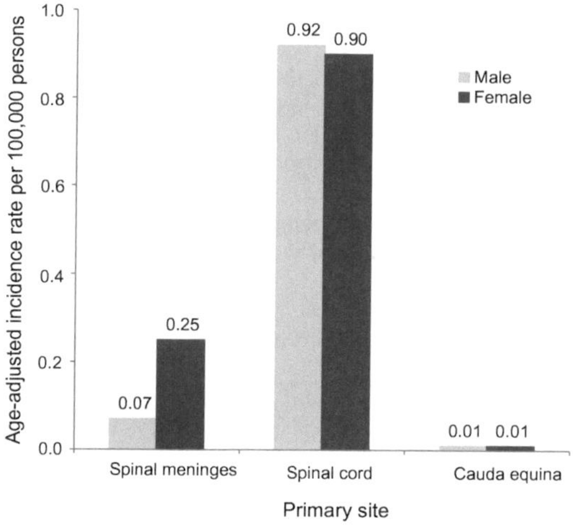

Fig. 1.1 Primary spinal cord and appendage tumor incidence rates by primary site and gender in Korea between 2006 and 2010 [8]

nonmalignant spine tumors, neoplasm of spinal meninges (D32.1) was significantly higher in females than in males ($P = <0.0001$, Table 1.2, Fig. 1.1).

The annual incidence rate of primary nonmalignant spine tumors increased significantly ($P = 0.005$, Table 1.1).

Among 3312 PSCATs cases, the most common histological type was neurilemomas (41.3%), followed by meningiomas (20.1%) and ependymomas (7.6%). Ependymomas were the most common histological type among malignant tumors (41.3%). Neurilemomas accounted for 47.7% of nonmalignant tumors.

Meningioma had the highest incidence among the spinal meninges (91.2%). Among tumors in the spinal cord, neurilemomas were the most common (49.3%, 0.43 per 100,000), followed by ependymomas and meningiomas.

1.4 Discussion

The incidence of PSCATs in our study (1.08 per 100,000 persons) was slightly higher than that observed in the United States (0.97 per 100,000 persons) [5] or Estonia (0.80 per 100,000 persons) [4], whereas it was slightly lower than that found in France (1.20 per 100,000 persons) [3] or Croatia (1.60 per 100,000 persons) [7]. When we consider all-cancer incidence rate in Korea it was 269.0 per 100,000 persons; PSCATs are very rare cancer group [15]. In our study, the most common site of PSCATs was the spinal cord (83.4%), followed by spinal meninges (16.1%) and cauda equina (0.5%). The spinal cord was more frequently cited as a tumor location in our study compared with studies in Western countries [7]. Studies in the United States reported the same order, whereas frequency of tumors of the spinal cord was less than that in Korea (60%–70%) [5, 6]. However, a study in Norway reported similar tumor rates in the spinal cord and spinal meninges, and a study in Croatia reported that the spinal meninges are the most common site with a rate of over 50% [4]. These differences may reflect population differences and small sample sizes.

1.5 Conclusion

Based on nationwide study during 2009–2012, 23.3% were malignant and 76.7% were nonmalignant. The most common tumor type was neoplasm of spinal cord among primary malignant (C72.0, 51.5%) and primary nonmalignant (D33.4, 66.2%) spine tumor. Differences in primary malignant, primary nonmalignant spine tumor incidence by sex were significant ($P = 0.004, <0.001$, respectively). Childhood tumors were more likely to be malignant than adult tumors. The common histological types were neurilemomas, meningiomas, and ependymomas.

References

1. Chi JG, Khang SK. Central nervous system tumors among Koreans–a statistical study on 697 cases. J Korean Med Sci. 1989;4:77–90.
2. Engelhard HH, Villano JL, Porter KR, et al. Clinical presentation, histology, and treatment in 430 patients with primary tumors of the spinal cord, spinal meninges, or cauda equina. J Neurosurg Spine. 2010;13:67–77.

3. Elia-Pasquet S, Provost D, Jaffre A, et al. Incidence of central nervous system tumors in Gironde. France Neuroepidemiology. 2004;23:110–7.
4. Liigant A, Asser T, Kulla A, et al. Epidemiology of primary central nervous system tumors in Estonia. Neuroepidemiology. 2000;19:300–11.
5. Duong LM, McCarthy BJ, McLendon RE, et al. Descriptive epidemiology of malignant and nonmalignant primary spinal cord, spinal meninges, and cauda equina tumors, United States, 2004–2007. Cancer. 2012;118:4220–7.
6. Schellinger KA, Propp JM, Villano JL, et al. Descriptive epidemiology of primary spinal cord tumors. J Neurooncol. 2008;87:173–9.
7. Materljan E, Materljan B, Sepcic J, et al. Epidemiology of central nervous system tumors in Labin area, Croatia, 1974–2001. Croat Med J. 2004;45:206–12.
8. Jung KW, Park KH, Ha J, et al. Incidence of Primary spinal cord, spinal meninges, and cauda equina tumors in Korea, 2006–2010. Cancer Res Treat. 2014.
9. Sohn S, Kim J, Chung CK, et al. A nationwide epidemiological study of newly diagnosed spine metastasis in the adult korean population. Spine J. 2016.
10. Sohn S, Kim J, Chung CK, et al. A nation-wide epidemiological study of newly diagnosed primary spine tumor in the adult Korean population, 2009–2011. J Korean Neurosurg Soc. 2017;60:195–204.
11. Sohn S, Kim J, Chung CK, Lee N-R, Park E, Chang U-K, Sohn MJ, Kim SH. Nationwide epidemiology and healthcare utilization of spine tumor patients in the adult Korean population, 2009–2012. Neuro-Oncology Practice. 2015;2:93–100.
12. Shin HR, Won YJ, Jung KW, et al. Nationwide cancer incidence in Korea, 1999–2001; first result using the national cancer incidence database. Cancer Res Treat. 2005;37:325–31.
13. Elixhauser A, Steiner C, Harris DR, et al. Comorbidity measures for use with administrative data. Med Care. 1998;36:8–27.
14. Charlson ME, Pompei P, Ales KL, et al. A new method of classifying prognostic comorbidity in longitudinal studies: development and validation. J Chronic Dis. 1987;40:373–83.
15. Jung KW, Won YJ, Kong HJ, et al. Cancer statistics in Korea: incidence, mortality, survival, and prevalence in 2016. Cancer Res Treat. 2019;51:417–30.

Pathology of the Spinal Cord Tumors

2

Sung-Hye Park

Abstract

The spinal cord is a continuum of the central nervous system (CNS), in which all tumors occur, which develops in the brain. Intradural spinal tumors are rare CNS tumors, comprising 22%–4% of CNS tumors. Here, a total of 892 adult spinal cord tumors from the archives of the Seoul National University Hospital, from January 2010 to December 2018, were analyzed and discussed. Among them, the most frequent primary spinal cord tumors were extra-axial tumors (68% of intradural spinal cord tumors [ID-SCT]), the second most common tumors were glioma ependymoma, subependymoma, myxopapillary ependymoma and astrocytic tumors (17.6% of ID-SCT), hemangioblastoma (5% of ID-SCT), and others including vascular malformation (5%), metastatic tumor (5% of ID-SCT), and chordoma (0.7% of ID-SCT). The most common extra-axial tumors were schwannoma (47% of ID-SCT), meningioma (16% of ID-SCT), neurofibroma (2% of ID-SCT) and malignant peripheral nervous tumor (<1% of ID-SCT) in order of frequency. The common gliomas were ependymoma (11% of ID-SCT), astrocytic tumors (4% of ID-SCT), myxopapillary ependymoma (3% of ID-SCT) and subependymoma (<1% of ID-SCT). The other tumor-like lesions were vascular malformation (5% of ID-SCT, n = 43) including cavernous, capillary. and arteriovenous malformation. Rare tumors were paraganglioma (1% of ID-SCT), chordoma (<1% of ID-SCT) and malignant melanoma (0.3% of ID-SCT). Metastatic tumors were similar incidence with hemangioblastoma (5%). The incidence of these spinal cord tumors of our hospital was similar to previously reported incidence. Intramedullary and extramedullary spinal cord tumors comprised approximately 5%–10% and 70%–80%, respectively.

Keywords

Spinal cord tumor · Pathology · Intradural extramedullary · Intramedullary · Glioma · Ependymoma · Neurogenic tumor · Meningioma

2.1 Introduction

The spinal cord is a continuation of the central nervous system, and all tumors that arise in the brain can develop. Intradural spinal cord tumors (ID-SCT) are rare central nervous system (CNS) tumors, comprising 2% to 4% of CNS tumors

S.-H. Park (✉)
Department of Pathology, Seoul National University College of Medicine, Seoul, South Korea
e-mail: shparknp@snu.ac.kr

C. K. Chung (ed.), *Surgery of Spinal Cord Tumors Based on Anatomy*,
https://doi.org/10.1007/978-981-15-7771-0_2

[1]. The present study analyzed and discussed a total of 892 adult spinal cord tumors and vascular malformation from the archives of the Seoul National University Hospital (SNUH), for 9 years, from January 2010 to December 2018 (Table 2.1). This article described the intradural spinal cord tumors about the frequency of tumors, age, gender difference, pathological features, and genetic abnormalities. The incidence of spinal cord tumors of SNUH is similar to the previously reported incidence [2]. Reported intra- and extramedullary spinal cord tumors (IM-SCT and EM-SCT) comprise approximately 5%–10% and 70%–80%, respectivel [1]. In SNUH, the most frequent tumors were extramedullary tumors [67.2% of ID-SCT] and gliomas (22.4% of ID-SCT) (Table 2.1). The most common extramedullary tumors were schwannomas (47% of ID-SCT, 70% of EM-SCT), followed by meningiomas (16% of ID-SCT), neurofibromas (2% of ID-SCT), paragangliomas (1% of ID-SCT), chordomas (<1% of ID-SCT), and malignant peripheral nerve tumors (<1% of ID-SCT). The common gliomas included ependymomas (10.5% of ID-SCT, 47% of IM-SCTs), astrocytic tumors (4% of ID-SCT, 16.5% of IM-SCT), myxopapillary ependymomas (3% of ID-SCT, 12.5% of IM-SCT), and subependymomas (<1% of ID-SCT, 2.7% of IM-SCT). The other tumorous lesions included vascular malformations (5% of ID-SCT) including cavernous, capillary, and arteriovenous malformations. The rare tumors included malignant melanomas (0.3%). Metastatic tumors to the spinal cord and adjacent spine had a similar incidence (5% of ID-SCT) as that of hemangioblastomas and vascular malformations. The order of frequency and percentage of the intradural spinal cord tumors are plotted in Fig. 2.1. Here, the author summarized the pathology of spinal cord tumors based on SNUH hospital cases.

Table 2.1 Incidence of spinal cord tumors in adults collected from the archives of Seoul National University Hospital, from 2000–2018

Tumors	% of ID-SPTs	No	% of EM-SCT or ID-SCT	Mean age	M:F ratio
Intradural extramedullary tumors	67.9%		100%		
Schwannoma	46.7	417	69.1	47.2 (20–75)	1:1
Meningioma	15.7	140	23.1	58.6 (21–82)	1:6
Neurofibroma	2.2	20	3.2	40 (17–72)	1:1
Paraganglioma	1.0	9	1.5	47.0 (28–71)	3.5:1
Solitary fibrous tumor	0.8	7	1.2	37.3 (18–61)	2.5:1
Chordoma	0.7	6	1.0	44 (20–67)	2:1
Malignant peripheral nerve sheath tumor	0.6	5	0.9	33.6 (19–46)	1.5:1
Intramedullary tumors	32.4%		100%		
Ependymoma	10.5	93	46.9	29 (23–81)	1.3:1
Hemangioblastoma	4.8	43	21.4	45.2 (16–81)	1.4:1
Astrocytoma	3.7	33	16.5	44.2 (16–75)	1.3:1
Myxopapillary ependymoma	2.8	25	12.5	44 (16–74)	1:1.5
Subependymoma	0.6	5	2.7	41 (21–56)	0.25:1
Vascular malformation	4.7	42		49.3 (16–75)	1.2:1
Metastatic tumor	5.3	47		57 (17–73)	0.9:1
Total	100%	892			

M:F: male to female, EM: extramedullary, IM: intramedullary, SCT: spinal cord tumor

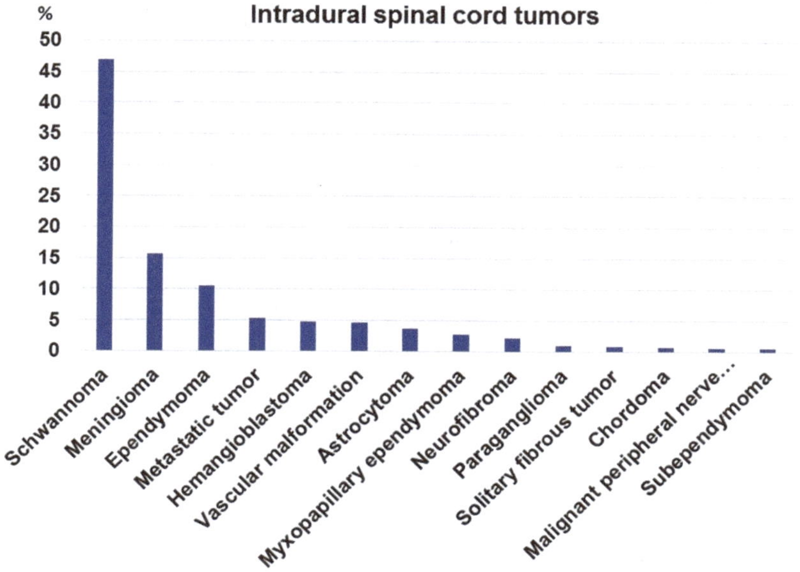

Fig. 2.1 The order of frequency and percentage of the intradural spinal cord tumors

2.2 Peripheral Nerve Sheath Tumors Including Schwannomas, Neurofibromas, and Malignant Peripheral Nerve Tumors

Schwannomas, the most common extramedullary benign nerve sheath tumor, grows eccentrically from nerve fascicles in the transition zone from the CNS to the PNS. Therefore, schwannomas often arise from the nerve root starting from the spinal cord. The mean age was 47.2 years with the age range was from 16 to 78 year old. Male to female ratio was 1:1. They are pure nerve sheath tumors composed of schwann cells surrounded by a fibrous capsule. The tumor cell nuclei are wavy eel-like, and bland-looking and taper at both ends. A biphasic pattern is characteristic; i.e., cellular Antoni A and loose, less cellular Antoni B-areas. Verocay bodies are banded eosinophilic acellular structures between the raw of the pseudopalisading nuclei in the Antoni A area (Fig. 2.2). Perivascular hyalinization is another characteristic microscopic finding. These tumors often show nuclear degenerative atypia, which is enlarged and somewhat hyperchromatic. Long-standing slowly growing schwannomas with degenerative nuclear atypia are called "ancient schwannoma." Cystic changes or macrophage infiltration are common findings. Mitoses or necrosis are very rare. Even if present, they do not indicate a malignant transformation. The shaving of tumor origin, which is the tumor attaching part, has peripheral nerve bundles, which is positive for neurofilament (NF) protein (Fig. 2.2). The tumor capsule has several layers of long slender, EMA-positive cells, which are the perineurial cells. Therefore, the capsule of the schwannoma is an extension of the perineurium (Fig. 2.2).

Malignant schwannomas are extremely rare, showing clear nuclear pleomorphism, high mitotic rate including atypical mitoses, and high proliferation indexes (Ki-67 index). Tumor cells of benign schwannomas are always positive for S-100 protein and vimentin. The prognosis is usually good when complete excision is conducted; however, without complete resection, continuous growth is usual.

Neurofibroma is a benign nerve sheath tumor composed of schwann cells, perineurial cells, and fibroblasts. The mean age was 40.0-year old with the age range from 17 to 72-year old. The male to female ratio was 1:1. The tumor cells

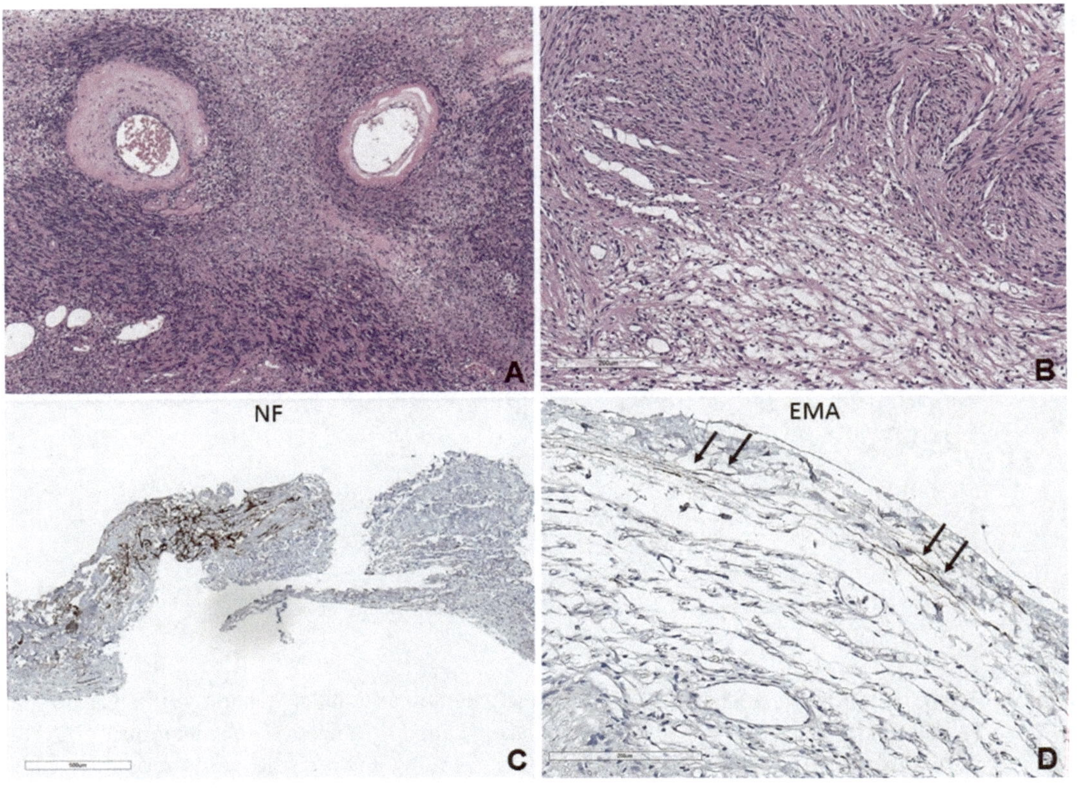

Fig. 2.2 **a** Schwannoma characteristically has hyalinized vasculature. **b** Schwannoma shows biphasic pattern composed of cellular Antoni A area (upper half) and loose less cellular Antoni B area (lower half). **c** The shaving of tumor origin, which is tumor attaching part has peripheral nerve bundles. Peripheral nerve bundles (tumor origin) are positive for neurofilament (NF) protein. **d** The capsule of the schwannoma has EMA positive thin and elongated perineurial cells; therefore, the capsule is the extension of the perineurium

are wavy spindle cells haphazardly arranged with loose intercellular matrix (Fig. 2.3). The tumor cell nuclei are characteristically eel-like with bilateral tapering ends. The tumor can be grossly nodular or diffuse without fibrous capsules. Mitosis is rare and necrosis or hemorrhage is usually absent. The schwann cells are positive for S-100 protein and vimentin. The Ki-67 proliferating index is generally very low. This tumor is mostly sporadic but can be associated with neurofibromatosis and neurofibromatosis type 1 (NF1) mutation or deletion [3].

If malignant transformation occurs, it is referred to as a malignant peripheral nerve sheath tumor (MPNST), which shows pleomorphic nuclei, high mitoses, and/or necrosis or hemorrhage [4]. Primary spinal MPNST is extremely rare, which comprises 0.65% of entire intradural spinal tumors [4]. MPNST usually has a loss of S-100 protein expression. The individual tumor cells are surrounded by external lamina; therefore, reticulin fibers surrounded individual tumor cells of the neurofibroma, while MPNST show less dense reticulin fibers than those of neurofibromas. MPNST is a very aggressive sarcoma, with five-year survival rates depending on surgical resectability and adjuvant treatment modality, but adjuvant therapy did not show any survival gain [5]. The prognosis and survival data have limitations due to the extremely low incidence of MPNST.

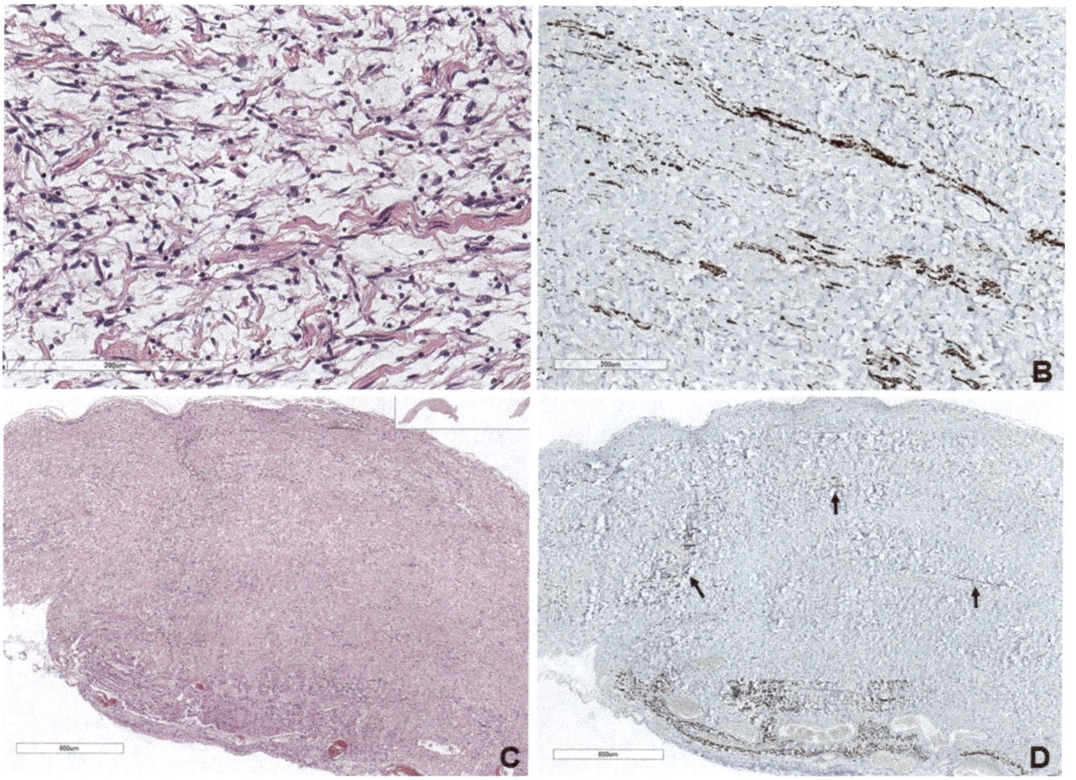

Fig. 2.3 **a** Neurofibroma shows loosely and haphazardly arranged wavy spindle cells and collagen bundles. The nuclei of tumor cells are also eel-like, similar to schwannoma cells. **b** There are some entrapped axons in the center of the tumors, here and there. This finding is the most distinguishing feature from Schwannoma. schwannoma also can have the entrapped axons that are usually located in the tumor periphery, which may be of the tumor origin because schwannoma grows eccentrically in the nerve. **c, d** The low power view of the nerve in that neurofibroma arose, showing diffuse bulbous enlargement of nerve and the axons of the origin nerve are present in the center of the origin nerve (arrows), therefore, the origin nerve cannot be saved when tumor removal is conducted

2.3 Meningiomas

Meningiomas were the second most common dural-based intradural extramedullary tumors (IDEMs). The incidence of meningioma was slightly more than one-third of that of schwannoma in SNUH. The mean age was 58.6-year-old with the age range from 21 to 82-year old. It occurs more commonly in women. The male to female ratio was 1:6. The order of frequency of the sites of meningiomas were thoracic, cervical, and lumbar levels, at 12:5.5:1, respectively. Spinal cord meningiomas are mostly benign and WHO grade I/II/III meningiomas comprised 82%, 17%, and less than 1% (0.7% in our hospital data) of the spinal cord meningiomas, respectively. Any histopathological subtype of meningiomas can occur in the spinal cord; however, psammomatous and meningothelial types were equally the most common. The psammomatous type characteristically occurs at the thoracic level [6]. Clear cell meningiomas are more common in the spinal cord than intracranially and show high recurrence rates [6] but are still extremely rare, comprising 2.1% of cases in the present study. Benign meningiomas are grossly well-circumscribed solid tumors with fibroma-like consistency, while the psammomatous type is stony hard and gritty on palpation or cut. The psammomatous subtype has extraordinary numerous psammoma bodies. Microscopically, benign meningiomas show a typical whirling (or whorl) pattern with syncytial growth of tumor cells, which is lost in higher grade meningiomas (Fig. 2.4). The nuclei of benign meningiomas commonly have vesicular chromatin with intranuclear inclusions due to nuclear irregularity. The six microscopic parameters suggesting high-grade meningioma are high cellularity, pattern-less growth with small cell high nucleocytoplasmic ratio, macronuclei, spontaneous necrosis, mitotic index, and brain invasion. If more than three of these parameters are present, the meningioma is categorized as atypical grade (WHO grade II). Anaplastic-grade meningiomas usually show overt malignant features such as pleomorphic nuclei, high mitoses, extensive necrosis, and invasive nature. Mitoses are the single most important parameter; the presence of four or more mitoses are present in 10 high-power fields (HPF) indicates atypical meningioma, while the presence of more than 20/10 HPF indicates anaplastic meningioma. Spinal cord invasion is another important prognostic factor; Morphologically WHO grade I meningioma with spinal cord invasion are considered atypical meningioma, grade II and morphologically WHO grade II meningiomas with spinal cord invasion are categorized as anaplastic meningioma, WHO grade III. The so-called spinal cord invasion is a finger-like invasion into the spinal cord parenchyma; however, pushing into the brain parenchyma or invasion along the Virchow Robin space are not considered as a true invasion. Regardless of the criteria

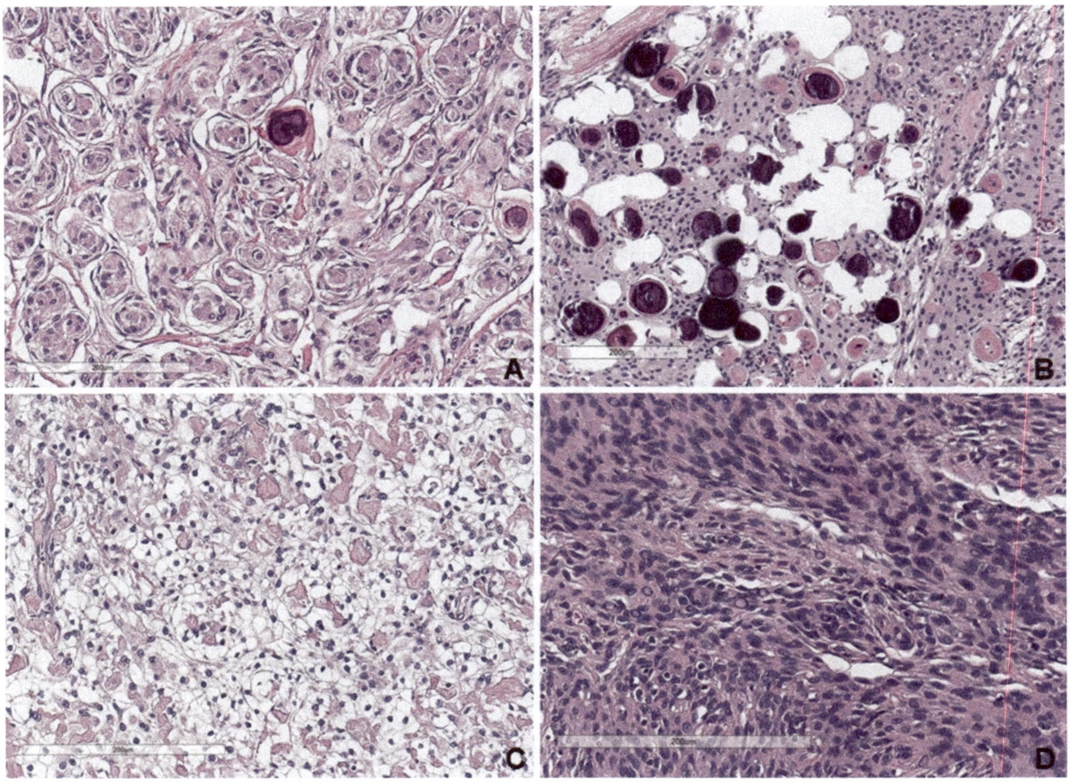

Fig. 2.4 **a** This meningioma shows a typical histopathological pattern of meningothelial meningioma, which is a whirling pattern. **b** Psammomatous meningioma is common in the spinal cord rather than in the intracranium and has numerous psammoma bodies. **c** Clear cell meningioma is atypical grade (WHO grade II) and common in the spinal cord and characteristically shows clear cytoplasm, which is filled with glycogen particles. **d** Atypical meningioma, WHO grade II shows high cellularity and frequent mitoses, 4 or more than 4/10 high-power fields. The nuclei of this tumor frequently have intranuclear pseudoinclusions, which are characteristics of the neoplastic meningothelial cells

suggesting high-grade, clear cell, and chordoid meningiomas are atypical meningioma, WHO grade II; papillary and rhabdoid subtypes are anaplastic meningioma, WHO grade III [6].

Meningiomas can be positive for epithelial membrane antigen (EMA), progesterone receptor, S-100 protein, and vimentin however, SSTR2 is the most sensitive marker for meningioma. The Ki-67 indexes of benign, atypical, and anaplastic meningiomas are usually less than 3%, 4%–10%, and more than 10%, respectively; therefore, while it is helpful for grading, the range of Ki-67 indices is wide and overlap between grades. Mitoses are a very important parameter for grading; however, mitosis count is not easy because they are usually small and not atypical. Phosphorylated histone H3 (pHH3) immunohistochemistry is very helpful to count mitoses.

Recently, the genomic landscape of meningioma has been revealed by whole exome sequencing or next-generation sequencing (NGS) using brain tumor targeted gene panel. The genetics differ according to the site of origin. The most common intracranial meningioma-associated genes are neurofibromin 2 (NF2), TNF receptor-associated factor 7 (TRAF7), Kruppel like factor 4 (KLF4), phosphatidylinositol-4,5-bisphosphate 3-kinase catalytic subunit alpha (PIK3CA), AKT serine/threonine kinase 1 (AKT1), smoothened, frizzled class receptor (SMO), RNA polymerase II subunit A (POLR2A), and SWI/SNF-related, matrix-associated, actin-dependent regulator of chromatin, subfamily B, member 1 (SMARCB1), while the gene associated with spinal cord meningiomas is SWI/SNF-related, matrix-associated, actin-dependent regulator of chromatin, subfamily E, member 1 (SMARCE1) [7]. High-grade meningiomas tend to have telomerase reverse transcriptase (TERT) promoter mutations, two hot spot mutations (C228T and C250T), are associated with histologic progression in grade and poor prognosis [8]. Loss of function mutations in SMARCE1 is associated with inherited multiple spinal and clear cell meningiomas [9].

2.4 Ependymomas Including Subependymomas and Myxopapillary Ependymomas

Ependymomas are the most common glial tumors of the spinal cord and arise from the ependymal cells of the spinal canal [10]. Ependymomas were three times more common (60% of spinal gliomas) than astrocytic tumors (21% of spinal gliomas) at SNUH. The order of frequency was ependymoma WHO grade II (73.0%), myxopapillary ependymoma (19.2%), and subependymoma (3.8%). The anaplastic subtype was extremely rare. Ependymomas were common in middle-aged men (male: female ratio 5:4). The mean age of patients with ependymomas was 46.1 years (range: 23–81 years) and they occurred most commonly in the fourth and seventh. The order of frequency levels in our hospital was cervical, lumbar, and thoracic (8.3:2.5:1).

Ependymomas are usually well-circumscribed tumors and have typical perivascular pseudorosettes composed of central blood vessels and a surrounding anuclear fibrillary zone (Fig. 2.5). The tumor cells are usually monotonous and small with uniformly round to oval nuclei showing salt and pepper chromatin patterns. The nucleoli are usually not conspicuous. Low-grade ependymomas have low mitotic rates but necrosis is possible; therefore, the latter is not a parameter of high-grade ependymomas. Rarely papillary and tanycytic ependymomas are seen in the spinal cord (Fig. 2.5). Papillary ependymomas show finger-like projections containing fibrovascular cores surrounded by multilayered tumor cells (Fig. 2.6). Tanycytic ependymomas show an astrocytoma-like fascicular appearance with indistinct perivascular pseudorosettes (Fig. 2.6). Tanycytic ependymomas have a predilection for the spinal cord.

Anaplastic ependymomas, WHO grade III, show high cellularity and brisk mitosis ($\geq$20/10

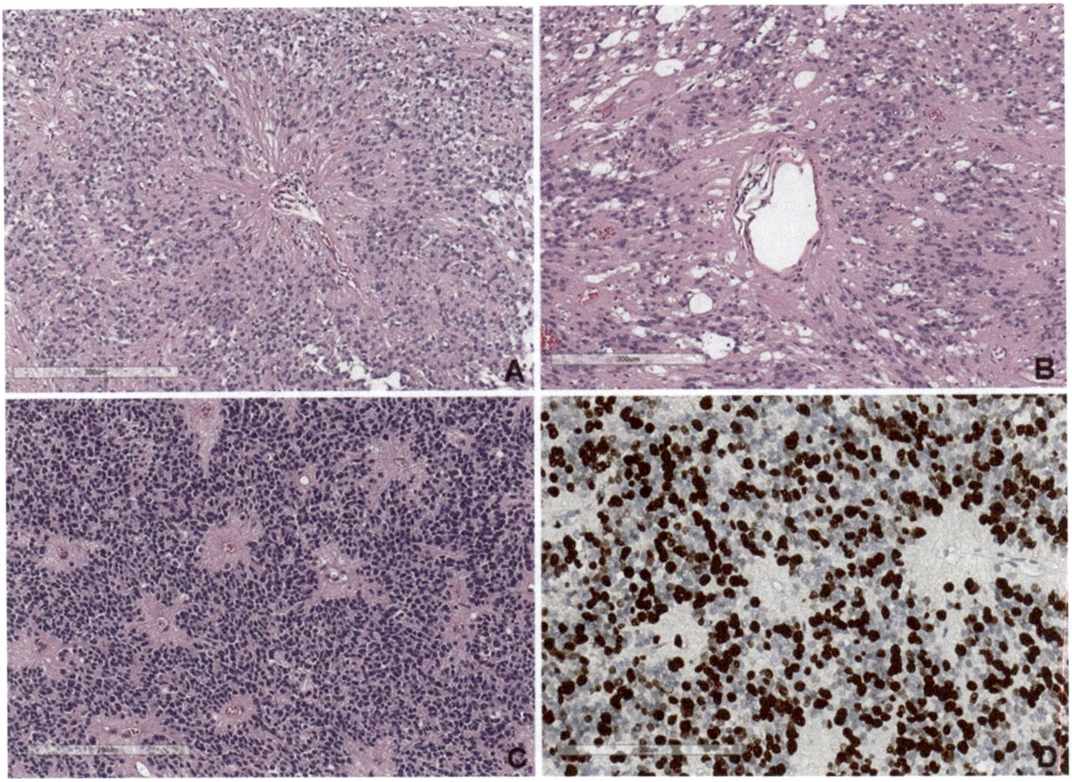

Fig. 2.5 **a** The perivascular pseudorosettes are one of the patterns of the ependymoma. **b** Some ependymomas have frequent vacuolar cytoplasm, which are the intercellular lumina. **c** Anaplastic ependymoma shows high cellularity and high mitoses. Well-preserved perivascular pseudorosettes are seen. **d** The Ki-67 labeling (proliferation) index of the tumor C, anaplastic ependymoma is very high (46%)

HPF) with microvascular proliferation; however, nuclear pleomorphism is not present or mild. Invasion to the brain tissue can be seen in anaplastic ependymoma. The most common genetic abnormalities of spinal cord ependymomas are one copy loss of NF2 or NF2 mutations [11, 12]. Anaplastic ependymomas can show chromosomal copy number variation.

Subependymomas are rare primary benign spinal cord tumors categorized as WHO grade I. They usually develop in the third to sixth decades (mean: 41.2 years, range 21–56 years) and are most common at the cervical and thoracic level. They are well-circumscribed or well-encapsulated tumors and show typical microscopic features, including alternative cellular and less cellular areas with micro-rosette-like aggregates of tumor cells composed of several cell clusters (Fig. 2.6). Mitoses are rare, and necrosis or brain invasion is absent. Degenerative nuclear atypia is rarely found but is not a high-grade feature, as described above. Genetic alteration of subependymoma is largely unknown, but TRS1 gene alteration was found in the familial subependymomas [13].

Myxopapillary ependymomas are not uncommon, which were typically benign spinal cord ependymomas that commonly developed at the lower thoracic to the lumbar levels (T12 to L2, 3), including the sacrum and filum terminale, and rarely occur at the upper thoracic or cervical levels of the spinal cord [14]. The mean age of patients in the present study was 44 years (range: 16–74 years). Grossly, these tumors are well-encapsulated and often dumbbell-shaped solid masses composed of hyalinized blood

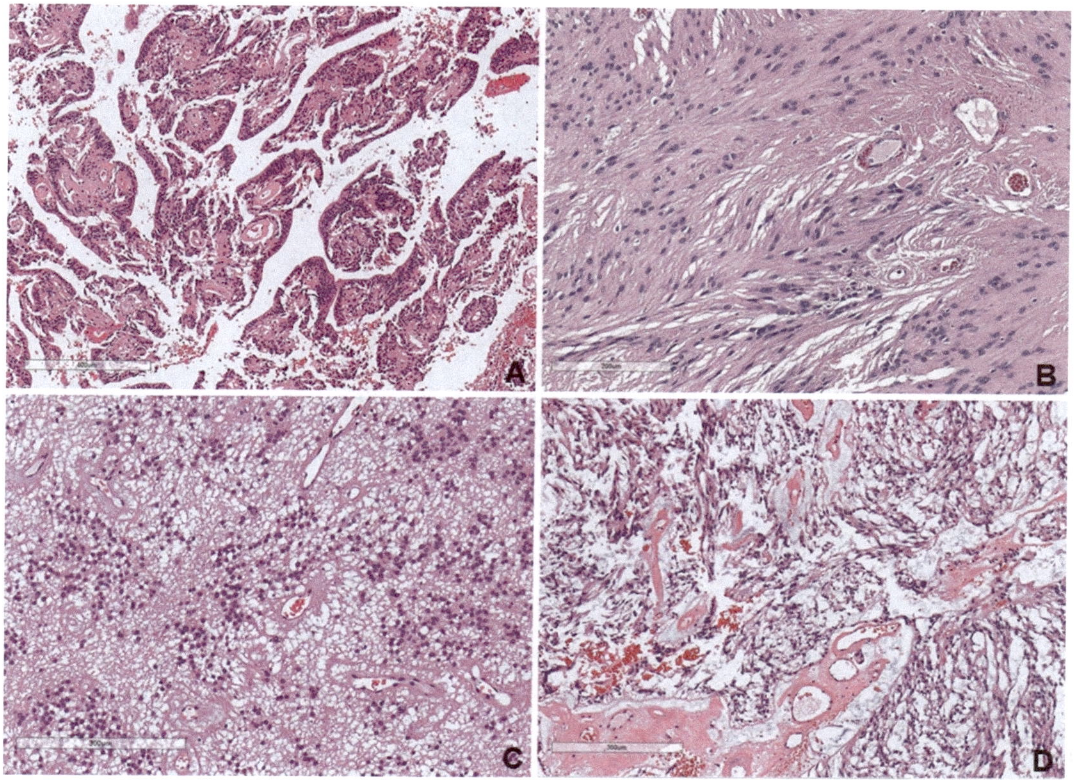

Fig. 2.6 **a** The papillary ependymoma shows finger-like projection containing fibrovascular cores surrounded by multilayered tumor cells. **b** Tanycytic ependymoma has the predilection to the spinal cord and have fascicular pattern with indistinct perivascular pseudorosettes. **c** Subependymoma shows a characteristic pattern, which is an alternating pattern of the clusters of cells and acellular areas. **d** Myxopapillary ependymoma shows perivascular hyalinization and myxoid intercellular space. The tumor cells usually have elongated cytoplasmic processes

vessels and myxoid or mucinous intercellular matrixes. The tumor cells are monotonous with a polygonal appearance and bland-looking nuclei but sometimes show bipolar elongated cytoplasmic processes (Fig. 2.6).

All types of ependymomas are positive for glial fibrillary acidic protein (GFAP), EMA, S100 protein, and vimentin [12]. GFAPs are usually more accentuated in the perivascular anucleated fibrillary zone. EMA positivity manifests as a dot-like or tiny ring-like appearance, which are ultrastructurally intracytoplasmic and intercytoplasmic micro-rosettes with microvilli and cilia. They are generally negative for oligodendrocyte transcription factor 2 (Olig2) and synaptophysin [12]. Myxopapillary ependymoma is positive for GFAP, S100, CD99 and CD56, but dot-like cytoplasmic EMA positivity or Olig2 positive nuclei are typically absent in this tumor.

The frequency of NF2 mutations in spinal and intracranial ependymoma was 32.1 and 4.4% in Lee et al.'s paper [15].

2.5 Astrocytic Tumors Including Other Astrocytomas (Pilocytic Astrocytomas)

Astrocytomas comprised 16.5% of intramedullary tumors and 25% of the spinal gliomas (one-fourth of ependymomas), including grade I pilocytic astrocytomas (n = 10, 33%), diffuse astrocytomas (10%), anaplastic astrocytomas (6.7%), glioblastomas (20%), and H3 K27M-mutant diffuse midline gliomas (30%)

in SNUH. H3 K27M-mutant diffuse midline gliomas were the most common adult high-grade glioma of the spinal cord in our hospital. Hamilton et al. reported that only 13% of spinal glioma was malignant, but it included pediatric tumors [16]. However, among adult primary spinal gliomas, malignant astrocytoma (Grade III and IV) was most common, and comprised about 57% in our series. There were 3 cases of glioneuronal tumors, WHO grade I, present. The distribution of spinal astrocytic tumors and glioneuronal tumors according to the WHO grade is shown in Fig. 2.7.

Astrocytic tumors show a characteristically pattern-less, sheet-like growth pattern with irregularly shaped hyperchromatic nuclei and fibrillary cytoplasmic processes (Fig. 2.8). According to the Dauma-Duport grading system, they are divided into four grades [17]. The male to female ratio was about 1:1, the same is for DMG H3, K27M-mutants. The age distributions were similar to those of grade I to III gliomas (mean age: 43.8, 53, and 41-year old for WHO grade I, II, and III astrocytomas, respectively). The age for grade IV GBM was 10 years less (mean age: 33.5 years, range: 16–60 years) than that for remained gliomas because half of GBMs in the spinal cord occurred in adolescents and young adults (< 40 years). Genetically, 80% of grade I spinal pilocytic astrocytomas harbored BRAF gene alteration, with 40% harboring the KIAA1549-BRAF fusion and the other 60% having a BRAF copy number gain. In addition, spinal pilocytic astrocytoma slightly more commonly has homozygous deletion of CDKN2A than cerebellar tumors (21.1%: 33.3%) [18]. Genetics of the spinal grade II astrocytoma is limited due to extreme rarity, but BRAF gene alteration like pilocytic astrocytoma has been reported [19]. Most spinal glioblastomas were IDH-wildtype de novo glioblastoma with EGFR amplification and/or PTEN or CDKN2A homozygous deletion in our series like Nakashi et al.'s cases [20].

Diffuse midline gliomas (DMGs), H3 K27M-mutants of the spinal cord, are relatively recently recognized aggressive gliomas that are categorized as WHO grade IV [21]. This tumor has somatic mutation of the H3F3A or HISTH3C or HISTH3B/C [21]. Morphologically, DMGs cannot be differentiated from astrocytic tumors (Fig. 2.9). The tumor cells are positive for GFAP and the nuclei are positive for K27M antibody, which is the H3 K27M-mutant-specific antibody. However, spinal cord DMG has a slightly better prognosis

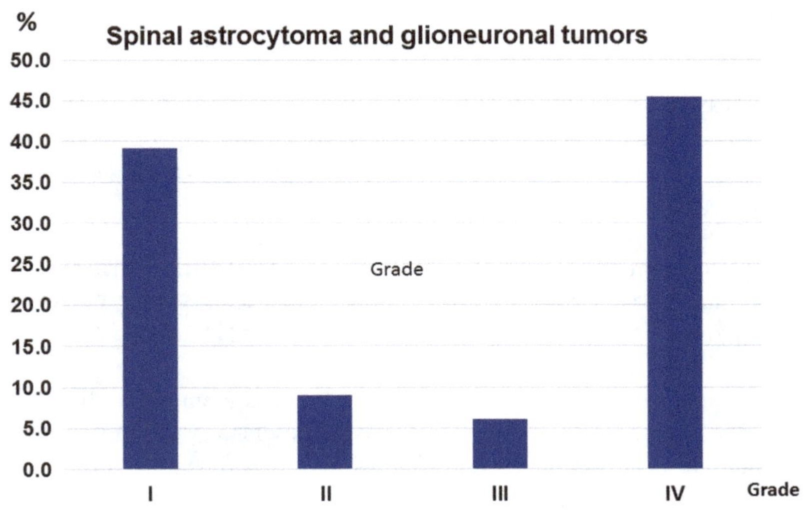

Fig. 2.7 The proportion of the adult spinal astrocytoma and glioneuronal tumors according to the WHO grade. The most common tumor was WHO grade IV, including glioblastomas and H3 K27M-mutant diffuse midline gliomas

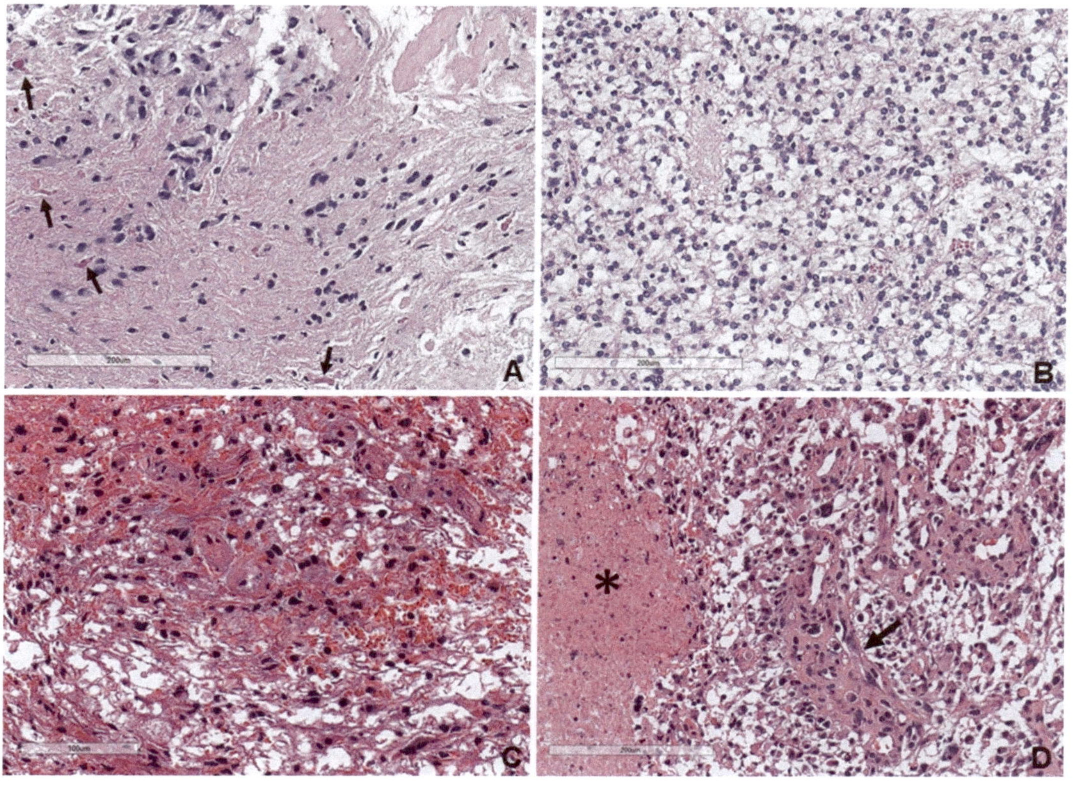

Fig. 2.8 **a** This picture shows pilocytic astrocytoma, WHO grade I. Rosenthal fibers (arrows) are present. These tumor cells show somewhat nuclear pleomorphism, which is the degenerative nuclear atypia, made by slowly growing and long-standing nature of the tumor. **b** Diffuse astrocytoma shows sheet of tumor cells in the background of the cytoplasmic processes. The mitoses are very rare and neither microvascular proliferation nor necrosis is present. **c** Anaplastic astrocytoma shows nuclear atypia and increased mitoses, more than 4/10 high-power fields. **d** This picture is glioblastoma, WHO grade IV showing tumor cell necrosis (*) and microvascular proliferation (arrow)

than that of spinal glioblastoma (WHO grade IV), contradictory to brainstem or thalamic H3 K27M-mutant diffuse midline gliomas.

2.6 Hemangioblastomas

Hemangioblastomas were also not uncommon benign intramedullary spinal cord tumors. They were 1.5 times more common than astrocytic tumors and one-third as common as ependymomal tumors. Hemangioblastomas occured in a wide range of patients aging (mean: 45.2 years, range 19–81 years). Hemangioblastomas comprised about 5% of spinal cord tumors. However, both intra- and extramedullary hemangioblastomas have been reported [22]. Male to female ratio was 1.4:1. Hemangioblastomas can occur at any level from the cervical to the lumbar spinal cord. The tumors are well-encapsulated by thin fibrous capsules and capillary-rich solid tumors (Fig. 2.10). The tumor cells are foamy stromal cells and the capillaries are accompanied by non-neoplastic cells. Immunohistochemically, the neoplastic stromal cells are positive for S100 protein, neuron specific enolase and GLUT-1. Ultrastructurally, the tumor cells have many fat vacuoles and intermediate filaments, resulting in foamy cytoplasm; however, the pathogenesis and origin cells remain unknown. Rarely, hyaline globules are present (Fig. 2.10). It can be associated with Von Hippel-Lindau disease [23]. The prognosis is good if the tumor is completely removed.

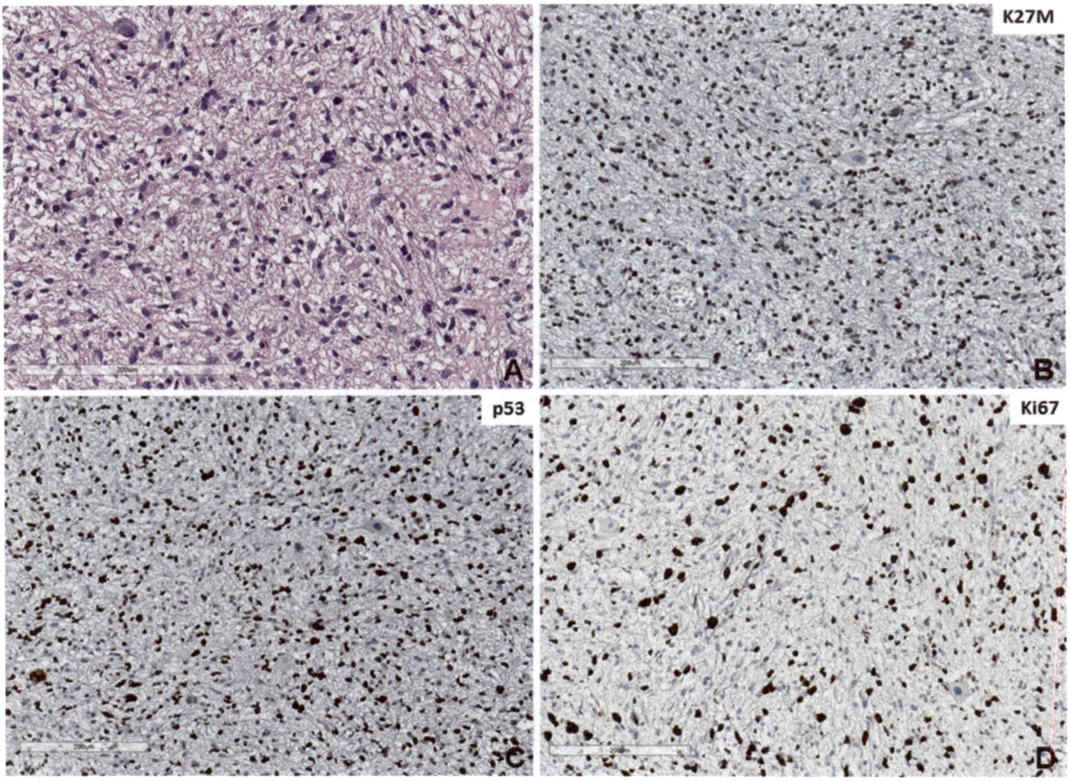

Fig. 2.9 **a** Diffuse midline glioma shows exactly astrocytoma-like feature. **b** H3F3A K27M-mutant-specific antibody, K27M is positive for the tumor cell nuclei, but negative in the entrapped neuronal cells and endothelial cell nuclei. **c** Half of the diffuse midline glioma, H3 K27M-mutant is positive for p53 or have TP53 mutation. **d** This tumor shows high Ki-67 labeling (proliferation) index, 35%

2.7 Solitary Fibrous Tumors

Solitary fibrous tumors (SFTs), formerly known as hemangiopericytomas, are rare intradural extramedullary mesenchymal tumors arising from dural mesenchymal cells. They occurred in the third to fifth decades of age (mean: 37.3 years, range: 18–61 years) and can develop at any level of the spinal cord from cervical to the lumbar levels. The male to female ratio of patients was 2.5:1. CNS SFTs are mostly malignant and WHO grade II (atypical) or III (anaplastic), while soft tissue or pleural SFTs are usually benign. Because of this aggressive behavior, the terminology of hemangiopericytomas is still used in parallel with that of SFTs.

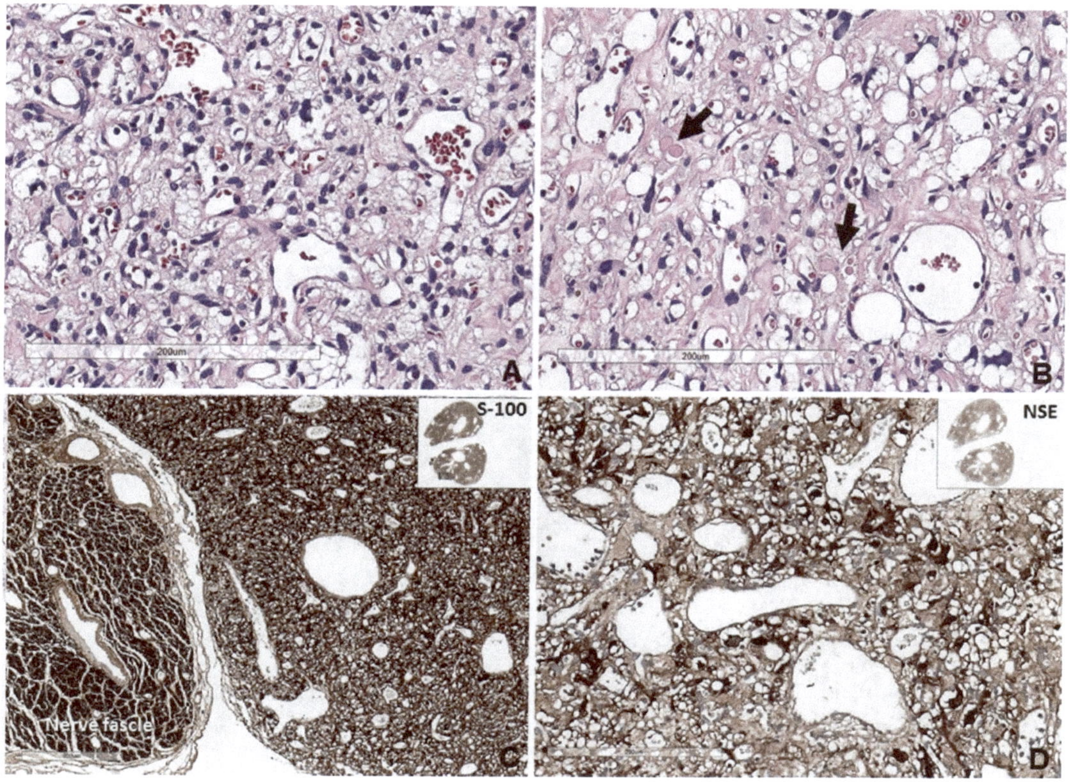

Fig. 2.10 **a**, **b** Hemangioblastoma shows rich thin-walled capillaries and stromal cells in between the capillaries. The stromal cells are the tumor cells and have foamy cytoplasm due to intracytoplasmic fat vacuoles. **c** The tumor cells are strongly positive for S100 protein, which is helpful to differentiate from metastatic renal cell carcinoma. On the left side of the picture, there is the nerve fascicles and the right side is the hemangioblastoma. **d** The stromal (tumor) cells of hemangioblastoma are positive for neuron-specific enolase (NSE)

SFTs are highly vascularized and relatively well-circumscribed. The cut surface may have a hemorrhagic firm appearance. Microscopically, this tumor shows highly cellular sheets of small to oval cells with rich vasculature (Fig. 2.11). These vasculatures show characteristically patent staghorn-shaped lumina with thin vascular walls. This tumor often has lace-like or keloid-type collagen.

This tumor is locally aggressive and late and remote extracranial metastasis is well known. A mitotic rate above 5, necrosis, and high cellularity are the most important parameters of anaplastic SFT, WHO grade III. Genetically, these tumors homogeneously have STAT6-NAB2 fusions; therefore, the nuclear expression of STAT6-protein is a diagnostic hallmark of this tumor [24, 25].

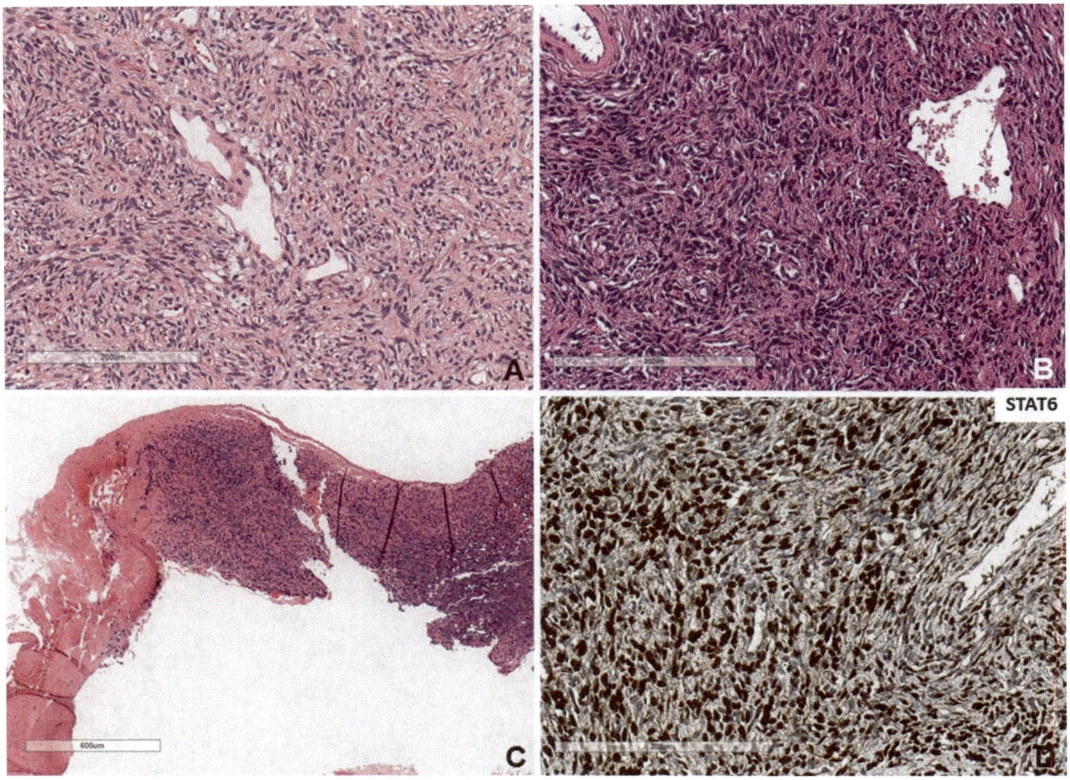

Fig. 2.11 **a** Solitary fibrous tumor (SFT) shows a sheet of oval to slightly spindle cells with minimal pleomorphism. Many dilated blood vessels are the hallmark of this tumor. **b** Anaplastic solitary fibrous tumor shows more cellular and more pleomorphic than grade II SFT. Grade III SFT usually has frequent mitoses (more than 5/10 high-power fields) than grade II SFT. **c** The original part of the SFT is dura, which is dense collagenous tissue. The tumor assumes to arise from the dural mesenchymal cells. **d** The tumor cell nuclei are positive for STAT6 because this tumor has STAT6-NAB2 gene fusion

2.8 Paragangliomas

Paragangliomas are rare benign neuroendocrine tumors of the spinal cord that mostly occur at the distal lumbar level as approximately 1–2 cm, well-encapsulated intradural and extramedullary masses. The mean age of patients with paragangliomas in the present study was 47.9 years (range: 28–71 years). M to F ratio was 3.5:1.

Microscopically, the monotonous polygonal-shaped tumor cells show "zellballen (cell balls)" due to sinusoids (Fig. 2.12). The tumor cells are positive for synaptophysin and CD56, and S-100 protein-positive sustentacular cells are often scattered or hug the nest of the cells; however, the number of sustentacular cells is very variable [26]. Pathogenic germ line variants in genes of the succinate dehydrogenase complex

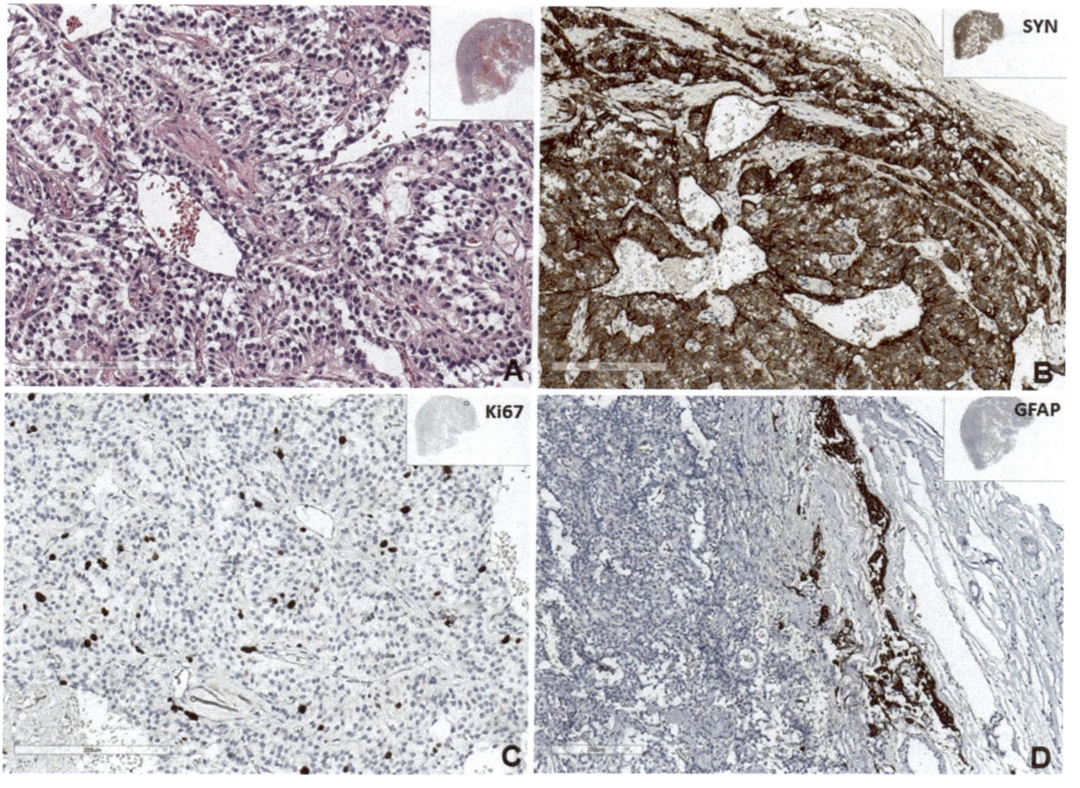

Fig. 2.12 **a** Paraganglioma shows the lobular arrangement, composed of monotonous cells. **b** The tumor cells are positive for synaptophysin. **c** Ki67 index is not high (3.5%). **d** The tumor has a well-developed fibrous capsule, the outside tissue of the tumor capsule is positive for GFAP

(SDHx), TMEM127 or MAX were found in approximately 20% of hereditary paragangliomas [27]. Most spinal paragangliomas are benign, but malignant paraganglioma rarely exists, which has to have metastases by definition [28, 29].

2.9 Chordomas

Chordomas are rare, slow-growing malignant bone tumors of the skull base and spine. The tumors arise from notochordal remnants and gradually extend into the bone and adjacent soft tissue with ill-defined and infiltrative margins. The chordomas can occur at any level of the spine but are common at the cervical level and less common in the sacrum. The mean age of patients with chordomas in the present study is 44 years (range: 20–67 years).

The tumors show lobular or trabecular growth of physaliphorous cells with intracytoplasmic bubbly vacuoles (Fig. 2.13). The nuclei are oval or round. Histologically, four

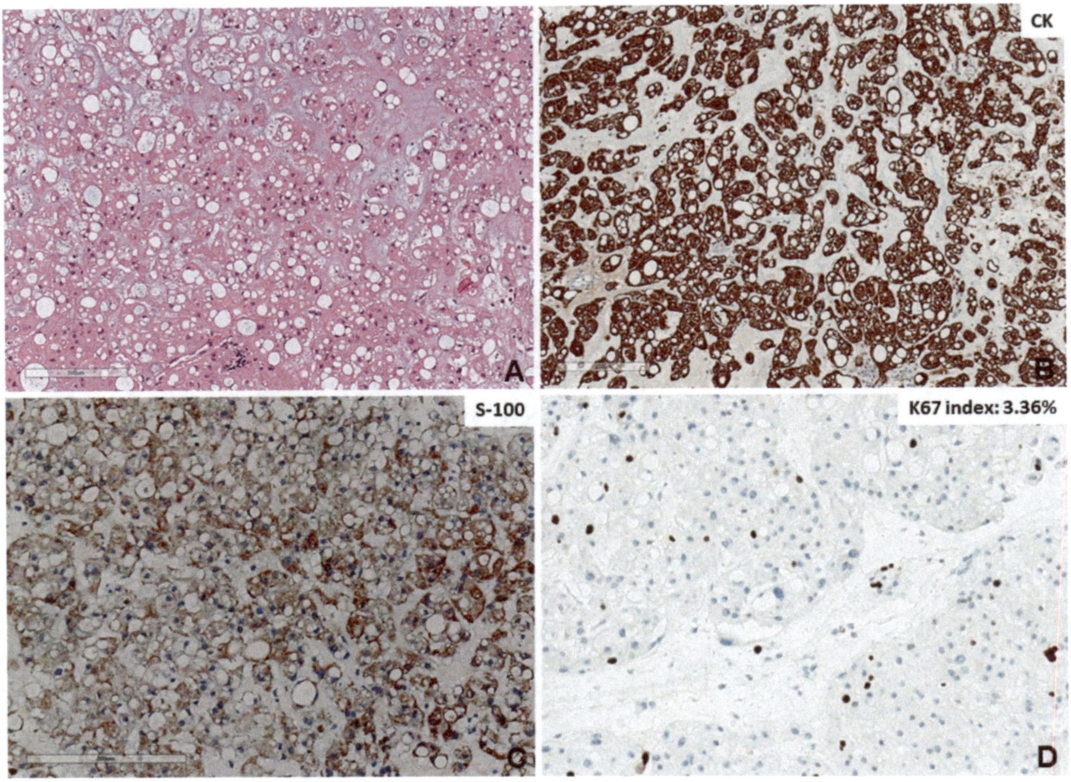

Fig. 2.13 **a**, Chordoma shows typical physaliphorus cells which have intracytoplasmic vacuoles. **b, c** The tumor cells are positive for cytokeratin and S-100 protein. **d** Ki-67 labeling (proliferative) index is usually not high, but this tumor is slowly growing malignant tumor

types are present; typical (NOS) (95%), chondroid (up to 4%), dedifferentiated types (less than 1%) and poorly differentiated (less than 1%). Dedifferentiated chordomas are biphasic tumours, comprising conventional chordoma juxtaposed to high-grade undifferentiated spindle cell sarcoma. The tumor cells are positive for cytokeratin, brachyury, S-100 protein, and vimentin [6]. Poorly differentiated chordomas show loss of nuclear INI1 expression.

The driver mutation of chordomas is *T* gene (brachyury) duplication (6q27). Familial chordoma is very rare but is associated with T gene duplication [30, 31]. Chordomas should be differentiated from benign notochordal cell tumors (BNCT), which are benign intraosseous lesions derived from notochordal cells [32].

2.10 Metastatic Tumors

Metastatic tumors have incidence rates similar to those of hemangioblastomas of the spinal cord, about 5% of spinal cord tumors. The most common metastatic tumors are lung adenocarcinomas, breast carcinomas, colon adenocarcinomas, hepatocellular carcinomas, and drop metastasis from brain tumors (Fig. 2.14) (Table 2.2). However, any carcinoma or sarcoma can metastasize to the spinal cord. The common sites of metastasis are vertebral bone, periverterbral soft tissue, and epidural space.

Conflict of Interest:
We have no conflicts of interest to declare.

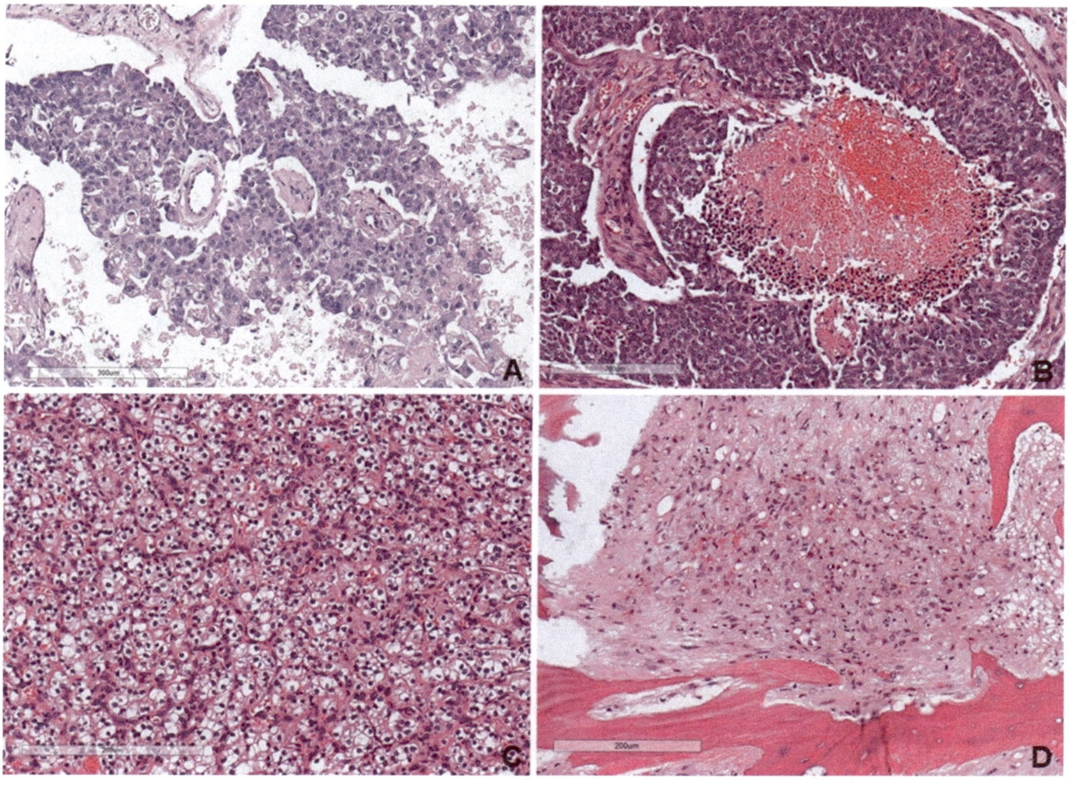

Fig. 2.14 **a** Metastatic carcinoma from lung is the most common metastatic tumor to the spine or adjacent soft tissue. **b** This is the metastatic invasive ductal carcinoma with central comedo necrosis. **c** This is the metastatic clear cell renal cell carcinoma. **d** This is the metastatic epithelioid hemangioendothelioma from the liver

Table 2.2 List of metastatic tumors to the spinal cord and adjacent tissue

Primary organ	%
Lung, adenocarcinoma	31.8
Liver, HCC, including epithelioid hemangioendothelioma	15.9
Kidney, renal cell carcinoma	9.1
Colon & rectum, adenocarcinoma and GIST	9.1
Breast, invasive ductal carcinoma	6.8
Prostate, adenocarcinoma	6.8
Brain, anaplastic solitary fibrous tumor	4.5
Uterus, endometrial adenocarcinoma	2.3
Thymus, thymoma	2.3
Thyroid, papillary carcinoma	2.3
Salivary gland, carcinoma	2.3
Bone osteosarcoma	2.3
Rhabdomyosarcoma	2.3
Malignancy of unknown primary (MUO)	2.3
Total	100

HCC: hepatocellular carcinoma, GIST: gastrointestinal stromal tumor, MUO: Malignancy of Unknown Origin

References

1. Abd-El-Barr MM, et al. Recent advances in intradural spinal tumors. Neuro Oncol. 2018;20(6):729–42.
2. Chamberlain MC, Tredway TL. Adult primary intradural spinal cord tumors: a review. Curr Neurol Neurosci Rep. 2011;11(3):320–8.
3. Ruggieri M, et al. The natural history of spinal neurofibromatosis: a critical review of clinical and genetic features. Clin Genet. 2015;87(5):401–10.
4. Ren X, et al. Clinical, radiological, and pathological features of 26 intracranial and intraspinal malignant peripheral nerve sheath tumors. J Neurosurg. 2013;119(3):695–708.
5. Chou D, et al. Malignant peripheral nerve sheath tumors of the spine: results of surgical management from a multicenter study. J Neurosurg Spine. 2017;26(3):291–8.
6. Mawrin C, Perry A. Pathological classification and molecular genetics of meningiomas. J Neurooncol. 2010;99(3):379–91.
7. Clark VE, et al. Genomic analysis of non-NF2 meningiomas reveals mutations in TRAF7, KLF4, AKT1, and SMO. Science. 2013;339(6123):1077–80.
8. Bi WL, Prabhu VC, Dunn IF. High-grade meningiomas: biology and implications. Neurosurg Focus. 2018;44(4):E2.
9. Smith MJ, et al. Germline SMARCE1 mutations predispose to both spinal and cranial clear cell meningiomas. J Pathol. 2014;234(4):436–40.
10. Lamszus K, et al. Molecular genetic alterations on chromosomes 11 and 22 in ependymomas. Int J Cancer. 2001;91(6):803–8.
11. Zemmoura I, et al. A deletion causing NF2 exon 9 skipping is associated with familial autosomal dominant intramedullary ependymoma. Neuro Oncol. 2014;16(2):250–5.
12. Leeper H, Felicella MM, Walbert T. Recent Advances in the classification and treatment of ependymomas. Curr Treat Options Oncol. 2017;18(9):55.
13. Fischer SB, et al. TRPS1 gene alterations in human subependymoma. J Neurooncol. 2017;134(1):133–8.
14. Acerbi F, et al. The role of indocyanine green videoangiography with FLOW 800 analysis for the surgical management of central nervous system tumors: an update. Neurosurg Focus. 2018;44(6):E6.
15. Lee CH, Chung CK, Kim CH. Genetic differences on intracranial versus spinal cord ependymal tumors: a meta-analysis of genetic researches. Eur Spine J. 2016;25(12):3942–51.
16. Hamilton KR, et al. A systematic review of outcome in intramedullary ependymoma and astrocytoma. J Clin Neurosci. 2019;63:168–75.
17. Kim TS, et al. Correlates of survival and the Daumas-Duport grading system for astrocytomas. J Neurosurg. 1991;74(1):27–37.
18. Horbinski C, et al. Association of molecular alterations, including BRAF, with biology and outcome in pilocytic astrocytomas. Acta Neuropathol. 2010;119(5):641–9.
19. Shankar GM, et al. BRAF alteration status and the histone H3F3A gene K27M mutation segregate spinal cord astrocytoma histology. Acta Neuropathol. 2016;131(1):147–50.
20. Nagaishi M, et al. Genetic mutations in high grade gliomas of the adult spinal cord. Brain Tumor Pathol. 2016;33(4):267–9.
21. Ebrahimi A, et al. High frequency of H3 K27M mutations in adult midline gliomas. J Cancer Res Clin Oncol. 2019;145(4):839–50.
22. Imagama S, et al. Rapid worsening of symptoms and high cell proliferative activity in intra- and extramedullary spinal hemangioblastoma: a need for earlier surgery. Global Spine J. 2017;7(1):6–13.
23. Li J. et al. Surgical management of a cervical intramedullary hemangioblastoma presenting with intracystic hemorrhage by hemi-semi-laminectomy via a posterior approach. J Int Med Res. 2019: 300060519847412.
24. Yao ZG. et al. Papillary solitary fibrous tumor/hemangiopericytoma: an uncommon morphological

form with NAB2-STAT6 gene fusion. J Neuropathol Exp Neurol. 2019.
25. Shukla P, et al. Reappraisal of morphological and immunohistochemical spectrum of intracranial and spinal solitary fibrous tumors/hemangiopericytomas with impact on long-term follow-up. Indian J Cancer. 2018;55(3):214–21.
26. Turkkan A, et al. Nuances to provide ideas for radiologic diagnosis in primary spinal paragangliomas: report of two cases. Br J Neurosurg. 2019;33(2):210–2.
27. Muth A, et al. Genetic testing and surveillance guidelines in hereditary pheochromocytoma and paraganglioma. J Intern Med. 2019;285(2):187–204.
28. Mei L, et al. Prognostic factors of malignant pheochromocytoma and paraganglioma: a combined SEER and TCGA databases review. Horm Metab Res. 2019;51(7):451–7.
29. Saavedra A, et al. Malignant paraganglioma and somatotropinoma in a patient with germline SDHB mutation-genetic and clinical features. Endocrine. 2019;63(1):182–7.
30. Sharifnia T, et al. Small-molecule targeting of brachyury transcription factor addiction in chordoma. Nat Med. 2019;25(2):292–300.
31. Meng T, et al. Molecular targeted therapy in the treatment of chordoma: a systematic review. Front Oncol. 2019;9:30.
32. Du J, et al. Benign notochordal cell tumour: clinicopathology and molecular profiling of 13 cases. J Clin Pathol. 2019;72(1):66–74.

Anatomy of Spinal Meninges and Meningeal Spaces: Relevant to Surgery of Spinal Cord Tumors

3

Young-Il Hwang

Abstract

Three layers of meninges, the pia mater, the arachnoid membrane, and the dura mater from inside out envelop the brain and the spinal cord. The relationship between these meninges and surrounding structures is somewhat different in the brain and spinal cord. In particular, understanding of the anatomical relationship in the spinal cord region is inevitable for surgical approaches to various disease conditions that occur in this region. Again, the anatomy can be more easily understood based on developmental knowledge. In this chapter, the development of the spinal meninges is briefly described first, followed sequentially by those for each meningeal membrane and the "spaces" associated with them.

Keywords

Embryology of the meninges · Meninx primitiva · Endomeninx · Ectomeninx · Dura mater · Dural border cell layer · Arachnoid membrane · Arachnoid barrier cell layer · Arachnoid reticular cell layer · Dura–arachnoid junction · Pia mater · Epidural space · Subarachnoid space · Ependyma

Y.-I. Hwang (✉)
Department of Anatomy and Cell Biology, Seoul National University College of Medicine, Seoul, South Koreae-mail: hyi830@snu.ac.kr

3.1 Embryology of the Meninges

Embryologically, meninges are derived from the meninx primitiva [1, 2]. After the neural tube is formed, cells derived from both the somite and the neural crest surround the neural tube and form the meninx primitiva. It soon divides into two layers. The inner layer, the endomeninx, is composed of cells derived from both the somite and neurectoderm and differentiates into the arachnoid and pia maters (leptomeninges). The outer layer, the ectomeninx, is composed of cells derived only from the somite and differentiates into the dura mater (pachymeninx), the neurocranium, and the vertebrae.

3.1.1 Morphological Development

The morphological development of the spinal [3] and the cranial [4] meninges has been described in detail in human embryos. Based on these works, the first sign of meningeal development appears in embryos of Carnegie stage

C. K. Chung (ed.), *Surgery of Spinal Cord Tumors Based on Anatomy*,
https://doi.org/10.1007/978-981-15-7771-0_3

11 (2.5–4.5 mm in length, ca 24 days old), as a single strand of cells migrating from the neural crest to the surface of the neural tube, initially at the level of caudal medulla oblongata and the cervical spine. Initially, the cells are morphologically distinguishable from somitic cells. However, soon, they become indistinguishable so that their origin cannot be assigned anymore. The sclerotomes persist until the next stages (Fig. 3.1) adding mesenchymal cells around the neural tube.

At stage 14 (5–7 mm, ca 32 days), vessels have been formed around the neural tube and begin to penetrate the neural tissue at the midbrain level. At stage 15 (7–9 mm, ca 33 days), the primordia of vertebrae become evident as condensed cell areas, leaving an intermediate zone of looser cells between them and the neural tube. This loose area is called "meninx primitiva" or "primary meninx" (Figs. 3.2 and 3.3), from which all the three meningeal layers are supposed to be derived. This change is especially prominent in the ventral aspect of the tube.

At stage 18 (13–17 mm, ca 44 days), the tissue of the meninx primitiva becomes looser, and spaces begin to appear in it, which are regarded as the primordium of the subarachnoid space. By the end of the embryonic period (stage 23, around 30 mm in CR length), these spaces become larger without cells but with occasional trabeculae. Another change that occurs in the meninx primitiva is its stratification. It begins first in the ventral area and extends laterally. At stage 19 (17–20 mm, ca 47–48 days), the meninx primitiva shows a reticular arrangement of its cells (Fig. 3.4). Now the distinction between the loose leptomeningeal tissue and denser pachymeninx becomes evident. Sensenig [3] described that "The epidural space is first indicated at about the 20-mm stage", which corresponds to the stage 20 embryos. However, other observations [5] showed an apparent epidural space at stage 18. At stage 23 (27–31 mm, ca 57 days), the end of the embryonic period,

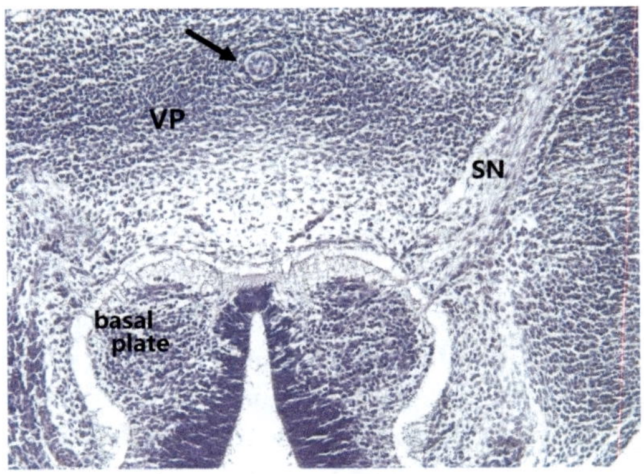

Fig. 3.2 A human embryo of stage 16 (7 mm, ca 37 days) (×200). The primordium of the vertebral body (VP) appears as a region with condensed cells in front of the neural tube, where the basal plate now forms. Between the neural tube and the vertebra primordium, cells are loosely arranged, representing the meninx primitiva, which is more or less confined to the ventral side of the neural tube. SN, ventral rootlet of the spinal nerve

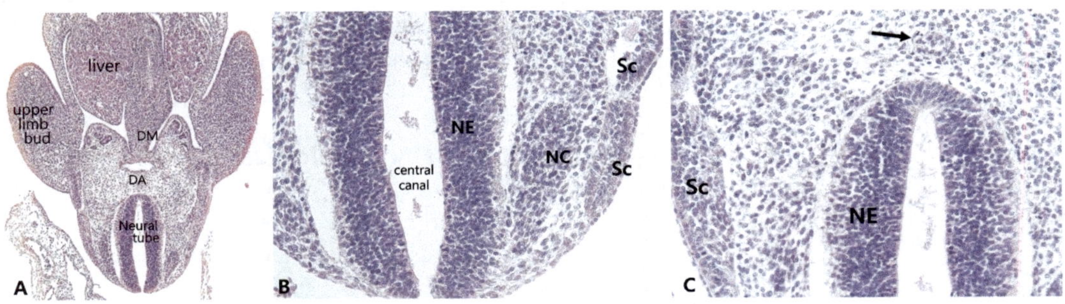

Fig. 3.1 A human embryo of Carnegie stage 13 (6 mm, 28 days). **A** Transverse section at the level of the upper limb bud (×100). **B** The neural crest is separated from the neural tube. The sclerotomes persist (×200) **C** The notochord (arrow) is located just ventral to the neural tube. (×200) DA, dorsal aorta; DM, dorsal mesentery; NC, neural crest; NE, neurectoderm; Sc, sclerotome

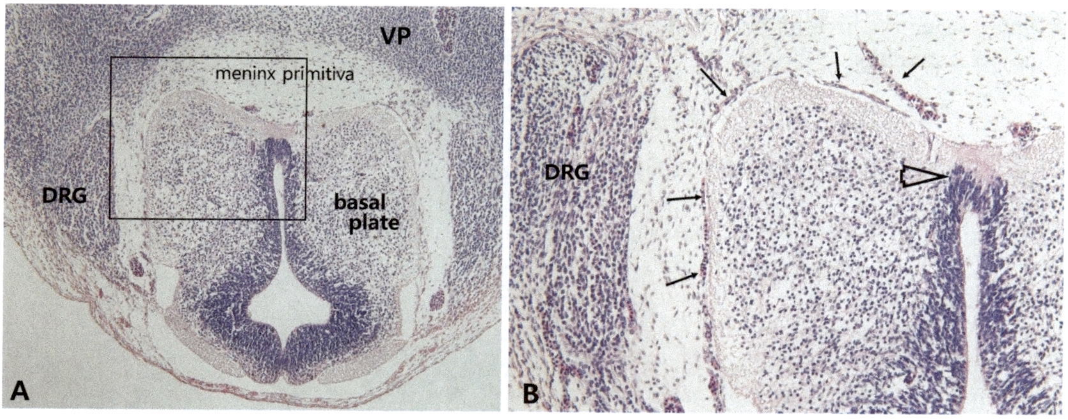

Fig. 3.3 A human embryo of stage 17 (13 mm, ca 41 days). **A** The boundary between the vertebral primordium (VP) and the meninx primitiva becomes more distinct. The latter now extends to the lateral side of the neural tube but not yet to the dorsal side of the tube (×100). **B** Higher magnification of the area indicated by a rectangle in figure A. Blood vessels are well developed around the neural tube close to its surface (arrows), where the pia mater is expected to be. The open arrowhead indicates the basal plate, which began differentiation, as indicated by the elongated shape of the cells (×200). DRG, dorsal root ganglion

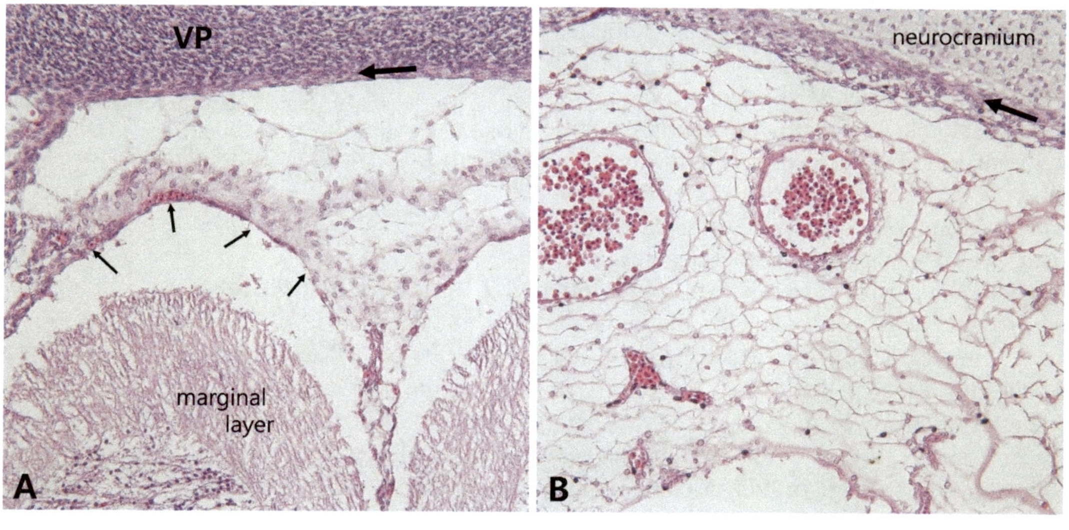

Fig. 3.4 A later stage human embryo (the specific stage has not been assigned to this embryo). **A** The neural tube has developed a substantial amount of the marginal layer. The presumptive pia mater (small arrows) with blood vessels in it is artificially peeled out from the surface of the neural tube. Intercellular spaces in the meninx primitiva are filled with amorphous substance. On the back of the vertebral primordia, a distinct layer of condensed meningeal cells (large arrow), the future pachymeningeal cells, are observed (×200). **B** In the more differentiated cephalic region, the pachymeningeal layer (arrow) is vividly distinguishing with both the anteriorly located neurocranium and posteriorly located leptomeninges. The leptomeningeal spaces look empty without amorphous substance (×400)

the dura mater is vividly separated from the neighboring perichondrial tissue.

3.1.2 Origin of the Meningeal Cells

As for the origin of the cells contributing to the formation of the meninges, there has been a long-standing debate between mesodermal tissue origin and neural crest origin.

Sensenig [3] concluded that meninges largely derived from the somatic mesoderm, with neural crest cells involving in the formation of the pia mater. This was based on their morphological observation that migrating cells from the neural crest to the vicinity of the neural tube could be distinguishable in the initial stages, stages 11 and 12 based on their shape and size, even though not anymore in later stages.

In animal experiments, quail-chick chimera and transgenic mice have been used to elucidate the origin of meningeal cells. As for the spinal meninges, transplantation of a quail somite [6] or a brachial segment of the neural tube [7] into chick embryos revealed no contribution of neural tissue cells to the meninges at all. An experiment using Wnt1-Cre/R26R transgenic mice, in which neural crest cells express β-galactosidase, showed that the meninges over the cerebral hemisphere were of neural crest origin, but not for those surrounding the midbrain and the hindbrain [8]. The experiment did not include the spinal region. Thus, the results of animal experiments seem to prefer no contribution of neural crest cells to the spinal meninges, against the observation in human embryos [3]. However, a recent experiment [9] reported contrary results to the previous ones. That is, both in quail-chick chimera and Wnt1-Cre/R26R mice, spinal meninges were observed to originate from neural crest cells. Thus, for now, a definite conclusion for the origin of the meninges should be reserved.

The development of the ependyma and related structures are discussed in "3.8. The Ependyma".

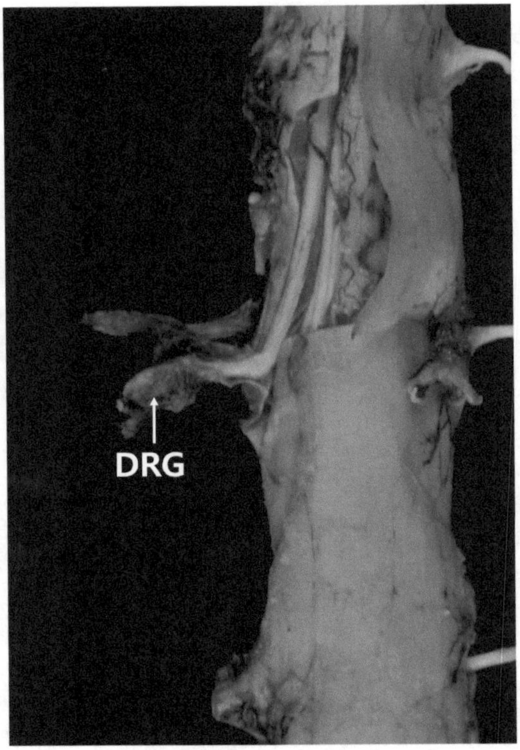

Fig. 3.5 The spinal dura mater. The dura is partially opened to show its thickness. Inside the dura, the spinal cord and some roots of the spinal nerves are seen. DRG, dorsal root ganglion

3.2 The Dura Mater

While the cranial dura mater is fused with the endosteum and thereby adherent to the inner surface of the skull, the spinal dura below the foramen magnum presents as a separate membrane from the periosteum lining the vertebral canal. The spinal dura mater is a white, thick, and tough membrane (Fig. 3.5), which forms the dural sac that contains the spinal cord in it and is surrounded by epidural space.

3.2.1 Attachments of the Dura Mater in the Vertebral Canal

The dural sac attaches cranially to the foramen magnum where the dura mater fuses with the endocranium around the foramen magnum. At the level of the second sacral vertebra, the sac contracts and caudally continues as a thin band which is named "the coccygeal ligament" or "the filum of the spinal cord." The ligament ensheathes the filum terminale and ends attaching to the dorsal surface of the first coccygeal vertebra. These attachments stabilize the sac in the vertebral canal. Another attachment of the sac can be found at the anterior surface of the sac. Anteriorly, through the vertebral canal, the dural sac loosely adheres to the posterior longitudinal ligament (PLL) on the dorsal surface of the vertebral bodies. This adhesion divides the anterior epidural space into the left and right compartments [10]. Again, the dural sac is fused with the PLL in any one of the C6 to T2 vertebral levels [11, 12]. These adhesions are inconsistent and, if present, usually appear at the intervertebral disc level, and the tissues from both structures are merged [13]. In addition to the adhesions, several fibrous bands extending from the anterior surface of the dura to the midline and lateral side of the PLL, named Hofmann ligaments, are present [11, 12]. These ligaments are thread-like fibrous bands, present through C7 to L5 vertebrae, 1–5 in number at a single level, and appear most frequently at the lower thoracic levels. Barbaix et al. [14] described another kind of ligament, the anterior sacrodural ligament or the Trolard's ligament, which are also fibrous connections between the anterior surface of the dural sac and the PLL from L3 to sacral vertebrae levels.

Similar ligaments, "the posterior epidural ligaments," were observed during lumbar laminectomy [15]. They were reported to be on the dorsal surface of the dura and extend dorsolaterally and dorsomedially to the vertebral laminae and ligamentum flavum.

On the lateral sides, the dura ensheathes spinal nerve roots like a sleeve as they pierce the sac. The sleeve forms separately for the dorsal and ventral roots each (Fig. 3.6A). Both sleeves unite at the dorsal root ganglion (Fig. 3.6B), and then distally continue as the epineurium of the ventral and dorsal rami of the spinal nerve. However, in the cauda equina, there is a single sleeve for both roots [13]. When these sleeves enter the intervertebral foramen, the dura attaches to the periosteum covering the foramen. These serial attachments also support the stability of the dural sac in the vertebral canal. The inner aspect of the dura mater is lined with the arachnoid membrane, and this relationship continues at the dural sleeve into the intervertebral foramen.

3.2.2 Histology of the Dura Mater

The dura mater appears as a single-layered thick membrane to the naked eye, with an average thickness of approximately 0.3 mm that varies depending on spinal levels and age [16]. However, it represents three different layers ultrastructurally [17].

The outermost layer, "the outer dural border layer," is less than 2 μm in thickness and mainly composed of less densely arranged extracellular collagen fibers intermingled with few elastic fibers and leptomeningeal cells with elongated processes.

The middle layer is the thickest and richly vascularized, consisting of approximately 80 layers of collagen fibers arranged in different directions. These collagen fibers partially interweave and intermixed with numerous elastic fibers, microfibrils, and infrequent fibroblasts.

The innermost layer is composed of one to several layers of cells and named as the "dural border cell (DBC) layer" by Nabeshima et al. [18]. Sometimes, this layer is regarded as a part of the arachnoid membrane by some authors [1, 2]. These cells, i.e., the dural border cells are flat and have long, twisty cytoplasmic extensions that interdigitate with those of surrounding cells. Among the cells and processes, there are occasional cell junctions, mainly desmosomes and infrequently gap junctions [19]. The pattern of the cytoplasmic extension is not constant so that the extracellular spaces created by connections of the extensions together are of irregular shape and size. Amorphous non-fibrillar materials fill these spaces, but collagen and elastic fibers and microfibrils are absent. Although these cells

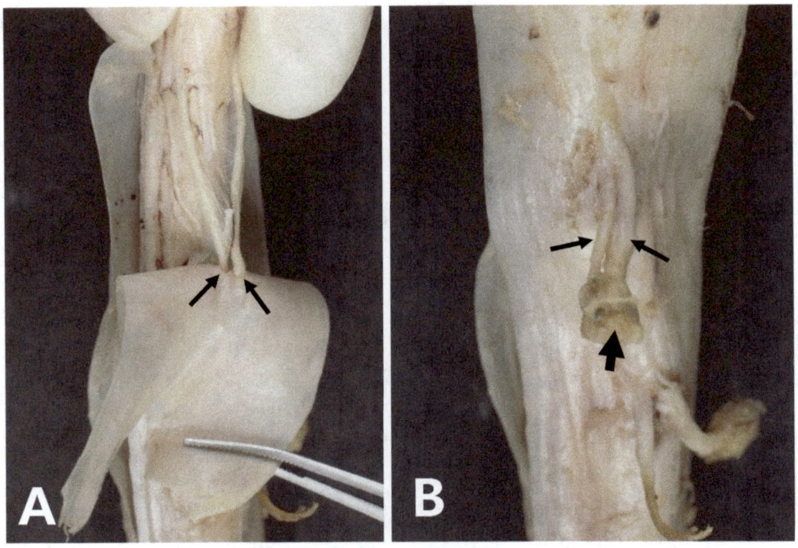

Fig. 3.6 The spinal root sleeve. The dorsal and ventral roots pierce the dura mater separately (**A**) and are enclosed in each sleeve (**B**). Both sleeves merge at the dorsal root ganglion (large arrow)

arrange like epithelium, no obvious basement membrane is observable and they are in direct contact with the fibers in the middle layer.

3.3 The Arachnoid Membrane

This translucent thin and avascular membrane is tightly attached to the dura mater, wraps the spinal cord with it, and continues with the cranial arachnoid membrane (Fig. 3.7). The arachnoid membrane extends laterally inside the dural sleeve that encloses the spinal nerve roots.

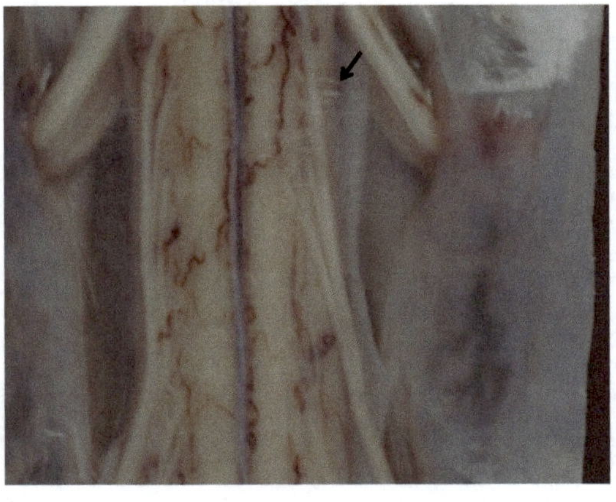

Fig. 3.7 The spinal dural sac is opened, leaving the translucent arachnoid membrane in situ. The presence of the membrane is easily recognizable by the light reflected on it (arrow)

3.3.1 Layers of the Arachnoid Membrane

Ultrastructurally, this membrane composes of two layers, the outer "arachnoid barrier cell (ABC) layer" and the inner "arachnoid reticular cell (ARC) layer" [17] with a distinct basement membrane in between. Some authors [2] include the dural border cell (DBC) layer to the arachnoid membrane, thus describes the arachnoid, being composed of three layers, the DBC layer, the ABC layer, and the innermost portion (or the ARC layer).

The outer ABC layer composes of tightly packed cells with numerous cell junctions, including desmosomes, tight junctions, and gap junctions. To be noted is that, tight junctions are absent in any other places of meninges than the ABC layer of the arachnoid membrane [19]. The number of cell layers varies depending on areas. No collagen and elastic fibers or microfibrils are present in the extracellular space. A continuous, but very thin basal lamina is present at the innermost aspect of the ABC layer, clearly demarcating it from the inner arachnoid reticular cell layer.

The outer side of the outer ABC layer tightly apposes to the DBC layer, and besides desmosomes and infrequent gap junctions are observed between the cells of the two layers [19]. That is, the DBC and ABC layers represent a continuity of cell layers from the dura to the arachnoid without significant extracellular space. However, this connection is very fragile and can easily be opened to make an artificial subdural space.

The inner reticular cell layer of the arachnoid composes of loosely arranged cells with elongated processes and extracellular collagen fibers. The processes are thin and surround collagen fiber bundles [19]. Collagen fibers are not uniform in their size, randomly orient, and intermingle with bundles of microfibrils. Some cellular processes penetrate the basal lamina to reach the ABC layer and connect to the cells in that layer by gap junctions and desmosomes.

From the inner surface of the arachnoid, many trabeculae come out to reach the pia mater across the subarachnoid space. Embryologically, both the arachnoid and pia mater derive from endomeninx [2]. Initially, there are no spaces between the future two membranes. Instead, the reticulated network of mesenchymal cells and gel-like ground substance stacking intercellular spaces (endomeninx) occupy the area around the neural tube. Fluid-filled cavities begin to appear in the ground substance of endomeninx, enlarge, and gradually coalesce to form a large space (Figs. 3.2 and 3.4), the subarachnoid space. This space splits the initial structure into the two leptomeningeal structures, the pia and arachnoid. During this differentiation process, cells and fibers between cavities remain as a rod or sheet which crosses the subarachnoid space to become the trabeculae. Thus, the arachnoid, the trabeculae, and the pia mater can conceptually be regarded as a continuum. In fact, core collagen fibers in the trabeculae are continuous with those of the arachnoid without interruption and again with those in the pia mater. Also, leptomeningeal cells wrapping the trabeculae are similar to those of the outer pia and inner arachnoid [2]. The arrangement of the trabeculae in the spinal subarachnoid space is somewhat different from that in the cranial cavity. Basically, there are sparse trabeculae in the anterior spinal subarachnoid space with few intermittent ones [20, 21].

3.3.2 The Posterior Midline Septum and the Intermediate Leptomeningeal Layer

In the posterior subarachnoid space, Nauta et al. [20] described a "posterior midline septum" from the inner surface of the arachnoid to the spinal cord extending from the mid-cervical down to the lumbar levels. This septum is not a continuous sheet but a "delicate layer of cells and collagen" [22]. To the naked eye [21], this septum is "single-strand or isolated, fenestrated septa" from C1 to C5 levels, and "spongy mass of interlacing fibrils" from C5 to lumbar levels. The attachment to the spinal cord is wider than that to the arachnoid membrane.

Meanwhile, Nicholas and Weller [22] reported the presence of a distinct "fenestrated intermediate leptomeningeal layer" in the posterior subarachnoid space of the thoracic and lumbar regions. This layer closely, but loosely attaches to the inner aspect of the arachnoid, is reflected on the posterior midline septum, covers its surface, and again reflects on the spinal cord extending laterally over the surface of the pia mater. It gradually becomes more fenestrated to be fine trabeculae and vanish. This tissue covers blood vessels over the surface of the spinal cord and nerve rootlets. Similar structures are not observed in the cerebral region. This intermediate layer is also present on the ventral surface of the spinal cord, but not as prominent as in the dorsal side, and no "ventral midline septum" is observable.

Another kind of septum, "the dorsolateral septum" is also described [20]. This septum, which is most evident from the lower cervical to thoracic levels, obliquely extends from the entry point of the dorsal rootlets into the spinal cord to the beginning point of the dural sleeve. During its course, this septum wraps the dorsal rootlets. No corresponding septum is found in association with the ventral rootlets so that they traverse the subarachnoid space without this kind of wrapping. Nicholas and Weller [22] described this septum as fenestrated and regarded it made of a fenestrated leptomeningeal layer.

3.3.3 Arachnoid Villi and Granulations

Some arachnoid mater pierces the wall of dural venous sinuses or veins adjacent to the spinal nerve roots to make microscopic arachnoid villi and macroscopic arachnoid granulations [23]. At the piercing point of the dura mater (or the venous wall), a relatively slender intradural stalk forms and it expands in the lumen of the sinus (or the vein) (Fig. 3.8). The boundary of a granulation (or a villus) is composed of arachnoid cells, the outer surface of which is covered with a fibrous membrane derived from the dura mater. Again, the outer surface of the fibrous membrane is covered with another layer of endothelial cells. However, these coatings do not completely cover the villus or granulation, leaving the apex devoid of the fibrous and

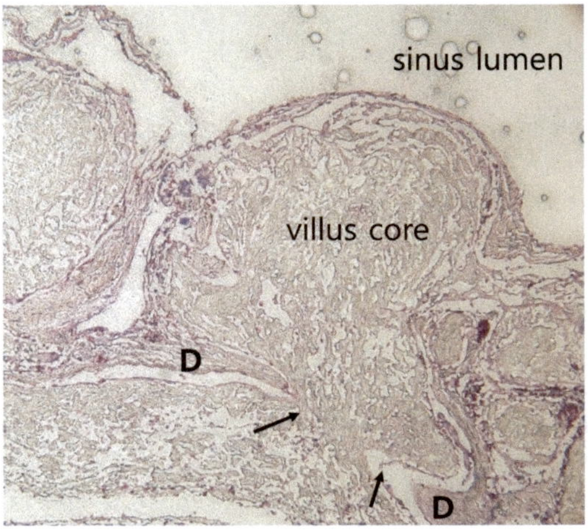

Fig. 3.8 An arachnoid villus in the superior sagittal sinus. Proliferated arachnoid tissue penetrates the dura mater (D) into the sinus lumen. The stalk (the area between arrows) is narrow, but the villus expands after entering the lumen. (×100)

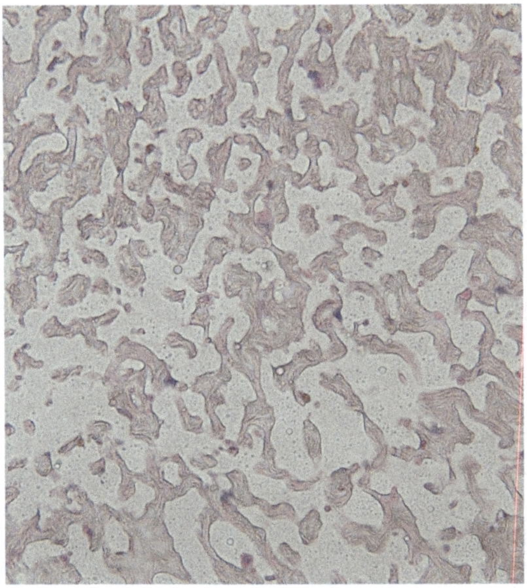

Fig. 3.9 Higher magnification of the villus core. The core composes of an irregularly arranged meshwork of connective tissue with intermingled spaces, where the cerebrospinal fluid is filtered into the sinus (or venous) lumen. (×400)

endothelial coverings so that the arachnoid cells make direct exposure to the lumen of the sinus or the vein [24]. In some areas of the arachnoid covering, there is a focal aggregation of arachnoid cells, which is called arachnoid cap cells. The core of the villus and granulation is composed of a meshwork of collagen fibers with intervening channels, through which CSF is filtered out into the venous lumen (Figs. 3.8 and 3.9).

3.3.4 The Dura–arachnoid Junction

This junction refers to the transitional zone between the dura mater and the arachnoid membrane, often called "the subdural space." Many textbooks state that this space is only a potential space between the normally closely adhered two membranes.

However, as previously described, the DBC and ABC layers are histologically continuous, even with occasional cell junctions between cells of the two layers. Reina et al. [25] used the term "dura–arachnoid interface" to refer to a structure consisting of 4–8 planes of neuroepithelial cells with intercellular spaces filled with amorphous substance and little collagen or elastic fibers. It seems likely that they mentioned the inner layer of the dura mater and the outer cell layer of the arachnoid membrane as a "dura–arachnoid interface." That means, it is difficult to distinguish these two layers of the dura and arachnoid, and thus there is no definite space between the two meninges. The subdural hematoma can be regarded as what is formed in an artificially created space due to the destruction of the connections between DBCs and are therefore actually "intradural." [26]

3.3.5 The Pia Mater

This relatively thin membrane is vascular and surrounds the entire spinal cord firmly adherent to the spinal cord surface, the glia limitans. The spinal pia mater is continuous with the cranial pia mater cranially, and it forms the filum terminale caudally as it leaves the spinal cord. The filum terminale continues downward in the terminal sac till the level of the lower border of the S1 vertebra, where it is wrapped by the spinal dura mater. Before the wrapping, it is 15–16 cm long and called the "filum terminale internum." After being wrapped, it is called the "filum terminale externum" or, with its dural wrapping, the "coccygeal ligament" or the "filum of the spinal cord." The ligament is about 8 cm long, passes through the sacral hiatus and adheres to the dorsal surface of the first coccygeal vertebra [27].

On the lateral side of the spinal cord between the ventral and dorsal nerve rootlets, the pia mater extends laterally to form a flat fibrous sheet extending from upper cervical to upper lumbar region (typically between the T-12 and L-1 nerve roots), the denticulate ligaments (Fig. 3.10). The ligaments form a series of triangular processes in between the two successive spinal nerves, the apex of which penetrates the dura matter. The number of these triangular processes counts approximately 20–22 unilaterally [28]. These ligaments incompletely separate the subarachnoid space into anterior and posterior compartments.

The core of the ligament consists of densely arranged collagen fibers that are continuous medially with subpial collagen and laterally with that in the dura mater [27]. The surface of the core is covered with leptomeningeal cells that are continuous with the cells covering the pia and arachnoid maters.

Histologically, the spinal pia mater is different from the cranial one. In the cranial region, the pia mater consists of a single interrupted layer of flattened cells, 1–2 cell layer thick, without basement membrane. The layer closely contacts the cortex, with a narrow interval of 6 nm thick that contains granular materials and a few collagen fibers [27, 29]. Meanwhile, the spinal pia mater consists of a cellular layer of pial cells and a subpial layer. The pial cells are flattened, 3–6 layers (8–15 μm in thickness) with intervening collagen fibers, and connected to each other with desmosomes and other specialized junctions. The subpial layer is 130–200 μm in thickness and mainly composed of collagen fibers. These fibers are arrayed randomly and are continuous with those in the arachnoid trabeculae core without interruption. In addition to large amounts of collagen fibers, a few elastic fibers, amorphous intracellular substances, small vessels, fibroblasts, and macrophages are present in the subpial layer [30]. As such, the spinal pia mater is much thicker than the cranial one and can be peeled off the surface of the spinal cord without destructing the cord parenchyma (Fig. 3.11) in contrast to the cranial one.

On the surface of the spinal pia mater in the pial cell layer, numerous fenestrations have been reported [30]. These fenestrations are found in the lumbar segments including conus medullaris and nerve roots, but not in the thoracic segments.

Meanwhile, the pia mater reflects from the surface of the spinal cord into the blood vessels where the vessels pass through the spinal parenchyma. Thus, the spinal subarachnoid space is separated from the perivascular or Virchow–Robin spaces by a layer of pia mater [22].

3.4 Coverings of the Spinal Nerve Rootlets

Dorsal and ventral rootlets of spinal nerves laterally converge into the intervertebral foramen from the spinal cord and join together to form the roots. During their pathway, nerve fibers are enveloped by the myelin sheath, and rootlets and roots are surrounded as a whole by membranes and spaces.

In general, nerve fibers are myelinated by oligodendrocytes and Schwann cells in the central and peripheral nervous systems, respectively. The roots or rootlets, either of the spinal and cranial nerves, by definition belong to peripheral nerves, and thus are myelinated by Schwann cells. However, there is a "transition zone" [31, 32] or, more specifically "central–peripheral transitional zone" [33], where Schwann cells and oligodendrocytes coexist to wrap the nerve fibers. The locations and lengths of this transitional zone for each cranial (and also for spinal) nerve are different from each other. For example, in the case of the nervus intermedius [33], the central myelin made by the oligodendrocytes extends in average 0.5 and 0.33 mm from the brain stem on the medial and lateral sides, respectively, out of which 0.279 and 0.134 mm in the medial and lateral sides are the transitional zones, where both the oligodendrocytes and Schwann cells co-exist.

At the point where the rootlets penetrate the pia mater, the pial layer surrounds the rootlet and is called the "pial sheath" or "root sheath." The dorsal rootlets are additionally covered with arachnoid material, while no such arachnoid coverings are found around the ventral rootlets [20]. Similar features were also observed in rats [34]. The arachnoid lining the dural sleeve turns back at "the subarachnoid angle (see below)" onto the dorsal root covering the pial sheath. However, on the ventral roots, the arachnoid mater joint to the pial sheath without turning back over the pial sheath.

The dorsal and ventral roots protrude from the dural sac being wrapped around by each dural sleeve, approach to each other, and enter the intervertebral foramen. Here, the two roots join together to the dorsal root ganglion and also the two sleeves. The dural sleeve gradually becomes thinner as it approaches the dorsal root ganglion [23] and adheres to the nerve roots [35]. Beyond this point, the dura covers the inner surface of the fibrous operculum, which closes the intervertebral foramen laterally and becomes the epineurium enclosing the nerve trunk [28, 35]. The arachnoid membrane follows the dural sleeve laterally, lining the inner surface of it, and fuses with the pial sheath wrapping the roots to be continuous with the perineurium of the spinal nerves [27].

Subarachnoid space also follows the dural sleeve making a CSF sleeve around the nerve roots and closes as blind ends just before the nerve trunk traverses the fibrous operculum [28]. These ends are bound by the fused arachnoid and pia mater, which forms the "subarachnoid angle" or "lateral recess." This angle extends laterally to the dorsal root ganglion.

3.5 The Epidural Space

The epidural space lies between the dura mater and the osteofibrous wall of the vertebral canal. Anteriorly, the space is bounded by the posterior longitudinal ligament, posteriorly by the spinal laminae and the ligamenta flava, and extends downward to the sacral hiatus.

Based on MRI observation [36], the posterior epidural space is mostly full of epidural fat. However, this fat pad is not continuous craniocaudal but incompletely segmented due to contact between the dura and the lamina. The spaces, as revealed by the shapes of the fat pad, differ in size and shape depending on the spinal levels. That is, the anterior–posterior length of the space is about 7 mm in the lumbar level, 2.6 mm in the midthoracic level (T7-8), and the space almost disappears in the cervicothoracic junction. The shape of the space varies from triangular in the lumbar to crescentic in the thoracic spine.

The epidural fat does not directly contact the periosteum lining the vertebral canal. Instead, a uniform, delicate, and translucent lining membrane made of thin connective tissue surrounds the fat pad, and this membrane is in contact with the lamina and the ligamenta flava [37]. Histological observations have revealed that the membrane surrounding the epidural fat is covered with a single cell epithelium. And, this membrane is tethered to the vertebral canal wall at the posterior midline where both ligamenta flava meet. There is no fibrous tissue or septum in the fat. Except at the sites where the membrane attaches to the midline, vessels are not noticeably present in the posterior epidural space [13].

Epidural fat is rarely present in the anterior epidural space. Instead, the internal vertebral venous plexus is present here. Furthermore, blood vessels, especially veins, are confined to the anterior epidural space, as revealed by epidural venography and CT imaging [13].

In addition to the epidural fat and the internal vertebral venous plexus, there are bands of fibrous tissues that cross the space, as mentioned above, to connect the dura mater and the periosteum. Hofmann's ligaments are representative examples [11, 12].

3.6 The Subdural Space

As mentioned above, many researchers consider the subdural space, not a real space. The traditional "subdural space" refers to an abnormal one resulting from splitting of the cells in the dural barrier cell layer, the innermost layer of the dura, not a potential space surrounded by epithelial tissue like the peritoneal and pleural cavities [19, 26]. When a hematoma was produced in experimental animals, the capsule surrounding the hematoma was composed of cells very similar to the DBCs [38]. Thus, nowadays, it is common to mention that a natural space is not present at the dura–arachnoid junction. This space is thought to be a "created" space in the structure that is most vulnerable of the dura mater [19, 26]. This vulnerability comes from the fact that there is little tight junction between the cells here, and there are not many other intercellular junctions. There is no fiber component in the intercellular space, which would play a structural role to reinforce the intercellular space. On the other hand, the cells firmly interweave in the dura mater just above this layer and in the ABC layer just below to it. Thus, when a shearing force is applied, a split is formed between the cells of the DBC layer. This is quite different from the spaces formed between the visceral and parietal layers of the pleural and pericardial cavities, which are real potential spaces. With the shearing force, cell damage accompanies [19, 26] in addition to the formation of space.

3.7 The Subarachnoid Space

Also known as the perimedullary space, the subarachnoid space occupies approximately one-third of the vertebral canal space [28]. The upper part

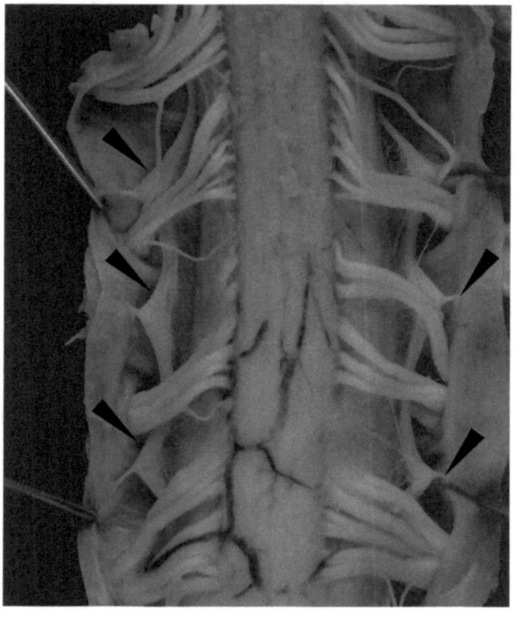

Fig. 3.10 Denticulate ligaments. Both the dura and arachnoid maters are reflected. A series of denticulate ligaments are indicated by arrowheads on the left side. These ligaments pierce the dura mater at the apex (arrowheads on the right side). Consider that the ligaments are somewhat pulled laterally because of their connection to the dura mater

is continuous with the cranial subarachnoid space and ends inferiorly at the lower part of the S2 vertebra. This space is filled with cerebrospinal fluid, and the main stems of the blood vessels lie in this space. The space is divided incompletely into ventral and dorsal compartments by the denticulate ligaments (Fig. 3.10), which laterally extend from the sides of the spinal cord [39].

Extension of the subarachnoid space into the dural sleeve is already described above (3.4. Coverings of the spinal nerve rootlets), in association with the subarachnoid angle or lateral recess. Also, the posterior midline septum and the intermediate leptomeningeal layer present in the subarachnoid space are described above (3.3. The arachnoid membrane).

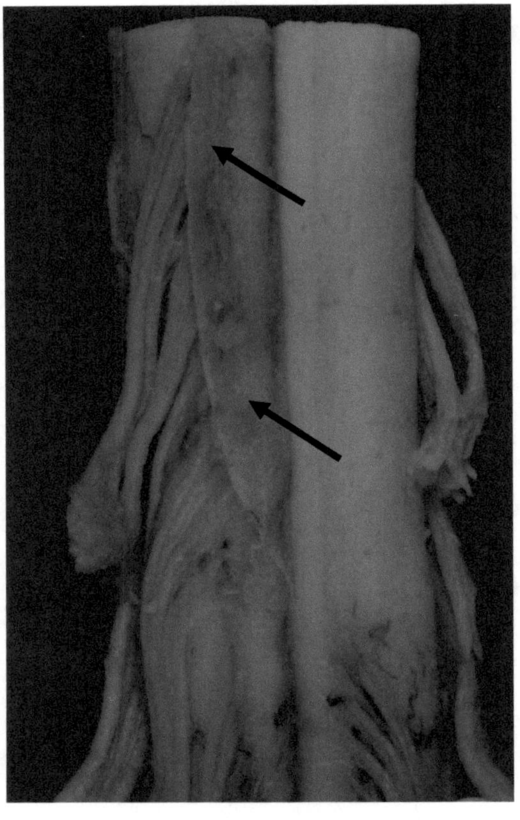

Fig. 3.11 The pia mater was peeled off the surface of the spinal cord on the right side (arrows)

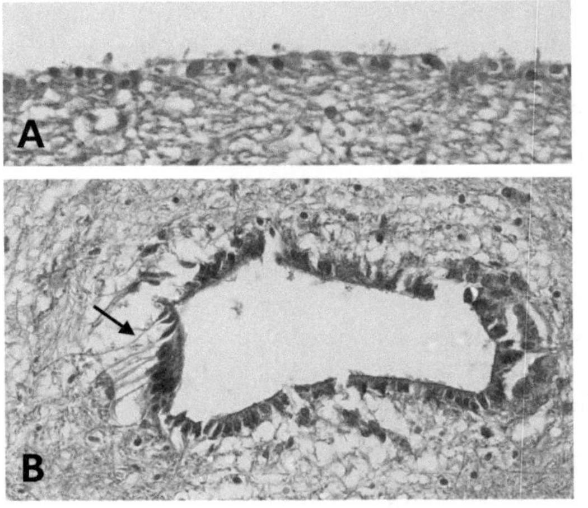

Fig. 3.12 The ependyma in the medulla oblongata (**A**) and spinal cord (**B**) (×400). Cells constitute a simple cuboidal epithelium. In B, the ependyma partially separates from the underlying neuropil as an artifact, which exposes the cytoplasmic processes of the ependymal cells to the neuropil evidently (arrow)

3.8 The Ependyma

The ependyma is a simple cuboidal to columnar epithelium lining the lumen of the central nervous system (Fig. 3.12), that is, the central canal, ventricles, and cerebral aqueduct. Ependymal cells, also called ependymocytes, are glial cells. They are ciliated and bear some microvilli on their apical surface [40, 41]. Among ependymal cells are present tanycytes, a specialized form of classical ependymocytes [42], which have cytoplasmic processes to the underlying neuropils or sometimes to the vessels [43] (Fig. 3.12B).

Characteristically, tight junctions, which are one of the typical characteristics of the ordinary epithelium, are hardly observed in the ependyma except for some areas such as circumventricular organs and the choroid plexuses [41]. That means that the ependyma functions as a selectively permeable sieve that permits CSF proteins to reach the extracellular space of the neural tissue. In addition, the basement membrane is not prominent. When stained with periodic acid-Schiff reagent, the ependyma did not show any PAS-positive basement membrane [44], which is also a usual finding for ordinary epithelium. In rats, a thin astrocytic cytoplasmic sheet, not a basement membrane, intervenes between the basal surface of ependymocytes and the underlying neuropil [44].

Embryologically, the ependyma develops from the pseudo-stratified neuroepithelium. The first differentiation, induced by the notochord, occurs at the floor plate at 4 weeks of gestation, followed by the roof plate during 8–10 weeks, and then by the basal and the alar plates [45]. At the beginning of the differentiation, the floor plate cells produce long cytoplasmic processes towards the surface of the spinal cord. Then, the processes gather and form a compact sagittal partition to form a ventral median septum [45, 46]. The same events happen in the roof plate resulting in a wedge-shaped posterior median partition composed of fibers (that is, the processes) (Fig. 3.13). With time, the wedge narrows to form a compact midline bundle and finally becomes the "posterior midline septum" of the spinal cord, which borders between the right and left posterior funiculi.

Once differentiated, the ependymal cells hardly proliferate, and possible defects in the ependyma would be covered by cytoplasmic processes of underlying astrocytes [47].

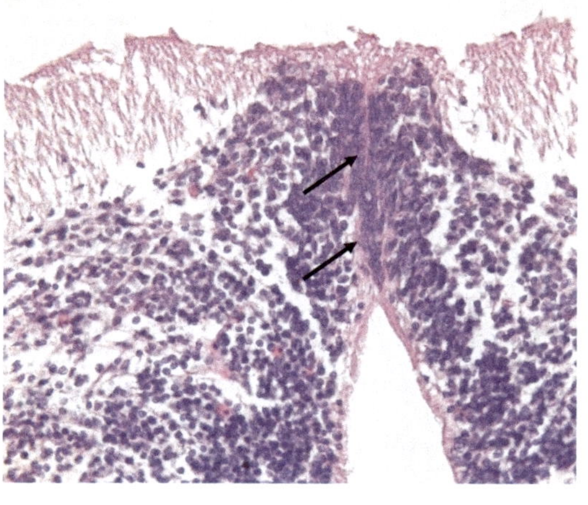

Fig. 3.13 The beginning of the differentiation of the roof plate in a human embryo of a later stage (a specific stage has not been assigned). Cells in the roof plate (arrows) become somewhat elongated and are compactly arranged in parallel

References

1. Patel N, Kirmi O. Anatomy and imaging of the normal meninges. Semin Ultrasound CT MR. 2009;30:559–64.
2. Mortazavi MM, Quadri SA, Khan MA, et al. Subarachnoid trabeculae: a comprehensive review of their embryology, histology, morphology, and surgical significance. World Neurosurg. 2018;111:279–90.
3. Sensenig EC. The early development of the meninges of the spinal cord in human embryos. In: Contributions to Embryology, No. 228, Carnegie Institution of Washington Publication, Washington pp 145–157. 1951.
4. O'Rahilly R, Müller F. The meninges in human development. J Neuropathol Exp Neurol. 1986;45:588–608.
5. Patelska-Banaszewska M, Woźniak W. The development of the epidural space in human embryos. Folia Morphol (Warsz). 2004;63:273–9.
6. Bagnall KM, Higgins SJ, Sanders EJ. The contribution made by cells from a single somite to tissues within a body segment and assessment of their integration with similar cells from adjacent segments. Development. 1989;107:931–43.
7. Halata Z, Grim M, Christ B. Origin of spinal cord meninges, sheaths of peripheral nerves, and cutaneous receptors including Merkel cells. An experimental and ultrastructural study with avian chimeras. Anat Embryol (Berl). 1990;182:529–37.
8. Jiang X, Iseki S, Maxson RE, Sucov HM, Morriss-Kay GM. Tissue origins and interactions in the mammalian skull vault. Dev Biol. 2002;241:106–16.
9. Batarfi M, Valasek P, Krejci E, Huang R, Patel K. The development and origins of vertebrate meninges. Bio Comm. 2017;62:73–81.
10. Newell RL. The spinal epidural space. Clin Anat. 1999;12:375–9.
11. Wadhwani S, Loughenbury P, Soames R. The anterior dural (Hofmann) ligaments. Spine. 2004;29:623–7.
12. Tardieu GG, Fisahn C, Loukas M, et al. The Epidural Ligaments (of Hofmann): A Comprehensive Review of the Literature. Cureus. 2016;8:e779.
13. Hogan Q, Toth J. Anatomy of soft tissues of the spinal canal. Reg Anesth Pain Med. 1999;24:303–10.
14. Barbaix E, Girardin MD, Hoppner JP, Van Roy P, Clarijs JP. Anterior sacrodural attachments - Trolard's ligaments revisited. Man Ther. 1996;1(2):88–91.

15. Kimmell KT, Dayoub H, Shakir H, Sincoff EH. Spinal dural attachments to the vertebral column: an anatomic report and review of the literature. Surg Neurol Int. 2011;2:97.
16. Hong JY, Suh SW, Park SY, et al. Analysis of dural sac thickness in human spine-cadaver study with confocal infrared laser microscope. Spine J. 2011;11:1121–7.
17. Vandenabeele F, Creemers J, Lambrichts I. Ultrastructure of the human spinal arachnoid mater and dura mater. J Anat. 1996;189(Pt. 2):417–30.
18. Nabeshima S, Reese TS, Landis DM, Brightman MW. Junctions in the meninges and marginal glia. J Comp Neurol. 1975;164:127–69.
19. Haines DE. On the question of a subdural space. Anat Rec. 1991;230:3–21.
20. Nauta HJ, Dolan E, Yasargil MG. Microsurgical anatomy of spinal subarachnoid space. Surg Neurol. 1983;19:431–7.
21. Parkinson D. Human spinal arachnoid septa, trabeculae, and "rogue strands." Am J Anat. 1991;192:498–509.
22. Nicholas DS, Weller RO. The fine anatomy of the human spinal meninges. A light and scanning electron microscopy study. J Neurosurg. 1988;69:276–82.
23. Kido DK, Gomez DG, Pavese AM Jr, Potts DG. Human spinal arachnoid villi and granulations. Neuroradiology. 1976;11:221–8.
24. Yamashima T. Ultrastructural study of the final cerebrospinal fluid pathway in human arachnoid villi. Brain Res. 1986;384:68–76.
25. Reina MA, De Leon CO, López A, De Andrés JA, Mora M, Fernández A. The origin of the spinal subdural space: ultrastructure findings. Anesth Analg. 2002;94(4):991–5.
26. Haines DE, Harkey HL, al-Mefty O. The "subdural" space; a new look at an outdated concept. Neurosurgey. 1993; 32:111–120.
27. Adeeb N, Mortazavi MM, Deep A, et al. The pia mater: a comprehensive review of literature. Childs Nerv Syst. 2013;29:1803–10.
28. Sakka L, Gabrillargues J, Coll G. Anatomy of the Spinal Meninges. Oper Neurosurg (Hagerstown). 2016; 12:168–188.
29. Lopes CA, Mair WG. Ultrastructure of the outer cortex and the pia mater in man. Acta Neuropathol. 1974;28:79–86.
30. Reina MA, Ode DLC, L, Villanueva MC, Lopez A, Maches F, De Andres JA, . Ultrastructural findings in human spinal pia mater in relation to subarachnoid anesthesia. Anesth Analg. 2004;98:1479–85.
31. Tarlov IM. Structure of the nerve root. I. Nature of the junction between the central and the peripheral nervous system. Archs Neurol Psychiat. 1937;37:555–83.
32. Fraher JP. The transitional zone and CNS regeneration. J Anat. 2000;196(Pt 1):137–58.
33. Alfieri A, Fleischhammer J, Strauss C, El P. The central myelin-peripheral myelin transitional zone of the nervus intermedius and its implications for microsurgery in the cerebellopontine angle. Clin Anat. 2012;25:882–8.
34. McCabe JS, Low FN. The subarachnoid angle: an area of transition in peripheral nerve. Anat Rec. 1969;164:15–33.
35. Wiltse LL. Anatomy of the extradural compartments of the lumbar spinal canal. Peridural membrane and circumneural sheath. Radiol Clin North Am. 2000;38:1177–206.
36. Hirabayashi Y, Saitoh K, Fukuda H, Igarashi T, Shimizu R, Seo N. Magnetic resonance imaging of the extradural space of the thoracic spine. Br J Anaesth. 1997;79:563–6.
37. Beaujeux R, Wolfram-Gabel R, Kehrli P et al. Posterior lumbar epidural fat as a functional structure? Histologic specificities. Spine (Phila Pa 1976). 1997; 22:1264–1269.
38. Frederickson RG. The subdural space interpreted as a cellular layer of meninges. Anat Rec. 1991;230:38–51.
39. Grassner L, Grillhösl A, Griessenauer CJ, et al. Spinal Meninges and Their Role in Spinal Cord Injury: A Neuroanatomical Review. J Neurotrauma. 2018;35:403–10.
40. Roy S, Hirano A, Zimmerman HM. Ultrastructural demonstration of cilia in the adult human ependyma. Anat Rec. 1974;180:547–50.
41. Del Bigio MR. The ependyma: a protective barrier between brain and cerebrospinal fluid. Glia. 1995;14:1–13.
42. Gould SJ, Howard S, Papadaki L. The development of ependyma in the human fetal brain: an immunohistological and electron microscopic study. Brain Res Dev Brain Res. 1990;55:255–67.
43. Bruni JE. Ependymal development, proliferation, and functions: a review. Microsc Res Tech. 1998;41:2–13.
44. Mathew TC. Regional analysis of the ependyma of the third ventricle of rat by light and electron microscopy. Anat Histol Embryol. 2008;37:9–18.
45. Sarnat HB. Regional differentiation of the human fetal ependyma: immunocytochemical markers. J Neuropathol Exp Neurol. 1992a;51:58–75.
46. Sarnat HB. Role of human fetal ependyma. Pediatr Neurol. 1992b;8:163–78.
47. Sarnat HB. Histochemistry and immunocytochemistry of the developing ependyma and choroid plexus. Microsc Res Tech. 1998;41:14–28.

4 Anatomical Compartment of Spinal Cord Tumors with Anatomical Classification

Jong-myung Jung and Chun Kee Chung

Abstract

Spinal cord tumors are uncommon neoplasms that, without treatment, can cause significant neurologic morbidity and mortality. Spinal cord tumors can be divided into intraependymal, intrapial extraependymal, pial, intraarchnoidal extrapial, extraarachnoidal intradural, dural, and transcompartmental based on anatomical compartment. In this chapter, we reviewed spinal cord tumors in terms of epidemiological, clinical, and radiographic characteristics. Surgical and adjuvant treatment options are also reviewed.

Keywords

Spinal cord tumors · Anatomical classification · Intraependymal · Intrapial extraependymal · Pial · Intraarchnoidal extrapial · Extraarachnoidal intradural · Dural · Transcompartmental

J. Jung
Department of Neurosurgery, Spine Center, Seoul National University Bundang Hospital, Seongnam, Republic of Korea
e-mail: beast2625@snu.ac.kr

C. K. Chung (✉)
Department of Neurosurgery, Seoul National University Hospital, Seoul National University College of Medicine, Seoul, Republic of Korea
e-mail: chungc@snu.ac.kr

Neuroscience Research Institute, Seoul National University Medical Research Center, Seoul, Republic of Korea

Clinical Research Institute, Seoul National University Hospital, Seoul, Republic of Korea

Department of Brain and Cognitive Sciences, Seoul National University College of Natural Sciences, Seoul, Republic of Korea

4.1 Introduction

Spinal cord tumors (SCTs) are uncommon lesions and affect only a minority of the population. However, these lesions can cause significant morbidity in terms of limb dysfunction and can be associated with mortality as well. SCTs are classified into three groups according to their anatomic location: intramedullary, intradural extramedullary, and extradural. Although this classification is somewhat of an oversimplification, since lesions can reside in several compartments, it is very useful in tumor characterization.

Intramedullary spinal cord tumors (IMSCTs) constitute 8%–10% of all primary spinal cord tumors composed of gliomas (80%–90%), of which 60%–70% are ependymomas, and 30%–40% are astrocytomas [1]. Oligodendrogliomas, mixed gliomas, neuron-derived tumors,

C. K. Chung (ed.), *Surgery of Spinal Cord Tumors Based on Anatomy*,
https://doi.org/10.1007/978-981-15-7771-0_4

Table 4.1 Classification of spinal cord tumors

Intraependymal (intra-central canal)	
	Ependymoma
Intrapial extraependymal	
	Astrocytoma
	Subependymoma
	Ganglioglioma
	Oligodendroglioma
Pial	
	Hemangioblastoma
Intraarachnoidal extrapial	
	Schwannoma
	Myxopapillary ependymoma
	Paraganglioma
	Dermoid and epidermoid cysts
Extrararachnoidal intradural	
	Meningioma
Dural	
	Solitary fibrous tumor
Trans-compartmental	
	Lipoma

gangliogliomas, hemangioblastomas, lipomas, and developmental tumors are uncommon.

Extramedullary spinal cord tumors (EMSCTs) account for more than 70% of adult intradural spinal cord tumors and are uncommon in children. The most common primary EMSCTs are derived from sheath cells covering the spinal nerve roots (schwannomas and neurofibromas) or meningeal cells located along the spinal cord surface (meningiomas). Myxopapillary ependymomas are extramedullary tumors arising from the conus medullaris and filum terminalis. Other tumor types such as hemangiopericytomas, lipomas, paragangliomas, epidermoid cysts, and dermoid cysts are less common.

Extradural lesions are the most common (60% of all spinal tumors), with the majority of lesions originating from the vertebrae. The most frequent extradural tumor is metastasis, while primary bone tumors are much less common. Concomitant intradural and extradural components are associated with roughly 10% of SCTs.

In 2000, the World Health Organization (WHO) ratified a new comprehensive classification of neoplasms affecting the central nervous system. This tumor classification is based on the premise that each type of tumor results from the abnormal growth of a specific cell type. The new WHO classification also provides a parallel grading system for each type of tumor. We classified the SCTs based on anatomical compartment (Table 4.1). To the extent that the behavior of a tumor correlates with the basic cell type, tumor classification dictates the choice of therapy and predicts prognosis.

Anatomic classification is particularly useful in this regard.

4.2 Intraependyma (Intracentral Canal) Tumors

4.2.1 Ependymoma

Intramedullary ependymomas represent almost 40%–60% of adults with IMSCTs with a peak incidence in the fourth to the fifth decade of life, and there is a slight male predominance [2–4]. Most intramedullary ependymomas arise in the cervical or cervicothoracic region; 67% of tumors occur or expand into this area [5, 6]. Ependymomas of the cord are solitary tumors arising from the ependymal lining of the central canal, causing a diffuse enlargement of the cord over multiple levels and related to syrinx in about 50% of the cases. Spinal cord ependymomas tend to infiltrate the adjacent neural tissue and have delicate capsules that form a cleavage plane that separates the tumor from the spinal cord.

MRI shows a lesion hypointense on T1-weighted images and hyperintense on T2-weighted images [7]. Intramedullary ependymomas homogeneously enhance with contrast [7]. Sometimes dark caps are seen, especially on T2WI, rostral and caudal of the tumor representing hemosiderin deposits.

Although not encapsulated, intramedullary ependymomas often show a distinct plane between the tumor and the adjacent spinal cord, despite the frequent association with cysts, syrinxes, and hemorrhage. Intramedullary ependymomas are mostly well-circumscribed tumors, which help with total surgical resection in 70%–100% of cases [8–11]. Tumor recurrence after gross total resection is less than 10% but can be delayed by the slow growth rate of ependymomas. With subtotal resection, tumor recurrence is seen in 50%–70% of cases [10, 11]. The extent of surgical resection was the only statistically significant factor in the aspect of disease progression [11]. Therefore, the prognosis for patients with intramedullary ependymomas is dependent on the extent of surgical resection. Postoperative radiation treatment remains controversial but could increase tumor-free survival rates of adult patients with high-grade or subtotally resected tumors [11–13]. Additionally, prior adjuvant radiotherapy might make subsequent surgical interventions more difficult and heighten postoperative neurological morbidity. Although there are little data to support the use of chemotherapy in the treatment of ependymoma, the high incidence of these tumors in children makes it an important option for therapeutic development. Chemotherapy has been studied in most cases of recurrent intracranial ependymoma and has shown some effect. However, its role in IMSCT has not been clarified yet [14]. The 5-year survival rates for low-grade intramedullary ependymomas range between 83 and 100% but decline rapidly with higher grade ependymomas [10, 12, 15, 16].

Preoperative functional status was the significant prognostic factors influencing the postoperative outcome, and the extent of surgical resection was the only statistically significant factor in the aspect of disease progression.

4.3 Intrapial Extraependymal Tumors

4.3.1 Astrocytoma

Astrocytomas account for 80%–90% of IMSCTs in childhood and roughly 60% of IMSCTs in adolescence [4, 8, 17–20]. In adults, intramedullary astrocytomas make up almost 25% of all IMSCTs [4]. Astrocytomas have a peak incidence in the third decade of life but are not as common as intramedullary ependymomas in this age group. The distribution of sex in patients is fairly even. The tumors occur in the cervical lesion in about 60% of patients [8, 17]. At the time of diagnosis, astrocytomas have usually extended to multiple bone levels and 30%–60% of tumors are associated with rostral, caudal, or intratumoral cysts [7, 17]. Elongated cysts extending several levels from the tumor location represent syringomyelia. Astrocytomas have an affinity to white matter tracts, which topographically are peripheral in the spinal cord. Thus, the asymmetric presentation is characteristic of these tumors. Statistically, about 85%–90% of astrocytomas are low grade (either fibrillary or pilocytic), and 10%–15% are a high grade (mostly anaplastic). Glioblastoma multiforme occurs in 0.2%–1.5% of all cord astrocytomas [21, 22].

MRI of low-grade astrocytomas reveals an enlarged homogeneous mass with a hypointense to isointense signal on T1-weighted images and a hyperintense signal on T2-weighted images [7]. There is little to no surrounding edema or hemorrhage with low-grade astrocytomas. Unlike most intracranial low-grade astrocytomas, spinal astrocytomas are enhanced with gadolinium [23]. The enhancement patterns are usually mild to moderate and patchy. However, the frequency of non-enhancing spinal cord astrocytoma is 18% [5, 6]. Similar to ependymomas, astrocytomas exhibit heterogeneous enhancement with contrast, making it difficult to distinguish between ependymomas and astrocytomas by MRI alone. For this reason, biopsy and histology can be considered the best way to distinguish astrocytomas from ependymomas and plan treatment options. Pilocytic astrocytomas can be well delineated and tend to displace rather than infiltrate the cord. However, fibrillary astrocytomas are poorly defined with irregular tumor margins and show widespread parenchymal infiltration and variable degrees of nuclear atypia and increased cellularity. Pilocytic astrocytomas typically contain Rosenthal fibers. On MRI, high-grade tumors often show heterogeneous enhancement due to the presence of intratumoral cysts, necrosis, and surrounding edema [23].

Treatment of intramedullary astrocytomas is directed at total surgical resection; however, less extensive surgical intervention could be considered with higher grade, more infiltrative tumors to avoid pronounced postsurgical morbidity. Gross total resection of pilocytic astrocytomas is achievable in many instances, as these tumors are often well circumscribed. However, because of the infiltrative nature of even low-grade fibrillary astrocytomas, gross total resection of these tumors is difficult with risking perioperative and postoperative morbidity and mortality. Gross total resection rates range between 30 and 70% [3, 17, 18]. Intramedullary fibrillary astrocytomas have a high recurrence rate, ranging from 25% in low-grade tumors to almost 100% in high-grade tumors [2, 17]. A previous study has shown that 47.6% of patients with primary spinal cord astrocytomas recurred, all of whom had originally undergone STR [24]. When recurrence of astrocytoma occurs, radiotherapy is the next treatment [25]. However, the radiotherapy for astrocytomas, especially low-grade astrocytomas, is generally controversial because they affect children and adolescents in general. The study of chemotherapeutic agents for astrocytomas is very limited, and further studies are warranted. In low-grade intramedullary astrocytomas, 5-year survival rates range from 80 to 100% [18]. Patients with intramedullary anaplastic astrocytomas or glioblastoma multiformes have an average life expectancy of 15 months [17, 18, 26]. Another study reported that the histological grade was the most significant predictor of survival in patients with astrocytoma of the spinal cord (184 months vs. 8 months, low- and high-grade astrocytoma, respectively) [27]. Neither the extent of resection nor radiation influenced the survival rate.

4.3.2 Subependymoma

Subependymomas of the spinalcord are rare representations of IMSCTs. These are benign, noninvasive, slow-growing spinal cord tumors. These tumors have a higher incidence in men and typically present in the fourth or fifth decade of life [28]. Intramedullary subependymomas are most commonly located in the cervical cord, although involvement of the thoracic cord has been reported [29].

On MRI, intramedullary subependymomas have characteristics similar to ependymomas, showing spinal cord enlargement with a hypointense signal on T1-weighted images and a hyperintense signal on T2-weighted images with heterogeneous enhancement [28, 30].

Treatment for intramedullary subependymomas is directed at total gross resection whenever possible. Because an intramedullary subependymoma is a benign and indolent WHO grade I tumor, gross total resection is not always necessary. Thus, a preoperative differential diagnosis of intramedullary subependymomas, especially from an ependymoma is important when devising an optimal surgical plan. Frequently, intramedullary subependymomas are eccentrically located in the spinal cord, which can help differentiate these tumors from the more centrally located ependymomas on a surgical basis [28, 30]. In a previous study, gross total resection of the tumor was performed in 50.0% (5 of 10 patients), whereas subtotal or partial resection was achieved in 50% (the other five patients) due to a poor dissection plane [31]. Among them, adjuvant radiotherapy was performed in two patients. No tumor recurrence or regrowth was observed during the mean follow-up period of 31.5 months. Considering the benign nature of subependymomas, subtotal removal without the risk of any neurological deficit can be a viable alternative.

4.3.3 Ganglioglioma

These tumors consist of ganglion cells as well as neoplastic glial elements. They account for approximately 1% of intramedullary spinal cord tumors [32]. They occur predominantly in the pediatric age group, with three-fourths of the patient's being younger than 16 years of age at the time of diagnosis [33]. There is a male dominance with a sex ratio of 1.7:1 [33]. Intramedullary gangliogliomas are located predominately at cervicothoracic or thoracic levels and can span multiple vertebral segments [33]. There could be a mild sex bias for men. In a large case series, the cervicothoracic segment was most commonly involved in about 37.5%, thoracic in 28.5%, cervicomedullary in 14.0%, cervical in 12.5%, and conus in 7.0% of patients with intramedullary spinal ganglioglioma [33]. These tumors favor eccentric locations [34]. They extend beyond an average of eight vertebral bodies compared with approximately four vertebral bodies in intramedullary astrocytomas and ependymomas [34].

Approximately 85% of these tumors show mixed signal intensity on the T1-weighted images [34]. They tend to be high signal intensity on T2-weighted images, although approximately 40% of them are heterogeneous on T2 as well as on contrast-enhanced images [32, 35]. The enhancement pattern is mostly patchy with pial surface enhancement. Approximately 20% of these tumors show focal enhancement and 15% of them are nonenhancing [34]. Vasogenic edema is rare and occurs only in less than 10% of tumors [34]. Tumoral cysts are seen in about 40% of patients [34]. Preoperative fluorodeoxyglucose positron emission tomography (FDG-PET) or a thallium-201 single-photon emission CT (201Tl-SPECT) scan may help distinguish a high-grade anaplastic ganglioglioma from a benign tumor [36].

Treatment of intramedullary gangliogliomas is directed at gross total tumor resection, which can be achieved in 80%–90% of cases, and tumor recurrence after resection ranges from 30 to 47% [33, 37, 38]. Adjuvant radiotherapy and chemotherapy with temozolomide are usually reserved for high-grade anaplastic tumors [39]. The 5-year survival rate is close to 90%, but the 10-year survival rate is about 80% [33, 40].

4.3.4 Oligodendroglioma

Intramedullary oligodendrogliomas represent a small percentage of spinal cord tumors and fewer than 2% of CNS oligodendrogliomas [41, 42]. These tumors have the highest incidence in the second or third decade of life with a slight male predominance. Intramedullary oligodendrogliomas are most often located at the thoracic levels [43].

Radiographically, intramedullary oligodendrogliomas present as an irregular mass with associated spinal cord enlargement and possible syrinx. MRI shows a lesion with an isointense signal on T1-weighted images and a hyperintense signal on T2-weighted images with heterogeneous enhancement [41]. As in the brain, bleeding and calcification are relatively common [42, 43].

Total surgical resection of intramedullary oligodendrogliomas is difficult as a result of their frequent infiltration of surrounding neural tissue. Additionally, these tumors frequently manifest leptomeningeal metastasis, which complicates management and worsens overall prognosis [44]. It is unclear whether chemotherapy adds any benefit. Also adjuvant radiotherapy has remained controversial. In a case report, a patient with WHO grade II spinal cord oligodendroglioma who underwent subtotal tumor removal and adjuvant radiotherapy showed good functional outcome and disease control [45]. Subtotal removal with adjuvant radiotherapy could be an acceptable treatment option for WHO grade II spinal cord oligodendrogliomas.

4.4 Pial Tumors

4.4.1 Hemangioblastoma

Hemangioblastomas of the spinal cord are predominantly intramedullary, although these tumors can be extramedullary and extradural. Intramedullary hemangioblastomas represent about 4% of spinal tumors [46]. The origin cells are uncertain but likely vascular endothelial growth factor (VEGF)-secreting cells of undifferentiated mesenchymal origin [47, 48]. They occur sporadically in about 75%, and the remaining 25% are associated with von Hippel–Lindau disease [49]. Mutations in the short arm of chromosome 3p25 are seen in patients with von Hippel–Lindau disease (VHL) with hemangioblastomas [50]. Sporadic intramedullary hemangioblastomas have a peak incidence in the third or fourth decade of life, and men are more prevalent than women. Hemangioblastomas associated with this syndrome occurs at a younger age than sporadic cases of hemangioblastoma [51]. Most are solitary tumors, although multiple lesions are not uncommon [51]. Cervical and thoracic segments are usually involved with a predilection for the dorsolateral surface of the spinal cord [52]. Most of the hemangioblastomas occur in the dorsal portion of the spinal cord. Thus, symptoms are usually sensory, especially slowly progressive proprioception deficits. There may be other long-tract signs and radicular symptoms. Rarely, subarachnoid or intramedullary hemorrhage can occur.

Grossly, they are well demarcated with a capsule and have characteristic abnormally dilated tortuous vessels on the surface [53]. On MRI, intramedullary hemangioblastomas often appear as cysts with enhancing mural nodules. Associated syringobulbia and syringomyelia are common. These tumors are isointense on T1-weighted images and hyperintense on T2 weighted images [54]. Contrast enhancement is usually homogenous and well demarcated, with superficial heterogeneous enhancement within the flow voids [7]. Feeding arteries and draining veins can also be visible with contrasted MRI. Because of the presence of dilated vessels, these tumors are often mistaken for a vascular malformation. The presence of a syrinx, which is uncommon in vascular malformations but appears in 30%–60% of patients with a hemangioblastoma, may help to distinguish between these two [53–55]. A spinal cyst with an enhancing mural nodule and a nonenhancing cyst rim is another characteristic of a hemangioblastoma. The cysts associated with the tumors tend to grow faster than the tumor itself. The symptomatic mass effect is predominantly caused by the cysts. The tumor alternates between a growth phase and a quiescent phase with no growth. Thus, the tumors may remain at the same size for several years in a quiescent phase [56]. For this reason, follow-up monitoring with serial imaging at regular intervals is recommended.

Surgical resection is the primary treatment because there are often well-defined margins that allow for complete resection and thus the potential to achieve long-term local cure [51, 52, 57]. In a previous study, gross total removal (GTR) was achieved in 76.9% (10 of 13 patients) [58]. All patients who underwent GTR showed clinical improvements. The statistical analysis showed that GTR produced a significantly better outcome than subtotal resection.

In patients with multiple hemangioblastomas of the spinal cord, tumor resection should be directed at the symptomatic neoplasm. When intramedullary hemangioblastomas are part of a systemic presentation of von Hippel–Lindau syndrome, tumor resection should be considered on a case-by-case basis. There has been growing interest in the use of the VEGF inhibitor, bevacizumab, which have demonstrated clinical and radiographic response [59, 60]. The prognosis is usually excellent, although the tumor recurrence is common in patients with von Hippel–Lindau disease [61].

4.5 Intraarachnoidal Extrapial Tumors

4.5.1 Nerve-Sheath Tumors

Schwannomas are more common than neurofibromas and usually present as solitary tumors. Occasionally, multiple spinal schwannomas are seen with schwannomatosis or neurofibromatosis type II. Neurofibromas are often multiplicative when associated with neurofibromatosis type I. Schwannomas and neurofibromas account for up to a third of intradural spinal cord tumors in the adult population but are less common in children. The peak incidence of nerve-sheath tumors is in the fourth to fifth decade of life, and there is an equal incidence in both men and women. About 60%–80% of nerve-sheath tumors arise from nerve roots before leaving the dural sac. A further 10% arise as the nerve root leaves the dural sac and becomes surrounded by the dural-root sleeve. These tumors, therefore, display both intradural and extradural components (dumbbell tumor). Nerve-sheath tumors that are entirely extradural or intramedullary are less common. Although intradural nerve-sheath tumors are most common in the lumbosacral region, cervical and thoracic tumors have also been reported [62]. Intradural nerve-sheath tumors may be more common in the lumbosacral region due to the longer intradural segment of the caudal spinal nerve roots in the neuraxis [63].

Nerve-sheath tumors are generally considered as benign tumors but can be malignant in a few cases, where they have designated the term malignant peripheral nerve-sheath tumors (MPNSTs). Although more than 50% of MPNSTs are associated with neurofibromatosis type I, only a small percentage of patients with this disease have malignant neoplasms. Anatomically, schwannomas tend to occur in the dorsal nerve root, while neurofibromas occur more commonly in the ventral root. In addition to this difference, schwannomas and neurofibromas cannot be distinguished from MRI. An understanding of the anatomy and growth pattern of these tumors is essential for successful removal of large ventral IDEM spinal cord tumors. Large ventral IDEM spinal cord tumors can be removed entirely using a posterior approach and conventional laminectomy. In a previous study, there were 11 cases of schwannomas and 7 of meningiomas [64]. Complete resection of the tumor was possible in 94.4% (17 cases). There were no cases of recurrence. The one residual tumor was stable for 62 months.

Nerve-sheath tumors have an isointense signal on T1-weighted images and a hyperintense signal on T2-weighted images. Gadolinium adds a variety of enhancement, from homogeneous to peripheral ring-like enhancement [7]. Although an irregular enhancement pattern is associated with malignant tumors, differentiation from benign entities is unreliable with radiographic methods.

The primary treatment of nerve-sheath tumors is directed at total surgical resection, which is obtainable in most cases. Subtotal resection of these tumors can be an option when the tumor is attached to the spinal cord or when the tumor shows an extradural component that is closely associated with vital structures, such as the vertebral artery in the cervical spine [63]. The ventral or dorsal roots are usually sacrificed to obtain total resection. However, resection of the nerve root is not usually associated with postoperative motor or sensory deficit [63]. Because schwannomas arise from dorsal nerve roots and are less invasive than neurofibromas, surgical resection less often results in pronounced motor deficits than does a resection of neurofibromas. Postoperative morbidity can be affected by the spinal location of nerve-sheath tumors, with cervical and thoracic lesions predicting worse neurological outcomes than more caudal sites [62]. Radiotherapy or chemotherapy is usually reserved for tumors with malignant histological characteristics. Tumor recurrence is less than 5% and may be highly associated with subtotal tumor removal [62].

4.5.2 Myxopapillary Ependymoma

Myxopapillary ependymomas are the most common subtype of ependymomas. Myxopapillary ependymomas account for roughly 40%–50% of spinal ependymomas and are more common in the adult population than in children [65]. Myxopapillary ependymoma is almost exclusively seen in the conus medullaris and the filum terminale (95%). More than half of all tumors of the filum terminale and conus medullaris are myxopapillary ependymomas. This variant is distinguished from other ependymomas by the mucinous changes undergone by the tumor cells. Patients normally present with a long history of radicular pain, lower extremity sensorimotor deficit, and sphincter dysfunction.

They usually span two to four vertebral segments and fill the lumbosacral thecal sac. There may be vertebral body scalloping as well as intravertebral foraminal widening. Myxopapillary ependymomas are typically benign, well-circumscribed tumors. MRI reveals a circumscribed mass with the hypointense signal on T1-weighted images and hyperintense signal on T2-weighted images. Contrast enhancement with gadolinium is usually homogeneous. On T1- and T2-weighted images, they sometimes may be hyperintense due to the accumulation of mucin. On T2-weighted images, they may be hypointense because the tumor margin is consistent with hemosiderin.

Total surgical resection of myxopapillary ependymomas is possible if the nerve roots in the cauda equina are not entrapped within the tumor. In an attempt to keep to a minimum postoperative neurological morbidity, subtotal resection is not uncommon. Focal fractionalized radiotherapy seems to be effective in improving neurological outcome and reducing tumor recurrence after subtotal tumor removal or piecemeal total removal [66]. Recurrence after total resection is generally rare, but the outcome is poor [67]. These tumors can seed the spinal subarachnoid space, in which case wider field radiation is used, but this is rare. Although chemotherapy is sometimes started for recurrent or disseminated myxopapillary ependymomas, the results are not convincing.

4.5.3 Paraganglioma

Paragangliomas are derived from autonomic-nervous-system paraganglion cells and areuncommon in the CNS. Spinal paragangliomas are generally nonsecreting, sympathetic neoplasms, which tend to occur in the fourth to fifth decade of life and show a male predominance [68]. The most frequent intradural location for paragangliomas is the cauda equina and lumbar spine regions [69, 70].

Paragangliomas show hypointense or isointense signal on T1-weighted images, which are relatively well delineated round, ovoid or lobulated masses with prominent flow voids. On T2-weighted images, there is isointensity to hyperintensity with hemosiderin rim as well as tumoral cyst formation [71]. Paragangliomas are characteristically hypervascular, and gadolinium contrast administration produces a heterogeneous salt and pepper pattern of enhancement [72]. Paragangliomas rarely occur in the cauda equina. In a previous study, four cases of paraganglioma of the cauda equina were misdiagnosed as neurinoma preoperatively [73]. On MRI, they were well demarcated, heterogeneously enhancing masses with a hypointense tumor margin, intratumoral hemorrhagic or cystic changes, intratumoral focal low signal intensity, and peritumoral loculated CSF spaces.

Intradural paragangliomas are mainly benign neoplasms, and gross total surgical resection is the preferred treatment. Catecholamine-secreting spinal paragangliomas are rare, but preoperative screening for a hyperadrenergic condition is necessary to prevent hypertensive crisis during tumor removal. The recurrence rate after total or subtotal resection of intradural paragangliomas is less than 5% and is not reduced by concurrent radiotherapy or chemotherapy. Although iodine-131 labeled mIBG (131I-mIBG) may slow progression and improve remission rate for metastatic paragangliomas, efficacy in primary intradural paragangliomas has not been demonstrated [74].

4.5.4 Dermoid and Epidermoid Cysts

Spinal dermoid cyst and epidermoid cyst are a relatively rare benign tumor. Spinal dermoid cyst accounts for less than 1% of spinal cord tumors in adult patients and fewer than 3% in pediatric patients [75]. Most of the spinal dermoid cysts are congenital neoplasms arising from heterotopic ectodermal-cell implantation into the neural tube in the early embryonic development. Some are acquired after lumbar puncture and other lumbar medical manipulations [76, 77]. These tumors most commonly affect the lumbosacral region, with rare reports of thoracic involvement [78]. Dermoid and epidermoid cysts are usually diagnosed in the first two decades of life, with dermoid cysts presenting earlier than epidermoid cysts [79].

On gross appearance, dermoid cysts can be differentiated from epidermoid cysts by the appearance of skin appendages such as hair follicles; however, the distinction between these tumors is often difficult by imaging. Both intradural dermoid and epidermoid cysts have variable MRI appearance, with hypointense to hyperintense signal on T1-weighted images and isointense to hyperintense signal on T2-weighted images. There is usually minimum enhancement with gadolinium.

The epidermoid cyst is a slow-growing benign tumor, but there is also a possibility of malignant tumors [80, 81]. Gross total resection of dermoid and epidermoid cysts are preferred when possible, but adhesion to neural tissue can prevent aggressive surgery. If subtotal resection is performed, it is better to empty the cystic contents and remove the capsule. Dissemination of the cystic contents spontaneously or during tumor removal can cause granulomatous meningitis, which can be treated with corticosteroids [82]. Recurrence of resected intradural dermoid and epidermoid cysts is uncommon, and malignant tumors are rare. Adjuvant radiotherapy or chemotherapy for nonoperative or malignant cases has not yet been fully studied.

4.6 Extraarachnoidal Intradural Tumors

4.6.1 Meningioma

Meningiomas are dural-based tumors that arise from arachnoid cap cells and consequently can be found at any location that dura is present. Spinal meningiomas account for up to 46% of spinal tumors and are more common intradural than extradural [83]. A small percentage of spinal meningiomas are located extradural, and extension of these tumors into the intradural compartment is common. In general, 80% of meningiomas are found in the thoracic region, 15% are cervical, and 5% are lumbosacral. The peak incidence for spinal meningiomas is in the fifth and sixth decades. About 70% is found in females. Intradural meningiomas are mostly located lateral or posterior to the spinal cord, with the anterior location being less frequent [83, 84]. Intradural meningiomas are usually solitary lesions, but multiple tumors can occur when these tumors are associated with neurofibromatosis type II.

On MRI, spinal meningiomas have a hypointense to isointense signal on T1-weighted images and a hyperintense signal on T2-weighted images. The addition of gadolinium contrast gives strong homogeneous enhancement. Calcifications are frequent and could preclude gadolinium enhancement [7].

These tumors are usually solitary and have a broad attachment to the dura. They are well circumscribed and delineated from the spinal cord.

Most intradural meningiomas are noninvasive benign tumors that help in gross total resection of the tumor. Despite the technical problem of anterior locations, total surgical resection of meningiomas is possible in more than 90% of patients [85]. The tumor recurrence rate with total or subtotal resection is between 3 and 7% [83–85]. Atypical and anaplastic spinal meningiomas have a higher tumor recurrence rate and rarely metastasize. For patients with incomplete resection or recurrence, conventional external beam fractionated radiotherapy or stereotactic radiosurgery is used [84, 86].

4.7 Dural Tumors

4.7.1 Solitary Fibrous Tumor

A solitary fibrous tumor (SFT) is a rare tumor of the central nervous system. Up to date, about 78 cases of SFT have been reported [87]. Most of these cases occurred in adults (94.8% in patients older than 21 years, mean 51.5 years). There is a slight male predominance (56.4% male vs. 43.6% female). Although SFT has been reported in all parts of the spinal column, the thoracic region (42.1%) is the most frequent site involved, followed by the cervical region (27.6%) and lumbar region (13.2%).

Most of the lesions were either hypointense or isointense on T1- and T2-weighted imaging. On contrast-enhanced MRI, they usually enhance homogeneously.

Gross-total resection (GTR) was achieved in 82.7% of patients, and subtotal resection (STR) was performed in 17.3%. Of 46 patients treated with GTR, 41 (89.1%) had no recurrence at a median of 1.2 years of follow-up. Four patients had a local recurrence. Another patient developed a local spinal recurrence (malignant transformation) and recurrent pulmonary and hepatic metastases. The beneficial role of postoperative radiotherapy in SFT has not yet been proven.

4.8 Transcompartmental

4.8.1 Lipoma

Lipomas are congenital, benign transcompartmental tumors. The incidence of lipoma is 1%–11% of spinal tumors [3]. Spinal lipomas are one of the most common spinal developmental anomalies encountered in pediatric neurosurgery and represent a group of disorders known as occult spinal dysraphism, which is often associated with "pathologic" spina bifida [88]. The embryonic background of spinal lipomas is marked by a premature disjunction between the neural and cutaneous ectoderm during the process of primary neurulation [89]. Failed primary neurulation allows invasion of mesenchymal tissue of mesodermic origin into the neural structure, leading to the formation of a spinal lipoma. Intradural extramedullary lipomas are usually located in the lower thoracic and lumbosacral levels. A tethered-cord syndrome present at birth or develop during infancy can be encountered with lipomas of the cauda equina. This syndrome consists of sensorimotor deficits, pain, skeletal deformities, and sphincter dysfunction and is less common in adults with lumbosacral lipomas [90]. When unrelated to spinal dysraphism, displacement of the spinal cord by lipomas can cause the early manifestation of symptoms.

MRI is the diagnostic study of choice for spinal lipomas, because of the characteristic hyperintense image produced by T1-weighted imaging and the relatively lower intensity on T2-weighted imaging and because of the characteristic imaging on fat-suppression sequences (e.g., T1 short tau inversion recovery). They are nonenhancing on postcontrast MRI.

Decompressive surgical resection is recommended for symptomatic intradural lipomas. Lack of cleavage plane and the intermingling of neural and fibrofatty tissue at the periphery of the tumor makes removal of the entire tumor extremely difficult. Surgical resection of symptomatic intramedullary lipomas aimed at the tumor debulking rather than gross total resection. Intraoperative electrophysiological stimulation with evoked EMG monitoring is often used to distinguish functional spinal cord from the mass. When unassociated with a tethered cord, prophylactic resection of asymptomatic lipomas of the filum terminalis can prevent subsequent neurological decline [91]. Congenital lipomas can impede the normal development of the surrounding neural tissue, and, therefore, postsurgical improvement is often absent [92].

4.9 Conclusion

Spinal tumors are relatively rare and affect only a minority of the population. Because they may cause significant morbidity in terms of pain and limb dysfunction and are associated with mortality as well, their correct diagnosis and prompt treatment can be very important. Primary treatment of primary spinal cord tumors is surgical resection, and predictors of outcome include preoperative functional status (limited to no neurologic deficit predicts for better outcome), the histologic grade of the tumor (lower grade predicts for improved survival), and extent of surgical resection (image-verified complete resection improves survival).

References

1. Parsa AT, Chi JH, Acosta FL Jr, et al. Intramedullary spinal cord tumors: molecular insights and surgical innovation. Clin Neurosurg. 2005;52:76–84.
2. Stein BM, McCormick PC. Intramedullary neoplasms and vascular malformations. Clin Neurosurg. 1992;39:361–87.
3. Kane PJ, el-Mahdy W, Singh A, et al. Spinal intradural tumours: part II-intramedullary. Br J Neurosurg. 1999; 13:558–63.
4. Miller DC. Surgical pathology of intramedullary spinal cord neoplasms. J Neurooncol. 2000;47:189–94.
5. Koeller KK, Rosenblum RS, Morrison AL. Neoplasms of the spinal cord and filum terminale: radiologic-pathologic correlation. Radiographics. 2000;20:1721–49.
6. Smith AB, Soderlund KA, Rushing EJ, et al. Radiologic-pathologic correlation of pediatric and adolescent spinal neoplasms: part 1, intramedullary spinal neoplasms. AJR Am J Roentgenol. 2012;198:34–43.
7. Van Goethem JW, van den Hauwe L, Ozsarlak O, et al. Spinal tumors. Eur J Radiol. 2004;50:159–76.
8. Innocenzi G, Raco A, Cantore G, et al. Intramedullary astrocytomas and ependymomas in the pediatric age group: a retrospective study. Childs Nerv Syst. 1996;12:776–80.
9. Epstein FJ, Farmer JP. Pediatric spinal cord tumor surgery. Neurosurg Clin N Am. 1990;1:569–90.
10. Raco A, Esposito V, Lenzi J, et al. Long-term follow-up of intramedullary spinal cord tumors: a series of 202 cases. Neurosurgery. 2005; 56:972–81; discussion-81.
11. Chang UK, Choe WJ, Chung SK, et al. Surgical outcome and prognostic factors of spinal intramedullary ependymomas in adults. J Neurooncol. 2002;57:133–9.
12. Stuben G, Stuschke M, Kroll M, et al. Postoperative radiotherapy of spinal and intracranial ependymomas: analysis of prognostic factors. Radiother Oncol. 1997;45:3–10.
13. Lin YH, Huang CI, Wong TT, et al. Treatment of spinal cord ependymomas by surgery with or without postoperative radiotherapy. J Neurooncol. 2005;71:205–10.
14. Chamberlain MC. Salvage chemotherapy for recurrent spinal cord ependymona. Cancer. 2002;95:997–1002.
15. McCormick PC, Torres R, Post KD, et al. Intramedullary ependymoma of the spinal cord. J Neurosurg. 1990;72:523–32.
16. Lee TT, Gromelski EB, Green BA. Surgical treatment of spinal ependymoma and post-operative radiotherapy. Acta Neurochir (Wien). 1998;140:309–13.
17. Constantini S, Houten J, Miller DC, et al. Intramedullary spinal cord tumors in children under the age of 3 years. J Neurosurg. 1996;85:1036–43.
18. Rossitch E Jr, Zeidman SM, Burger PC, et al. Clinical and pathological analysis of spinal cord astrocytomas in children. Neurosurgery. 1990;27:193–6.
19. Nadkarni TD, Rekate HL. Pediatric intramedullary spinal cord tumors. Critical review of the literature. Childs Nerv Syst. 1999; 15:17–28.
20. Innocenzi G, Salvati M, Cervoni L, et al. Prognostic factors in intramedullary astrocytomas. Clin Neurol Neurosurg. 1997;99:1–5.
21. Tinchon A, Oberndorfer S, Marosi C, et al. Malignant spinal cord compression in cerebral glioblastoma multiforme: a multicenter case series and review of the literature. J Neurooncol. 2012;110:221–6.
22. Santi M, Mena H, Wong K, et al. Spinal cord malignant astrocytomas. Clinicopathologic features in 36 cases. Cancer. 2003; 98:554–61.
23. Runge VM, Muroff LR, Jinkins JR. Central nervous system: review of clinical use of contrast media. Top Magn Reson Imaging. 2001;12:231–63.

24. Karikari IO, Nimjee SM, Hodges TR, et al. Impact of tumor histology on resectability and neurological outcome in primary intramedullary spinal cord tumors: a single-center experience with 102 patients. Neurosurgery. 2011; 68:188–97; discussion 97.
25. Chamberlain MC, Tredway TL. Adult primary intradural spinal cord tumors: a review. Curr Neurol Neurosci Rep. 2011;11:320–8.
26. Ciappetta P, Celli P, Palma L, et al. Intraspinal hemangiopericytomas. Report of two cases and review of the literature. Spine (Phila Pa 1976). 1985; 10:27–31.
27. Kim MS, Chung CK, Choe G, et al. Intramedullary spinal cord astrocytoma in adults: postoperative outcome. J Neurooncol. 2001;52:85–94.
28. Sarkar C, Mukhopadhyay S, Ralte AM, et al. Intramedullary subependymoma of the spinal cord: a case report and review of literature. Clin Neurol Neurosurg. 2003;106:63–8.
29. Matsumoto K, Nakagaki H. Intramedullary subependymoma occupying the right half of the thoracic spinal cord–case report. Neurol Med Chir (Tokyo). 2002;42:349–53.
30. Jallo GI, Zagzag D, Epstein F. Intramedullary subependymoma of the spinal cord. Neurosurgery. 1996;38:251–7.
31. Yuh WT, Chung CK, Park SH, et al. Spinal cord subependymoma surgery: a multi-institutional experience. J Korean Neurosurg Soc. 2018;61:233–42.
32. Lee JC, Glasauer FE. Ganglioglioma: light and electron microscopic study. Neurochirurgia (Stuttg). 1968;11:160–70.
33. Jallo GI, Freed D, Epstein FJ. Spinal cord gangliogliomas: a review of 56 patients. J Neurooncol. 2004;68:71–7.
34. Patel U, Pinto RS, Miller DC, et al. MR of spinal cord ganglioglioma. AJNR Am J Neuroradiol. 1998;19:879–87.
35. Cheung YK, Fung CF, Chan FL, et al. MRI features of spinal ganglioglioma. Clin Imaging. 1991;15:109–12.
36. Kincaid PK, El-Saden SM, Park SH, et al. Cerebral gangliogliomas: preoperative grading using FDG-PET and 201Tl-SPECT. AJNR Am J Neuroradiol. 1998;19:801–6.
37. Park CK, Chung CK, Choe GY, et al. Intramedullary spinal cord ganglioglioma: a report of five cases. Acta Neurochir (Wien). 2000;142:547–52.
38. Lang FF, Epstein FJ, Ransohoff J, et al. Central nervous system gangliogliomas. Part 2: Clinical outcome. J Neurosurg. 1993; 79:867–73.
39. Schneider C, Vosbeck J, Grotzer MA, et al. Anaplastic ganglioglioma: a very rare intramedullary spinal cord tumor. Pediatr Neurosurg. 2012;48:42–7.
40. Hamburger C, Buttner A, Weis S. Ganglioglioma of the spinal cord: report of two rare cases and review of the literature. Neurosurgery. 1997; 41:1410–5; discussion 5–6.
41. Nam DH, Cho BK, Kim YM, et al. Intramedullary anaplastic oligodendroglioma in a child. Childs Nerv Syst. 1998;14:127–30.
42. Fountas KN, Karampelas I, Nikolakakos LG, et al. Primary spinal cord oligodendroglioma: case report and review of the literature. Childs Nerv Syst. 2005;21:171–5.
43. Traul DE, Shaffrey ME, Schiff D. Part I: spinal-cord neoplasms-intradural neoplasms. Lancet Oncol. 2007;8:35–45.
44. Ushida T, Sonobe H, Mizobuchi H, et al. Oligodendroglioma of the "widespread" type in the spinal cord. Childs Nerv Syst. 1998;14:751–5.
45. Yuh WT, Chung CK, Park SH. Primary spinal cord oligodendroglioma with postoperative adjuvant radiotherapy: a case report. Korean J Spine. 2015;12:160–4.
46. Lonser RR, Weil RJ, Wanebo JE, et al. Surgical management of spinal cord hemangioblastomas in patients with von Hippel-Lindau disease. J Neurosurg. 2003;98:106–16.
47. Morii K, Tanaka R, Washiyama K, et al. Expression of vascular endothelial growth factor in capillary hemangioblastoma. Biochem Biophys Res Commun. 1993;194:749–55.
48. Frank TS, Trojanowski JQ, Roberts SA, et al. A detailed immunohistochemical analysis of cerebellar hemangioblastoma: an undifferentiated mesenchymal tumor. Mod Pathol. 1989;2:638–51.
49. Neumann HP, Eggert HR, Scheremet R, et al. Central nervous system lesions in von Hippel-Lindau syndrome. J Neurol Neurosurg Psychiatry. 1992;55:898–901.
50. Latif F, Tory K, Gnarra J, et al. Identification of the von Hippel-Lindau disease tumor suppressor gene. Science. 1993;260:1317–20.
51. Murota T, Symon L. Surgical management of hemangioblastoma of the spinal cord: a report of 18 cases. Neurosurgery. 1989; 25:699–707; discussion 8.
52. Cristante L, Herrmann HD. Surgical management of intramedullary hemangioblastoma of the spinal cord. Acta Neurochir (Wien). 1999; 141:333–9; discussion 9–40.
53. Na JH, Kim HS, Eoh W, et al. Spinal cord hemangioblastoma : diagnosis and clinical outcome after surgical treatment. J Korean Neurosurg Soc. 2007;42:436–40.
54. Chu BC, Terae S, Hida K, et al. MR findings in spinal hemangioblastoma: correlation with symptoms and with angiographic and surgical findings. AJNR Am J Neuroradiol. 2001;22:206–17.
55. Bostrom A, Hans FJ, Reinacher PC, et al. Intramedullary hemangioblastomas: timing of surgery, microsurgical technique and follow-up in 23 patients. Eur Spine J. 2008;17:882–6.
56. Wanebo JE, Lonser RR, Glenn GM, et al. The natural history of hemangioblastomas of the central nervous system in patients with von Hippel-Lindau disease. J Neurosurg. 2003;98:82–94.

57. Spetzler RF, Detwiler PW, Riina HA, et al. Modified classification of spinal cord vascular lesions. J Neurosurg. 2002;96:145–56.
58. Lee DK, Choe WJ, Chung CK, et al. Spinal cord hemangioblastoma: surgical strategy and clinical outcome. J Neurooncol. 2003;61:27–34.
59. Schuch G, de Wit M, Holtje J, et al. Case 2. Hemangioblastomas: diagnosis of von Hippel-Lindau disease and antiangiogenic treatment with SU5416. J Clin Oncol. 2005; 23:3624–6.
60. Benesch M, Windelberg M, Sauseng W, et al. Compassionate use of bevacizumab (Avastin) in children and young adults with refractory or recurrent solid tumors. Ann Oncol. 2008;19:807–13.
61. Garces-Ambrossi GL, McGirt MJ, Mehta VA, et al. Factors associated with progression-free survival and long-term neurological outcome after resection of intramedullary spinal cord tumors: analysis of 101 consecutive cases. J Neurosurg Spine. 2009;11:591–9.
62. Conti P, Pansini G, Mouchaty H, et al. Spinal neurinomas: retrospective analysis and long-term outcome of 179 consecutively operated cases and review of the literature. Surg Neurol. 2004; 61:34–43; discussion 4.
63. Jinnai T, Koyama T. Clinical characteristics of spinal nerve sheath tumors: analysis of 149 cases. Neurosurgery.2005; 56:510–5; discussion -5.
64. Kim CH, Chung CK. Surgical outcome of a posterior approach for large ventral intradural extramedullary spinal cord tumors. Spine (Phila Pa 1976). 2011; 36:E531–7.
65. Celli P, Cervoni L, Cantore G. Ependymoma of the filum terminale: treatment and prognostic factors in a series of 28 cases. Acta Neurochir (Wien). 1993;124:99–103.
66. Schweitzer JS, Batzdorf U. Ependymoma of the cauda equina region: diagnosis, treatment, and outcome in 15 patients. Neurosurgery. 1992;30:202–7.
67. Gagliardi FM, Cervoni L, Domenicucci M, et al. Ependymomas of the filum terminale in childhood: report of four cases and review of the literature. Childs Nerv Syst. 1993;9:3–6.
68. Walsh JC, O'Brien DF, Kumar R, et al. Paraganglioma of the cauda equina: a case report and literature review. Surgeon. 2005;3:113–6.
69. Sundgren P, Annertz M, Englund E, et al. Paragangliomas of the spinal canal. Neuroradiology. 1999;41:788–94.
70. Silverstein AM, Quint DJ, McKeever PE. Intradural paraganglioma of the thoracic spine. AJNR Am J Neuroradiol. 1990;11:614–6.
71. Faro SH, Turtz AR, Koenigsberg RA, et al. Paraganglioma of the cauda equina with associated intramedullary cyst: MR findings. AJNR Am J Neuroradiol. 1997;18:1588–90.
72. Shin JY, Lee SM, Hwang MY, et al. MR findings of the spinal paraganglioma: report of three cases. J Korean Med Sci. 2001;16:522–6.
73. Yang SY, Jin YJ, Park SH, et al. Paragangliomas in the cauda equina region: clinicopathoradiologic findings in four cases. J Neurooncol. 2005;72:49–55.
74. Noorda RJ, Wuisman PI, Kummer AJ, et al. Nonfunctioning malignant paraganglioma of the posterior mediastinum with spinal cord compression. A case report. Spine (Phila Pa 1976). 1996; 21:1703–9.
75. Watanabe E, Tanaka K, Takeda N, et al. Surgical technique to prevent spillage of cyst fluid during operation for cystic ovarian tumors. Pediatr Surg Int. 2013;29:645–9.
76. Suocheng G, Yazhou X. A review on five cases of intramedullary dermoid cyst. Childs Nerv Syst. 2014;30:659–64.
77. Park JC, Chung CK, Kim HJ. Iatrogenic spinal epidermoid tumor. a complication of spinal puncture in an adult. Clin Neurol Neurosurg. 2003; 105:281–5.
78. Scarrow AM, Levy EI, Gerszten PC, et al. Epidermoid cyst of the thoracic spine: case history. Clin Neurol Neurosurg. 2001;103:220–2.
79. Shikata J, Yamamuro T, Mikawa Y, et al. Intraspinal epidermoid and dermoid cysts. Surgical results of seven cases. Arch Orthop Trauma Surg. 1988; 107:105–9.
80. Seif B, Pourkhalili R, Shekarchizadeh A, et al. Malignant transformation of an intracranial extradural epidermoid cyst into squamous cell carcinoma presented with cerebrospinal fluid leakage. Adv Biomed Res. 2017;6:16.
81. Shah A, Patil M, Goel A. Recurrent craniospinal epidermoid: a case report. J Craniovertebr Junction Spine. 2016;7:59–61.
82. Lunardi P, Missori P, Gagliardi FM, et al. Long-term results of the surgical treatment of spinal dermoid and epidermoid tumors. Neurosurgery. 1989;25:860–4.
83. Roux FX, Nataf F, Pinaudeau M, et al. Intraspinal meningiomas: review of 54 cases with discussion of poor prognosis factors and modern therapeutic management. Surg Neurol. 1996; 46:458–63; discussion 63–4.
84. Gezen F, Kahraman S, Canakci Z, et al. Review of 36 cases of spinal cord meningioma. Spine (Phila Pa 1976). 2000; 25:727–31.
85. Solero CL, Fornari M, Giombini S, et al. Spinal meningiomas: review of 174 operated cases. Neurosurgery. 1989;25:153–60.
86. Ryu SI, Chang SD, Kim DH, et al. Image-guided hypo-fractionated stereotactic radiosurgery to spinal lesions. Neurosurgery. 2001;49:838–46.
87. Albert GW, Gokden M. Solitary fibrous tumors of the spine: a pediatric case report with a comprehensive review of the literature. J Neurosurg Pediatr. 2017;19:339–48.
88. Gabbe SG, Mintz MC, Mennuti MT, et al. Detection of open spina bifida by the lemon sign: pathologic correlation. J Clin Ultrasound. 1988;16:399–402.

89. Pang D, Zovickian J, Wong ST, et al. Surgical treatment of complex spinal cord lipomas. Childs Nerv Syst. 2013;29:1485–513.
90. Gupta SK, Khosla VK, Sharma BS, et al. Tethered cord syndrome in adults. Surg Neurol. 1999; 52:362–9; discussion 70.
91. Pierre-Kahn A, Zerah M, Renier D, et al. Congenital lumbosacral lipomas. Childs Nerv Syst. 1997; 13:298–334; discussion 5.
92. Lee M, Rezai AR, Abbott R, et al. Intramedullary spinal cord lipomas. J Neurosurg. 1995;82:394–400.

How to Approach Anatomical Compartment; Extradural Nerve Plexus Tumor

5

Sung Bae Park and Chun Kee Chung

Abstract

Although extradural nerve plexus tumors in brachial and lumbosacral plexuses are rare, the removal of the tumors should be considered. The surgical strategy requires not only the anatomical understanding but also the appropriate surgical approach according to tumor characteristics. In the present chapter, we describe the general concepts for the tumors and show the way how to surgically approach the tumors.

Keywords

Extradural · Nerve · Plexus · Tumor · Schwannoma

Electronic supplementary material The online version of this chapter (https://doi.org/10.1007/978-981-15-7771-0_5) contains supplementary material, which is available to authorized users.

S. B. Park
Department of Neurosurgery, Seoul National University Boramae Hospital, Seoul, South Korea
e-mail: ddolbae01@naver.com

C. K. Chung (✉)
Department of Neurosurgery, Seoul National University Hospital, Seoul National University College of Medicine, Seoul, Republic of Korea
e-mail: chungc@snu.ac.kr

Neuroscience Research Institute, Seoul National University Medical Research Center, Seoul, Republic of Korea

Clinical Research Institute, Seoul National University Hospital, Seoul, Republic of Korea

Department of Brain and Cognitive Sciences, Seoul National University College of Natural Sciences, Seoul, Republic of Korea

5.1 Introduction

Thirty-one pairs of spinal nerves are formed by convergence of dorsal and ventral roots within the intervertebral foramen. Then, each spinal nerve divides into a dorsal and ventral rami. The ventral rami, except T2–T12, form interlacing nerve networks called plexuses, which include the cervical, brachial, and lumbosacral plexus [1]. The peripheral nerve, consisting of the plexus, is composed of motor and sensory neurons in the spinal canal and axons, which signal with a distant target organ [2]. The axons are surrounded by thin collagen fibers forming an endoneurium and are sorted into fascicles separated by a discrete connective tissue sheath known as the perineurium. There is internal epineurium between these fascicles and a connective tissue sheath, external epineurium encompasses all the fascicles that group together to form a single nerve (Fig. 5.1).

C. K. Chung (ed.), *Surgery of Spinal Cord Tumors Based on Anatomy*,
https://doi.org/10.1007/978-981-15-7771-0_5

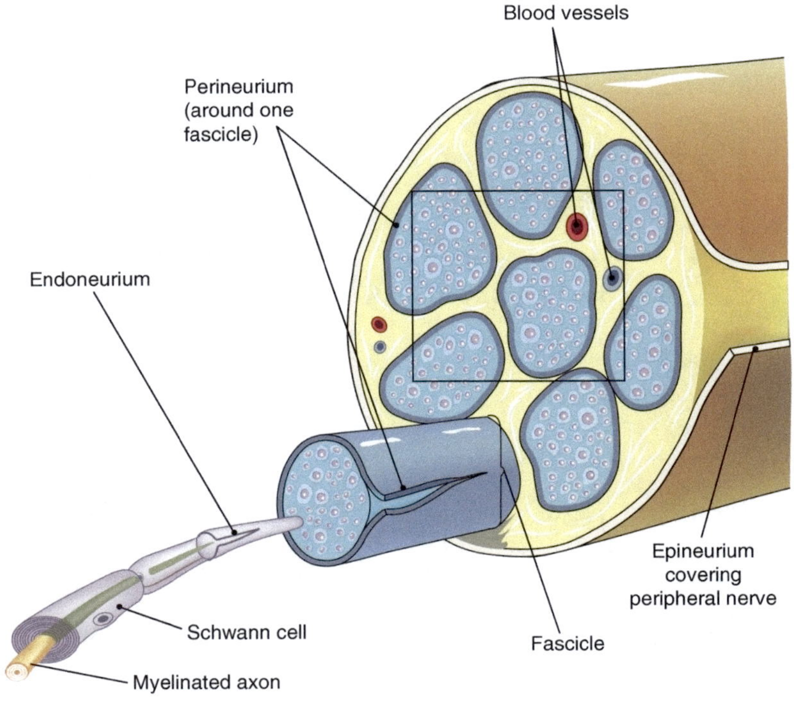

Fig. 5.1 Peripheral nerve anatomy

Primary tumors of the brachial and lumbosacral plexuses are rare [3, 4]. The tumors can be divided into two groups such as peripheral neural sheath tumors (PNSTs) and peripheral nonneural sheath tumors (PNNSTs), each of which could be benign or malignant [5]. PNNSTs are rarer than PNSTs [6, 7]. PNSTs including schwannomas and neurofibromas are the most common tumors arising from peripheral nerve and rarely affect brachial and lumbosacral plexuses [3]. Most publications on brachial and lumbosacral plexus tumors are case reports or small series of patients [3, 4, 7, 8]. Schwannomas are thought to arise from an intraneural Schwann cell and neurofibromas are heterogeneous tumors that arise from the connective tissue of peripheral nerve sheaths [9, 10]. PNSTs present as a local slowly growing mass and manifest clinically with symptoms of nerve compression [3, 4]. Malignant PNSTs affect only 0.001% of the general population and are known as neurogenic sarcomas including malignant schwannomas and neurofibrosarcomas [10]. These lesions are rapidly growing, firm, and fixed; patients with malignant PNST may present with rapidly progressive loss of function or severe pain [10]. Most common presenting symptom in nerve sheath tumors was generally palpable mass, pain, followed by sensory change [3].

Although MR imaging is unable to differentiate between schwannoma and neurofibroma, the MRI has become a critical tool in making a presumptive diagnosis and in surgical planning of nerve sheath tumors [11]. Typical MRI findings of benign PNSTs are a well-defined oval mass with the long axis in line with the nerve of origin, homogeneous intermediate signal intensity (SI) on T1-weighted images and hyperintense on T2-weighted images with inhomogeneous central low SI (Fig. 5.2a). Also, the mass is of strong enhancement following contrast administration (Fig. 5.2b).

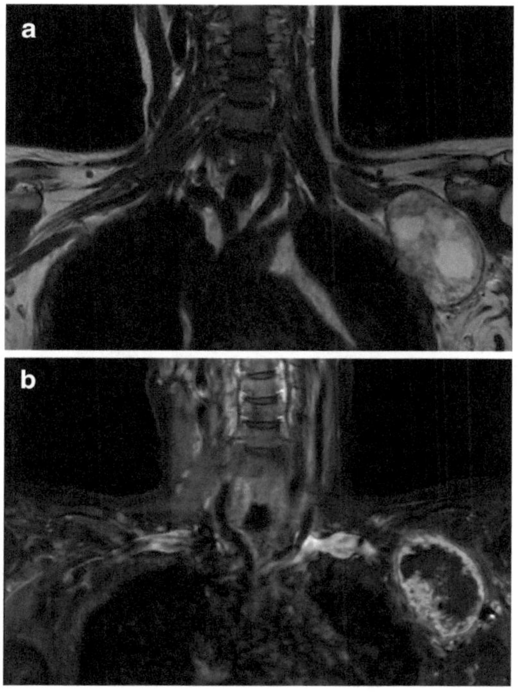

Fig. 5.2 MRI imaging of schwannoma arising from the left brachial plexus. **a** Coronal MRI imaging showing schwannoma arising from the left brachial plexus. A) T2 image shows well-delineated, inhomogeneous hyperintense mass. **b** Following gadolinium administration, the tumor shows inhomogeneous enhancement

Because the normal anatomical locations of neurovascular structures around these lesions may be changed, tumor removal may cause neurological deficit. Therefore, the planning of surgical approach may be changed according to the origin, characteristics, extension, and pathology. PNST can be completely resected for relatively small and medium-size tumors and that kinds of gross total resection can be expected good postoperative outcome and prognosis. However, wide local resection of the tumor and adjacent soft tissues in malignant PNST is unavoidable, followed by radio and chemotherapy [10].

We describe the surgical steps in the removal of PNSTs and illustrate our cases of PNSTs arising from brachial and lumbar plexuses as follows.

5.1.1 Strategy of Surgical Treatment

Schwannomas tend to displace the surrounding fascicles, whereas neurofibromas involve the nerve [12]. Therefore, the schwannoma can be resected with sparing the involved nerve, whereas the underlying nerve is sacrificed in the removal of the neurofibroma (Fig. 5.3). Surgical steps are introduced as follows:

1. The longitudinal incision on skin usually is more advantageous than a short or transverse incision. Surrounding neurovascular structures should be mobilized and preserved. The neural structures should be identified and protected.
2. The proximal and distal poles of tumor and tumor are isolated followed by direct dissection of tumor. Because the intraneural mass usually spans between fascicles, the longitudinal epineurotomy should be made to devoid of fascicles in the spanned area by Fig. 5.4a. Nerve action potential (NAP) monitoring may help identify the safe zones between fascicles (Fig. 5.5).
3. In schwannomas, there are mostly one or two entering and exiting fascicles into the tumor. Therefore, the proximal and distal poles of mass should be identified. In dissection of tumor, the NAP recording can provide information for the functional or non-functional traversing fascicles across the tumor capsule and non-functional fascicles entering and exiting the tumor (Fig. 5.4b). The tumor is then removed en bloc after the sectioning of proximal and distal exiting fascicle into the tumor (Fig. 5.4c).

5.1.2 Case Reviews

Case 1. Schwannoma in brachial plexus (Video 1).

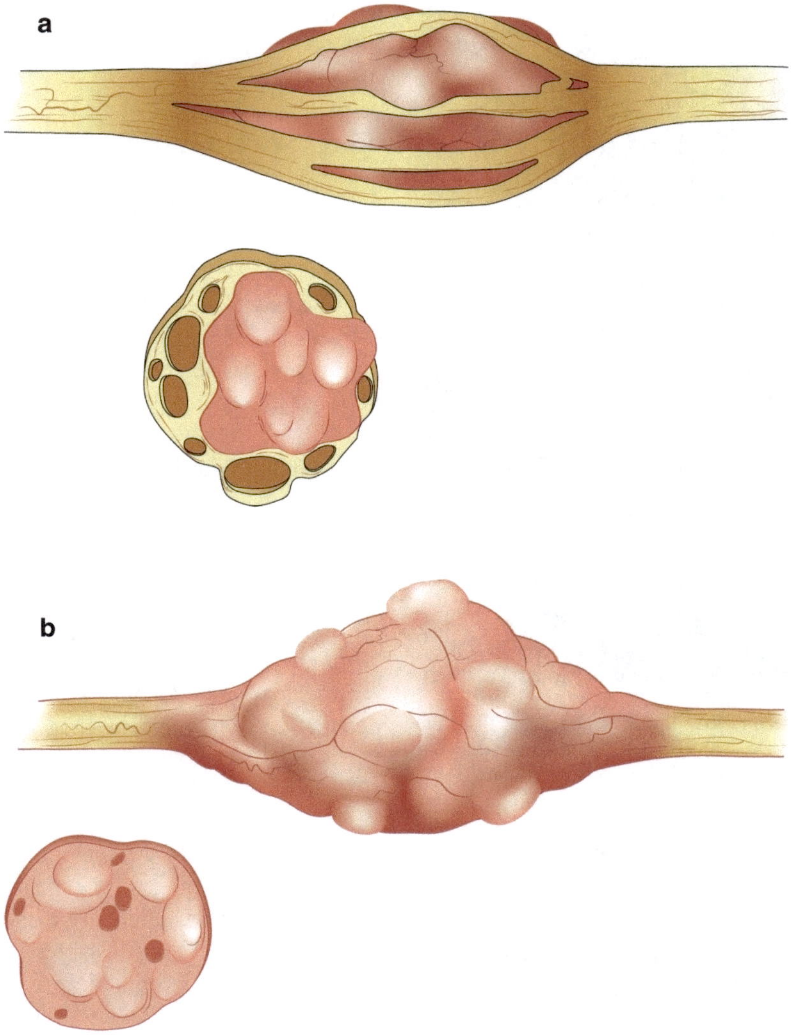

Fig. 5.3 Illustration of schwannoma and neurofibroma appearance **a** Schwannoma appearance with cross-sectional view. Unaffected normal fascles are displaced by tumor mass. **b** Neurofibroma appearance with cross-sectional view. All fascicles are affected and intermingled within the mass

A 39-year-old female patient complained of mass in left axillary area. The patient also complained of pain for the palpable mass on left axillary area. Magnetic resonance (MR) images showed an ovoid mass along brachial plexus (Fig. 5.1). The patient underwent brachial plexus tumor removal. The thinned epineurium was opened between fascicles and the tumor was

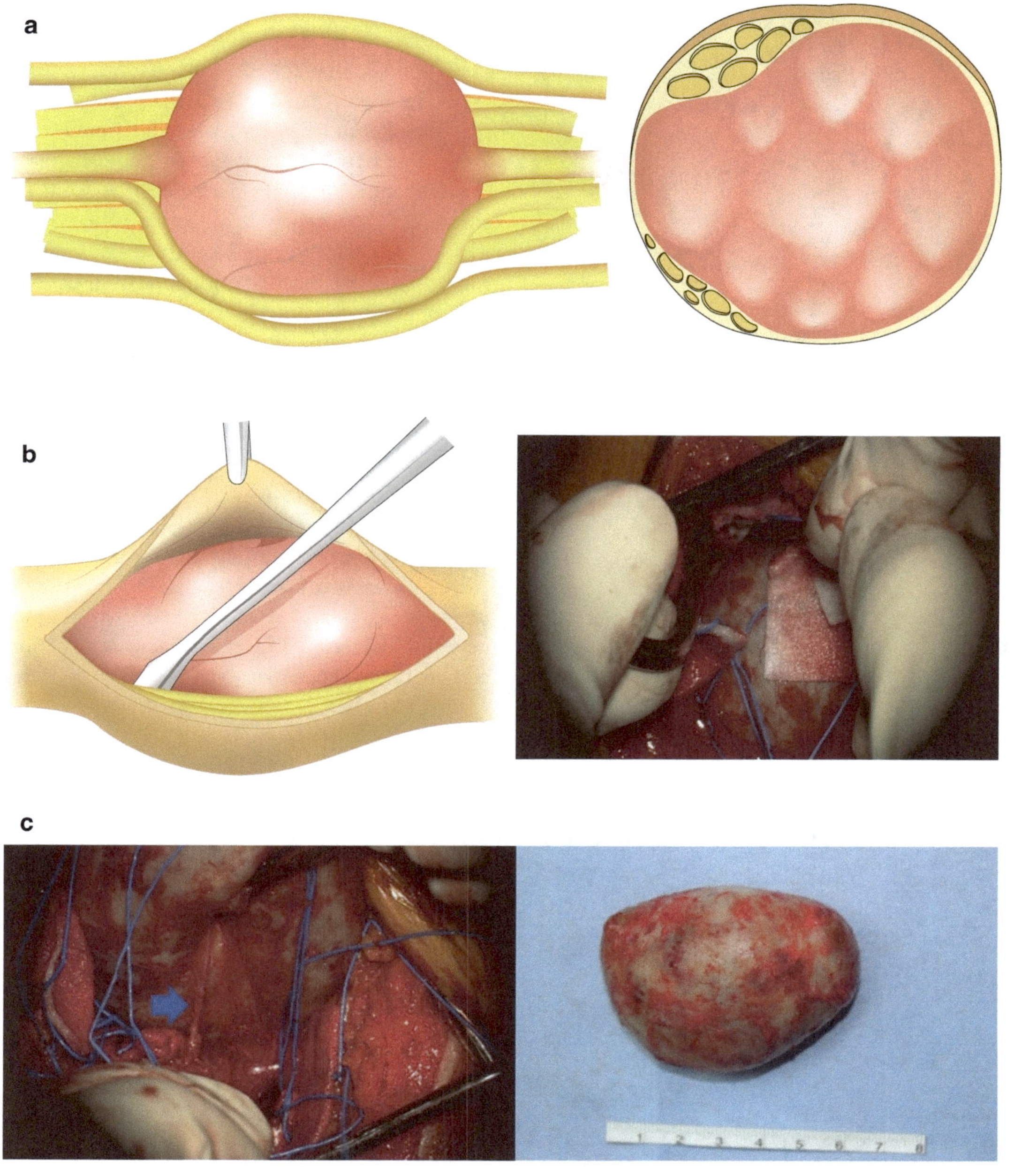

Fig. 5.4 Illustration of surgical steps for removal of benign peripheral nerve sheath tumor. **a** Adjacent nerves, vessels, and other structures must be dissected away and the lesion with proximal and distal parts of lesion should be isolated. **b** Because a tumor spans other normal fascicles, epineurotomy is performed over the tumor capsule. **c** In isolation of tumor, other fascicles are dissected free from the tumor. **d** After the identification of proximal and distal poles of tumor (arrow), the tumor is removed at a time

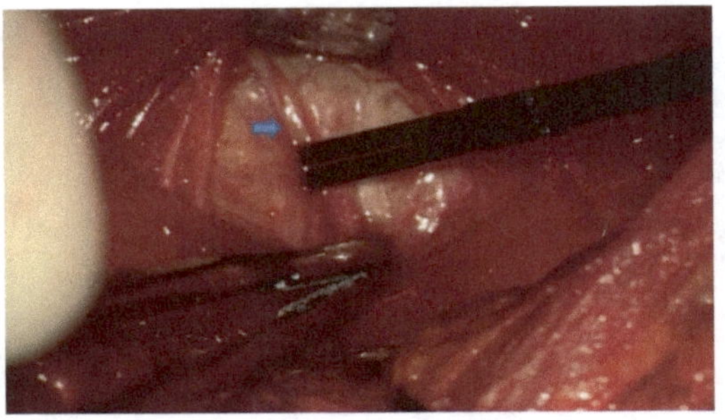

Fig. 5.5 Intraoperative nerve action potential monitoring. Nerve action potential monitoring was performed to identify safe zones between fascicles and preserve the traversing fascicle (arrow)

dissected free from the adjacent fascicles and connective tissues. The tumor was removed en bloc.

Case 2. Schwannoma in lumbar plexus (Video 2).

A 48-year-old female patient complained of left back pain and paresthesia on thigh and leg. The pain has increased over time. Magnetic resonance (MR) images showed an ovoid mass encompassed by left psoas muscle (Fig. 5.6). The patient underwent lumbosacral plexus tumor removal. After dissection of psoas muscle, the tumor mass was easily found. The thinned epineurium was opened between fascicles and the tumor was dissected free from the adjacent fascicles and connective tissues. The tumor was removed en bloc. The epineurotomy was done, with nerve action potential recording to avoid the traversing fascicle (Fig. 5.5). After identification of distal and proximal pole of tumor, isolated tumor from adjacent structure was removal.

5.1.3 Conclusion

In conclusion, extradural nerve plexus tumor such as peripheral nerve sheath tumors can be removed as a single mass without additional neurological deficits. The outcome is excellent and the recurrence is very rare.

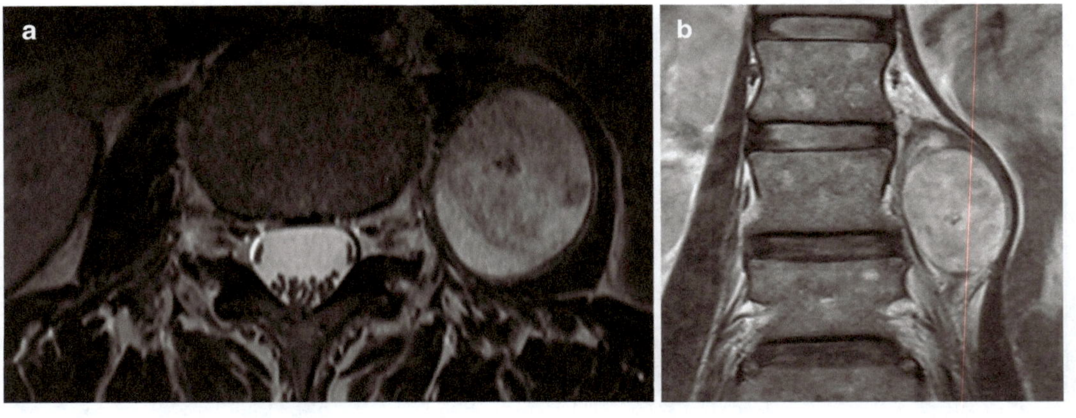

Fig. 5.6 MRI imaging of schwannoma arising from the left lumbar plexus. The MRI images showing schwannoma arising from the left lumbar plexus. **a** T2 image axial (A) and coronal images **b** show well-delineated, homogenous hyperintense mass within left-side psoas muscle

References

1. Darby SA, Daley DL. Neuroanatomy of the spinal cord. In: Cramer GD, Susan AD, editors. Basic and clinical anatomy of the spine, spinal cord, and ANS. St. Louis: Mosby. publ; 1995. p. P251-303.
2. Grinsell D, Keating CP. Peripheral nerve reconstruction after injury: a review of clinical and experimental therapies. Biomed Res Int. 2014:698256.
3. Go MH, Kim SH, Cho KH. Brachial plexus tumors in a consecutive series of twenty one patients. J Korean Neurosurg Soc. 2012 Aug;52(2):138–43.
4. Benjamin CG, Oermann EK, Thomas JA, Distaso CT, Sandhu FA. Minimally invasive direct lateral transpsoas approach for the resection of a lumbar Plexus Schwannoma: technique report. Surg J (N Y). 2016 Aug;2(3):e66–9.
5. Montano N, D'Alessandris QG, D'Ercole M, Lauretti L, Pallini R, Di Bonaventura R, La Rocca G, Bianchi F, Fernandez E. Tumors of the peripheral nervous system: analysis of prognostic factors in a series with long-term follow-up and review of the literature. J Neurosurg. 2016 Aug;125(2):363–71.
6. Huang JH, Zaghloul K, Zager EL. Surgical management of brachial plexus region tumors. Surg Neurol. 2004 Apr;61(4):372–8.
7. Kim DH, Murovic JA, Tiel RL, Moes G, Kline DG. A series of 146 peripheral non-neural sheath nerve tumors: 30-year experience at Louisiana state university health sciences center. J Neurosurg. 2005 Feb;102(2):256–66.
8. Vučemilo L, Lajtman Z, Mihalj J, Plašćak J, Mahović Lakušić D, Mužinić D. Brachial Plexus Schwannoma—case report and literature review. Acta Clin Croat. 2018 Jun;57(2):366–71.
9. Kline DG, Hudson AR, Tiel R, Guha A: Management of peripheral nerve tumors, in Winn HR (ed): Youmans neurological surgery. Philadelphia: Elsevier, 2004, vol 4, pp 3941–3957.
10. Das S, Ganju A, Tiel RL, Kline DG. Tumors of the brachial plexus. Neurosurg Focus. 2007 Jun;22(6):E26.
11. Cerofolini E, Landi A, DeSantis G, Maiorana A, Canossi G, Romagnoli R. MR of benign peripheral nerve sheath tumors. J Comput Assist Tomogr. 1991; 15: 593–597.
12. Kline DG, Hackett ER, Happel LH. Surgery for lesions of the brachial plexus. Arch Neurol. 1986 Feb;43(2):170–81.

How to Approach Anatomical Compartment; Extradural Paraspinal Tumor

6

Nam Hun Yu and Chun Kee Chung

Abstract

Paraspinal tumors are defined as any soft tissue mass that comes into contact with the vertebral column. Paraspinal tumors without intraspinal involvement can be treated with one surgical approach. The surgical goals are complete tumor resection without neurovascular injury. The optimal surgical approach for tumor resection mainly depends on several factors including location, extension, size, involvement of the bony spinal canal. The paraspinal tumors can be better reached through outside-in approach. Lateral extracavitary retroperitoneal approach is useful for extraforaminal tumors deep to the psoas muscle.

Keywords

Tumor · Paraspinal · Approach

Electronic supplementary material The online version of this chapter (https://doi.org/10.1007/978-981-15-7771-0_6) contains supplementary material, which is available to authorized users.

N. H. Yu
Department of Neurosurgery, Suhgwang General Hospital, Gwangju, South Korea
e-mail: nhyoo00@hanmail.net

C. K. Chung (✉)
Department of Neurosurgery, Seoul National University Hospital, Seoul National University College of Medicine, Seoul, Republic of Korea
e-mail: chungc@snu.ac.kr

Neuroscience Research Institute, Seoul National University Medical Research Center, Seoul, Republic of Korea

Clinical Research Institute, Seoul National University Hospital, Seoul, Republic of Korea

Department of Brain and Cognitive Sciences, Seoul National University College of Natural Sciences, Seoul, Republic of Korea

6.1 Introduction

Paraspinal tumors are defined as any soft tissue mass that comes into contact with the vertebral column. Paraspinal tumors are mostly nerve sheath tumors. Schwannomas are the most common paraspinal tumors, followed by neurofibromas and ganglioneuromas. Paraspinal tumors may involve any portion of the vertebral column and extend through the adjacent neural foramen to enter the epidural space.

Eden presented a classification in 1941 based on radiological findings for spinal schwannomas (Table 6.1) [1]. Paraspinal tumors correspond to Eden types III and IV. Type III is purely extradural growth with a paravertebral tumor mass. Type IV is a tumor limited to the paravertebral and intraforaminal spaces.

McCormick categorizes paraspinal tumors depending on axial relation to spinal canal [2]. Paraspinal tumors correspond to McCormick's

C. K. Chung (ed.), *Surgery of Spinal Cord Tumors Based on Anatomy*,
https://doi.org/10.1007/978-981-15-7771-0_6

types 2, 3, and 5. Type 2 is confined to anterior spinal region and near spinal canal without foraminal or intraspinal extension. Type 3 is anterior paraspinal tumors with minor foraminal or intraspinal extension. Type 5 involves paraspinal soft tissue only.

Paraspinal tumors usually remain asymptomatic until they reach a large size and extend into the adjacent organ or spinal cord. Surgical tumor excision is preferred in tumors showing rapid growth or causing the neurologic deficit. The surgical goals are to complete tumor resection and to prevent neurovascular injury. Preoperative selection of surgical approaches is critical. The size and position of the tumor and extraspinal components are the most important factors in deciding the surgical approach [3, 4].

Various approaches have been reported for paraspinal tumors. For paraspinal tumors, two-stage approaches have been used in the past. Traditional approaches for resection of retroperitoneal tumors are usually multidisciplinary, involving a general surgeon using an anterior retroperitoneal approach.

The classic lateral extracavitary approach (LECA) has been the gold standard for many years. The advantage of this procedure is that it provides the surgeon with access to both the posterior and lateral aspects of the spinal canal through a single incision. The LECA allows for the placement of posterior instrumentation without a second incision [5].

In recent years, a single-stage posterior approach has been preferred to remove paraspinal tumors that have an extraforaminal tumor component. The posterior approaches to the spine are the most commonly employed surgical exposure and familiar techniques. This approach may not require posterior fixation and less invasive for foraminal and extraforaminal tumor removal [6, 7].

Table 6.1. Eden classification [1]

Type I	Intra and extradural type
Type II	Intra and extradural and paravertebral type
Type III	Extradural and paravertebral type
Type IV	Foraminal and paravertebral type

The posterior approach is divided into inside-out and outside-in approach. Inside-out approach is to remove the intraspinal–extradural component first, followed by the extraforaminal tumor component. Inside-out approach would have necessitated hemilaminectomy, unilateral facetectomy, and intertransverse approach. Fusion may be required to correct postlaminectomy deformity. For paraspinal tumor, inside-out approach is some demerit, such as inadequate exposure or large incision. Approaching extraforaminal tumors from a midline exposure requires extensive muscular retraction and extensive removal of facet joint. Inside-out approach may be not a suitable for extraforaminal tumor without intradural components.

Outside-in approach is to remove the extraforaminal tumor component first, followed by the intraspinal–extradural component. Paraspinal tumors are located in the far lateral zone. The far lateral zone is difficult to approach from the midline but easily reaches through a paramedian access. The paraspinal tumors with or without intraforaminal involvement can be better reached through outside-in approach. In case of intraforaminal tumor involvement, the approach can be extended to a foraminal decompression and tumor excision in the neuroforamen. It is possible to perform total resection with costotransversectomy in case of thoracic paraspinal tumors [8].

But, outside-in approach is difficult to remove a tumor extending anteriorly and inside the iliopsoas muscle. Akawasi reported the lateral transpsoas approach, which can be performed in a minimally invasive or open fashion for resection of retroperitoneal, paravertebral nerve sheath tumors within the psoas muscle [9].

More recently, mini open or minimally invasive techniques without stabilization have been reported. Minimally invasive techniques reduce bony destruction, blood loss, and postoperative pain. Tumor size and locations are the critical factors for the application of the minimally invasive surgery approach [10–13].

Traditionally, thoracic paraspinal tumor resection by posterolateral thoracotomy is the standard treatment, which offers excellent outcomes. A costotransversectomy approach can be used to remove small to moderate-sized thoracic paraspinal tumors. For a large thoracic paraspinal tumor extending into the chest cavity, a thoracotomy or thoracoscopic approach may be needed to allow visualization and access. Recently, thoracoscopic surgery has been documented as a good alternative method for excision of thoracic paraspinal tumors [14, 15].

6.2 Strategy of Surgical Treatment

The surgical goals are complete tumor resection without neurovascular injury. The optimal surgical approach for tumor resection mainly depends on several factors including location, extension, size, involvement of the bony spinal canal, and the relation with neural compartments. In recent years, paraspinal tumors without intraspinal involvement can be treated with one surgical approach. Approaches to paraspinal tumors are classified in Table 6.2 [2, 7].

The lateral extracavitary approach to the thoracic and lumbar spine can be used for the removal of paraspinal tumors, causing anterior or lateral spinal cord compression. The posterior approach provides a direct view of the tumor mass through only one surgical route. The intraforaminal tumor part could be excised out of the foramen without injuring the spinal dura.

Outside-in approach was performed using paramedian or far lateral skin incision as an entry point. The paraspinal muscle-splitting approach can provide a good exposure for the foramen. Skin incision is performed using the cleavage plane of the multifidus and longissimus muscles. A lateral vertical skin incision is made about 30–40 mm lateral to the spinous process at the corresponding level and the fascia is opened longitudinally. After blunt dissection between the multifidus and longissimus muscles, the transverse process, isthmus, and facet joint are exposed. The transverse process and isthmus are important landmarks for the exact location. Partial drilling of the transverse process is accomplished to widen the intervertebral foramen for removal of the extraforaminal tumor. The isthmus is may be removed for enlarging the intervertebral foramen during the removal of extracanalicular tumor. The paraspinal tumor was identified between the transverse processes.

Outside-in approach is difficult to remove a tumor extending anteriorly and inside the psoas muscle. Lateral mini-open transpsoas approach can be performed for resection of paraspinal tumors within the psoas muscle. Direct visualization in lateral extracavitary approach allows for identification of nerve branches and thus minimizes intraoperative injury. The patient was positioned in a lateral decubitus position. Electrodes for electromyography and monitoring of somatosensory-evoked potentials are placed. A small lateral skin incision is made and the underlying fascia is incised. The transversalis fascia is opened bluntly to enter the retroperitoneal space. Digitally sweeping the retroperitoneal fat from posterior to anterior, moving the peritoneum anteriorly, allows palpation of the psoas muscle. The retractor is placed through the psoas muscle with continuous EMG monitoring. Under direct vision, the psoas muscle is split bluntly, protecting any visualized nerves. The tumor can then be detected.

Table 6.2 Paraspinal tumor approach

1. Lateral extracavitary approach
2. Posterior approach a. Inside out approach b. Outside-in approach
3. Minimally invasive approach

6.3 Case Review

Case 1. Lateral extracavitary retroperitoneal approach (Video 1).

A 48-year-old male patient complained of low back pain. The patient also complained of leg paresthesia. Magnetic resonance (MR) images showed a large mass within the psoas muscle at the level of L3–L4 (Fig. 6.1). The patient underwent a lateral extracavitary retroperitoneal approach. The patient was positioned in a left lateral decubitus position. A lateral skin incision is made and the underlying fascia is incised. The transversalis fascia is opened bluntly to enter the retroperitoneal space.

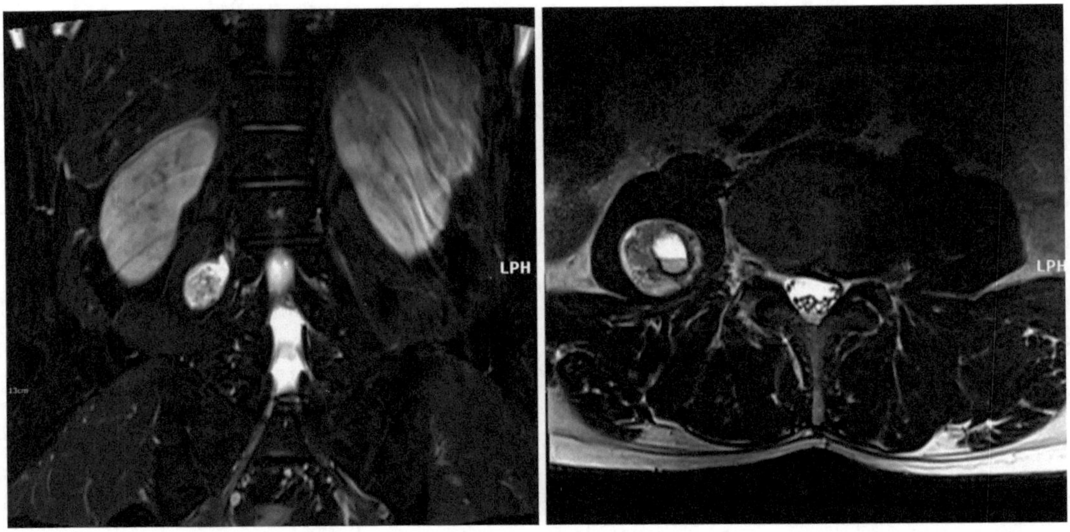

Fig. 6.1 Magnetic resonance images (MRI) showed the paraspinal tumor imbedding in the psoas muscle on the right side at the level of L3–L4

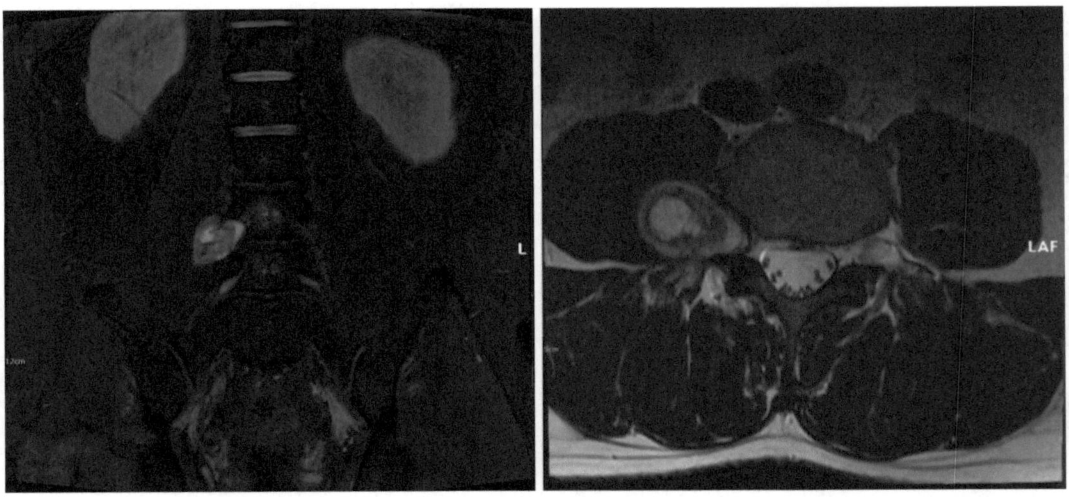

Fig. 6.2 Axial section showed a paraspinal tumor with a small extension into the right L3–L4 foramina without foraminal widening

Digitally sweeping the retroperitoneal fat from posterior to anterior, moving the peritoneum anteriorly, allows palpation of the psoas muscle. The retractor is placed through the psoas muscle. Under direct vision, the psoas muscle is split bluntly, protecting genitofemoral nerve. The tumor can then be detected and was totally excised.

Case 2. Outside-in approach (Video 2).

A 41-year-old male patient suffered from progressive low back pain for 1 year without any neurological deficits. MR imaging revealed an extradural tumor on right of L3 and L4 body with small foraminal component (Fig. 6.2). Surgery for the patient was performed outside-in approach. After blunt dissection between the multifidus and longissimus muscles, the transverse process and facet joint are exposed. Internal debulking allowed a progressive collapse of the tumor capsule, which was then easily dissected off the surrounding tissues. The origin of the tumor was confirmed, followed by cutting and tumor removal with no response on the electromyography.

6.4 Conclusion

In conclusion, the paraspinal tumor can be excised using either a lateral extracavitary approach or an outside-in approach. The paraspinal tumors can be better reached through outside-in approach. Lateral extracavitary retroperitoneal approach is useful for extraforaminal tumors deep to the psoas muscle.

References

1. Eden K. The dumb-bell tumors of the spine. Br J Surg. 1941;28:549–70.
2. McCormick PC, Stein BM. Spinal cord tumors in adults. In: Youmans JR, editor. Neurological surgery. Vol. 6. 5th ed. Philadelphia: WB Saunder: 1996. P. 3102–22.
3. Spitzer AL, Ceraldi CM, Wang T-N, Granelli SG. Anatomic classification system for surgical management of Paraspinal Tumors. Arch Surg. 2004;139(3):262–9.
4. Arjun Dhar, Sumeet Pawar, Apurva Prasad, P.S. Ramani. Approaches to paraspinal tumours-a technical note. Neurological Research. 2017; 39(4):315–22.
5. Schmidt MH, Larson SJ, Maiman DJ. The lateral extracavitary aprroach to the thoracic and lumbar spine. Neurosurg Clin N Am. 2004;15:437–41.
6. Seungcheol Lee. Surgical management of Giant Lumbar extradural schwannomas: report of 3 cases. International Journal of Spine Surgery. 2018; 9:18. https://doi.org/10.14444/2018.
7. Suat Canbay, Askin Esen Hasturk, Mehmet Basmaci, Fuat Erten, Ferhat Harman. Management of thoracal and Lumbar Schwannomas using a unilateral approach without instability: an analysis of 15 cases. Asian Spine Journal. 2012; 6(1);43–9.
8. Hong-tao Rong, Yue-shan Fan, Si-peng Li, Zheng-shan Zhang, Hui Liu, Tong Liu, Tao Zhu, Jian-ning Zhang. Management of Dumbbell and paraspinal tumors of the thoracic spine using a single-stage posterolateral approach: case series. Orthopaedic Surgery. 2018 November; 10:4.
9. Akwasi Ofori Boah, Noel I. Perin. Lateral access to paravertebral tumors. J Neurosurg Spine. 2016; 24:824–28.
10. Vergara P. A novel less invative technique for the excision of large intradural and extradural Dumbbell Lumbar Schwannomas: the "Dual Approach" . World Neurosurgery. 2016;95:171–6.
11. Li C, Ye Y, Yutong Gu, Dong J. Minimally invasive resection of extradural dumbbell tumors of thoracic spine: surgical techniques and literature review. Eur Spine J. 2016;25:4108–15.
12. Kratzig T, Dreimann M, Klingenhofer M, Floeth FW, Krajewski K, Eicker SO. Treatment of large thoracic and lumbar paraspinal schwannoma. Acta Neurochir. 2015;157:531–8.
13. Japhet Gideon Ngerageza, Kiyoshi Ito, Tatsuro Aoyama, Takahiro Murata, Tetsuyoshi Horiuchi, Kazuhiro Hongo. Posterior laminoplastic laminotomy combined with a paraspinal transmuscular approach for removing a Lumbar Dumbbell-shaped schwannoma: a technical note. Neurol Med Chir (Tokyo). 2015; 55:756–60.
14. Ruth Prieto, Xavier Santander, Jose Manuel Naranjo, Esperanza Marin, Cesareo Corbacho. Giant dumbbell-shaped thoracic Schwannoma in an Elderly patient resected through a single-stage combined laminectomy and video-assisted thoracoscopy: surgical strategy and technical nuances. World Neurosurgery. 2018 November; 119:155–62.
15. Li Y, Wang B, Lv G, Li L. Thoracoscopy-assisted mini-open approach for resection of neurogenic tumors arising at the thoracic apex. Int J Clin Exp Med. 2017;10(3):5175–81.

How to Approach Anatomical Compartment; Extradural Foraminal Tumor

7

Jun Ho Lee and Chun Kee Chung

Abstract

Spinal extradural foraminal neoplasms are uncommon lesions that are constricted at the point they penetrate the intervertebral foramina or dura mater. Because of their varied locations, extradural foraminal neoplasms have features, clinical symptoms, and pathological characteristics that are unique compared with the more common intradural extramedullary (IDEM) tumors, consequently, their surgical approach and treatment should be also differentiated. Surgically, extradural extension into the foramen necessitates a more or less important resection of the facet joints. This raises the question of spinal stability and the need for additional fixation. However, recent progression of anatomy-preserving minimally invasive surgical techniques along with the concomitant evolution of their tools allows for excellent exposure while limiting damage to surrounding tissues through a minimized surgical corridor or modified approach method, followed by safe and completed resection of these extradural foraminal neoplasms.

Keywords

Extradural tumor · Intervertebral foramen · Minimally invasive approach · Laminectomy · Facetectomy

J. H. Lee
Department of Neurosurgery, Kyung Hee University Medical Centre, Seoul 02447, Republic of Korea
e-mail: moo9924@khu.ac.kr

C. K. Chung (✉)
Department of Neurosurgery, Seoul National University Hospital, Seoul National University College of Medicine, Seoul, Republic of Korea
e-mail: chungc@snu.ac.kr

Neuroscience Research Institute, Seoul National University Medical Research Center, Seoul, Republic of Korea

Clinical Research Institute, Seoul National University Hospital, Seoul, Republic of Korea

Department of Brain and Cognitive Sciences, Seoul National University College of Natural Sciences, Seoul, Republic of Korea

7.1 Introduction

As defined by Heuer [1], spinal extradural foraminal neoplasms are uncommon lesions that are constricted at the point they penetrate the intervertebral foramina or dura mater and assume an hourglass (dumbbell) shape. Currently, the term 'dumbbell tumors' does not refer to the hourglass shape but is used as a conceptual term meaning separate tumors that connect and have two or more separate regions such as intradural space, epidural space, and locations outside the paravertebral space [2, 3].

C. K. Chung (ed.), *Surgery of Spinal Cord Tumors Based on Anatomy*,
https://doi.org/10.1007/978-981-15-7771-0_7

Because of their varied locations, extradural foraminal neoplasms have features, clinical symptoms, and pathological characteristics that are unique compared with the more common intradural extramedullary (IDEM) tumors, consequently, their surgical approach and treatment should be also differentiated. These lesions are traditionally resected via an open laminectomy and facetectomy approach and in cases requiring complete facetectomy (e.g., a nerve sheath tumor extending both medial and lateral to the facet joint), prior reports have rather recommended concomitant fusion for stabilization [4, 5]. However, recently, the use of mini-open surgical technique for the resection of these extradural spinal foraminal neoplasms that extend through the foramen and lateral to the facet have been reported [6]. In this chapter, the author describes about the features, surgical approaches, and their preceded considerations for these 'extradural-foraminal' tumors.

7.2 Classification and Epidemiology

In 2007, Ozawa et al. have featured and classified these 118 spinal extradural foraminal neoplasms from their 674 spinal cord tumors that were encountered at the Tohoku University School of Medicine during the period between 1988 and 2002 [5]. The pathological diagnoses included 81 schwannomas (69%), 14 neurofibromas (12%), nine neuroblastomas/ganglioneuromas (8%), six meningiomas (5%), and two hemangiomas (2%). Six tumors (5%) were of miscellaneous diagnoses, including an angiolipoma, a paraganglioma, a malignant peripheral nerve sheath tumor, a malignant lymphoma, a melanoma, and a rhabdomyosarcoma.

Neurogenic tumors consisting of schwannomas and neurofibromas accounted for 80% of the dumbbell tumors [5, 7]. Malignant tumors were found in 10 cases (8.5%). These malignant dumbbell tumors accounted for 64% of cases in pediatric patients and 2.8% in adult patients.

While the usual IDEM tumors appeared more commonly in the thoracic and lumbar spine than the cervical spine, these extradural foraminal neoplasms had more prevalence in the cervical spine (44%), followed by the thoracic spine (27%), and the lumbar spine (21%) [8–10]. Fifteen (18%) of 81 schwannomas were observed in the C-2 nerve root, thus having a higher rate than those in the other nerve roots [9, 11–13]. According to Eden classification [14], 9% of tumors were classified as Type 1, 33% as Type 2, 53% as Type 3, and 5% as Type 4 (Fig. 7.1). The tumors classified as Type 3 were most frequent. In the cervical spine, Type 2 was most frequent; however, in the thoracic spine, Type 3 was most frequent. In the schwannomas, Eden Type 3 accounted for 48% and was most frequent. In the neurofibromas, Type 2 accounted for 52% of the lesions. All neuroblastomas and anglioneuromas were Type 3. In the meningiomas, there were two Type 2 tumors and two Type 3 tumors. The Type 3

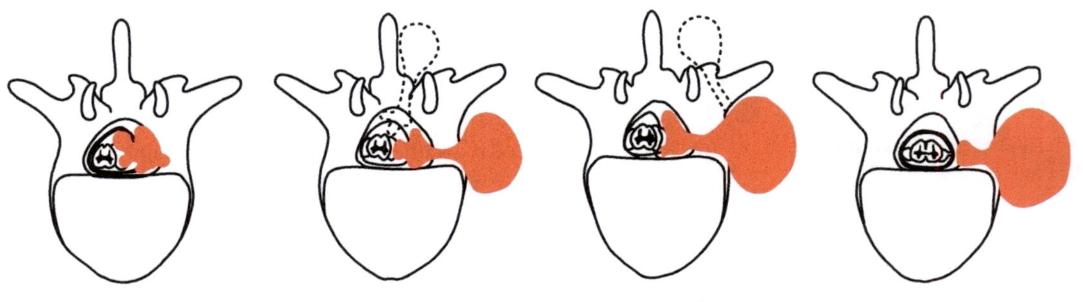

Fig. 7.1 A diagram of Eden's classification for dumb-bell shaped tumors of the spine

meningiomas had been recurrent at the epidural space and paravertebral region after excision of the intradural tumors.

7.3 Diagnosis

Pain is the most common presenting symptom being either local (50%) or radicular (30%). Very rarely patients present with symptoms due to raised intracranial pressure associated with papilledema [15] or hydrocephalus [16, 17]. At the time of diagnosis, motor deficit is rare and usually moderate including 30% and 15% of radicular and medullary deficits, respectively [9, 11]. Sphincter disturbances are exceptionally observed.

MRI is the best imaging tool as it offers all the relevant information for diagnosis, localization, and surgical strategy. It permits to define any type of extension (intradural, extradural, foraminal, and extraspinal). It shows very well the cystic and hemorrhagic forms [18]. Conversely, it is generally difficult to differentiate schwannomas from solitary neurofibromas. MRI is also quite sufficient to demonstrate the relationship between the schwannoma and the vertebral artery (VA). In case of foraminal extension, the VA is most of the important to evaluate the size of both VAs.

A computerized tomography (CT) scan may still be useful to appreciate the bony erosion in foraminal and extraspinal types. It varies from a limited widening of the intervertebral foramen to a large defect in one or several vertebral bodies and/or facet joints.

7.4 Strategy of Surgical Treatment

7.4.1 Conventional Midline Access

In the vast majority of neoplasms with an intradural location, there is a common agreement to use the midline posterior approach through a single- or two-level laminectomy, hemilaminectomy, or laminoplasty [19], followed with a vertical paramedian incision of the dura, curved laterally at both extremities and an en bloc excision can be achieved after a limited number of rootlets (one or two) that give origin to the schwannoma are separated from the others and sacrificed (Fig. 7.2).

In case of concomitant extra- and intradural components (dumbbell form), some modifications must be added;

- The laminectomy is extended laterally toward the facets [20].
- A dural contraincision perpendicular to the paramedian incision directed to the foramen is performed. The dura always adheres to the tumor capsule and has to be cut around the tumor at the level of intra-/extradural communication. This might result in an unrepairable dural defect, which needs to be closed with a patch after tumor removal.
- The extradural component is resected until the distal root is reached. It may be necessary to resect some more bone toward the neural foramen (medial aspect of the facet joint).

This hemilaminectomy combined with the medial partial facetectomy had a great advantage for excising the dumbbell tumor. Because most tumors were located unilaterally in the spinal canal and paravertebral space, the tumors could be excised easily from the posterolateral enough large space provided by the hemilaminectomy and facetectomy. In addition, the spinal stability can be reconstructed or augmented easily by either wiring or contralateral facet fusion, because the hemilaminectomy and facetectomy can minimize damage to spinal stability by preserving the spinous process, supra- and intraspinous ligaments, and contralateral facet joint.

7.4.2 Modification for Dominantly Extradural and Foraminal Component

The above-mentioned posterior approach with facetectomy [3, 21] might necessitate an additional fixation procedure and sometimes a complementary anterior or lateral approach if the extraspinal component is large. Lu et al. have demonstrated a mini-open treatment of

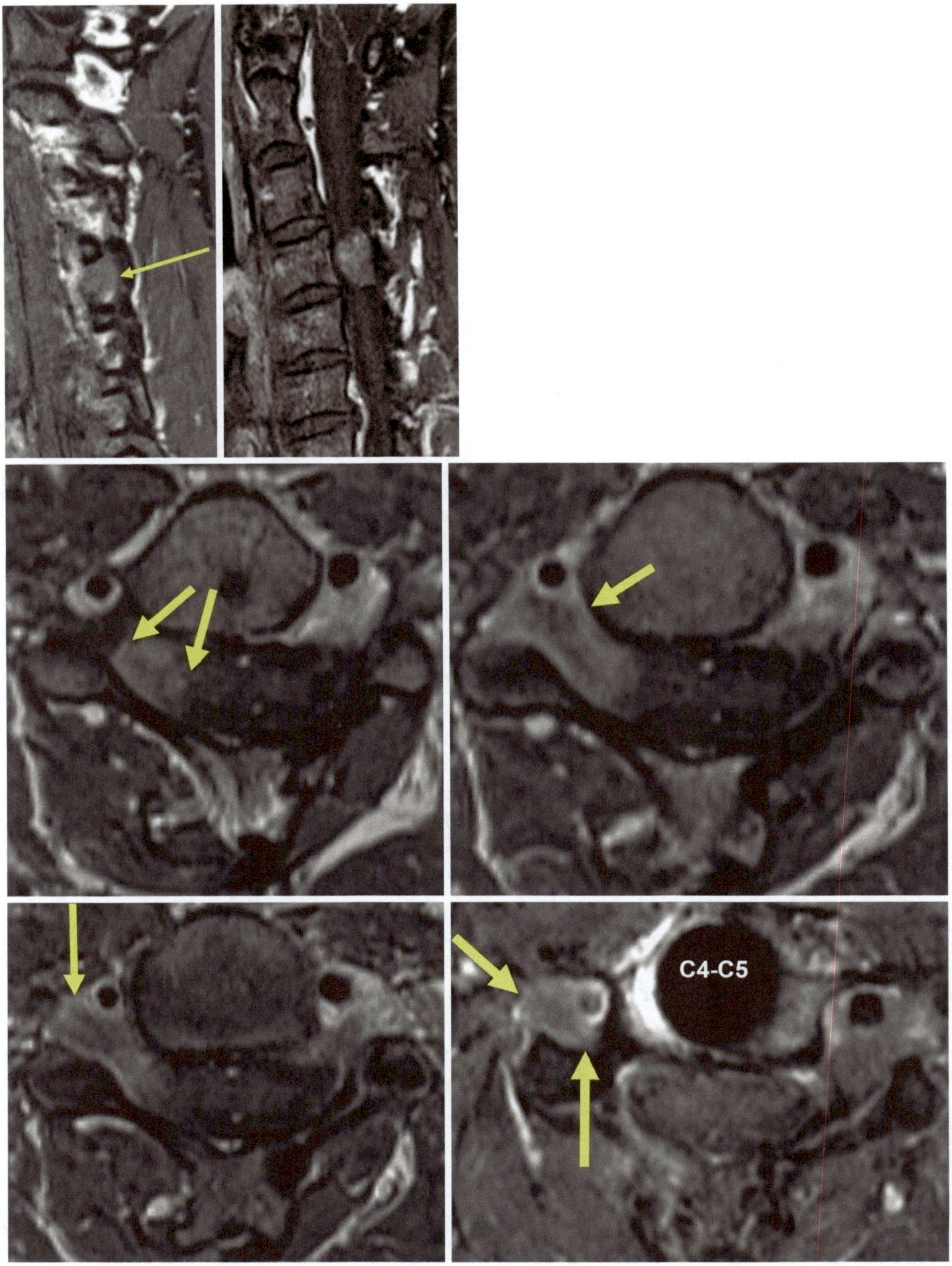

Fig. 7.2 An illustrative case of 40-year-old male with neurofibroma existing at intradural—extramedullary portion of the right side inside of the spinal canal at the C4-5 level, with extension to neural foramen as well as to the dorsal aspect of vertebral artery (VA) and its groove. Ipsilateral hemilaminectomy—medial partial facetectomy through a paramedian surgical access directed to the foramen was performed to evacuate the compacted lesion. Despite a considerable elaboration to remove the whole portion of the neurofibroma, still a remnant portion of the tumor at the most lateral portion inside the VA groove could be noted

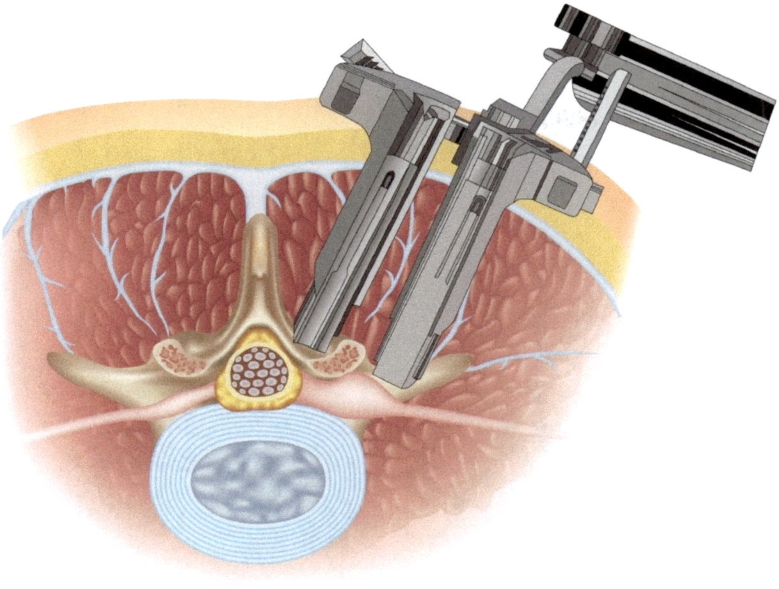

Fig. 7.3 Illustration of a foraminal nerve sheath tumor being removed through a mini-open approach with an expandable tubular retractor. (courtesy from Lu D et al. J Neurosurg Spine 2009)

extradural spinal nerve sheath tumors that extend through the intervertebral foramen and lateral to the facet that it is performed through the Wiltse's plane, approximately 3–4 cm lateral to the conventional midline access (Fig. 7.3). They found that, especially for foraminal lumbar nerve sheath tumors, this mini-open approach is feasible with acceptable amount of blood loss and operative time. Additionally, this can be applied for reoperative cases who harbor such foraminal tumors but had undergone prior midline surgery.

The advantage is that, since it is performed in the Wiltse plane, lateral to the scar tissue from the prior operation, this de novo approach through a relatively virgin tissue plane reduces the time for untoward dissecting scar tissue from the dura in patients who have undergone prior laminectomies. Furthermore, this lateral approach allows for same surgical route for concomitant pedicle screw placement and posterolateral fusion.

However, especially at the cervical level, it does not permit a proper visualization of the important vital structures and control of the vertebral artery (VA), which may be hazardous. In the case of huge extension to outside of foramen, the posterior approach might be adjunct with an concomitant anterior approach [2, 3]. George et al. have proposed as the other option is to use the anterolateral approach which, in their experience, is more advisable since any component from extraspinal to intradural can be resected with a perfect control of the VA and no need for additional fixation (Fig. 7.4) [12, 13, 22, 23]. Their suggested surgical steps would be;

- The skin incision is vertical along the medial border of the sternocleidomastoid (SM) muscle at the corresponding level and extended over 6–7 cm.
- The field is opened by first exposing the medial aspect of the sternocleidomastoid muscle (SM), which is then retracted laterally until the internal jugular vein (IJV) is reached. The lateral aspect of the IJV is separated from the SM and retracted medially. The retractors are progressively moved down into the field. In contrast to a classical anterior cervical approach, all the

Fig. 7.4 Illustration showing the dissection plane. The neurovascular package is retracted medially and the cervical spine is reached anterolaterally. (courtesy from Kiris T et al. Neurosurgery 2008)

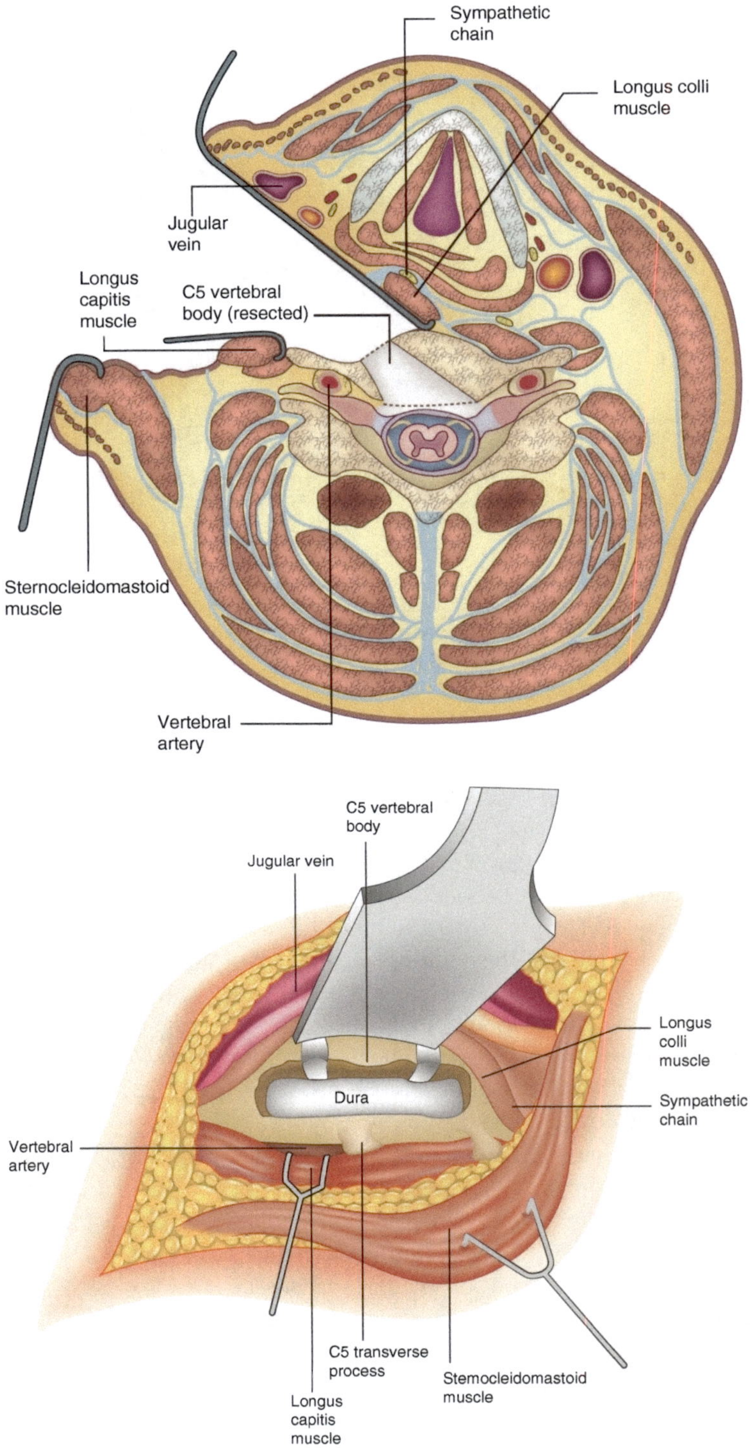

vasculo-nervous elements are kept undissected in their sheath and retracted medially together with the trachea and esophagus using a malleable blade.

- The anterolateral aspect of the vertebral bodies becomes apparent. In the depth of the field, there is a fatty and lymphatic sheath, which is retracted medially to expose the prevertebral muscles (longus colli and longus capitis).
- The sympathetic trunk running over these muscles is retracted medially. This trunk is in close relationship with the fascia. As such, it is safe to dissect the fascia away from the underlying muscles and retract medially along with the trunk [24].
- The longus colli muscle is retracted medially above the transverse processes and then longitudinally along the vertebral bodies so that the transverse processes come onto view with the tumor in between the two of them [24].
- The VA is controlled above and below the tumor after resection of the transverse processes.
- The far lateral retraction of the longus capitis muscle permits the exposure laterally of the distal root. The nonfunctional, distal root is cut after coagulation and the tumor can then be debulked progressing from lateral to medial, underneath the VA.
- Then the VA is mobilized laterally and the tumor remnants, medial to it, are removed.
- Sometimes a little amount of the bone on the posterolateral aspect of the vertebral bodies needs to be drilled away; this realizes an enlargement of the intervertebral foramen whenever it has not been sufficiently done by the tumor itself.
- After having resected the extradural part of the tumor, the dura is cut around the tumor where it goes intradurally. The intradural component can then be pulled out and removed progressively until the proximal root becomes visible.
- The root is cut and the last intradural piece of tumor is removed.
- The dural defect is covered using artificial dural or can be packed with a piece of fat taken from the fatty sheath, and onlayed with fibrin glue [25].

7.5 Potential Complications

Extradural extension into the foramen necessitates a more or less important resection of the facet joints. This raises the question of spinal stability and the need of additional fixation.

The extraspinal extension of those tumors, displacing the VA, can better be resected with adequate exposure of the VA using the anterolateral approach. The VA must be controlled above and below so that any injury can be easily repaired. In this view, evaluation of the size of the VA on preoperative MRI is essential.

There is a potential complication, related to the injury of a radiculomedullary artery arising at the tumoral level, without supply of the medulla by a collateral network, causing medullary ischemia.

Horner's syndrome due to damage of the sympathetic trunk (during the anterolateral approach) may be transiently observed after excessive manipulations but should recover, except if the sympathetic trunk has been cut.

7.6 Conclusion

Spinal extradural neoplasms that traverse the intervertebral foramen can be safely resected using a minimized surgical corridor or approach modification, which allows for excellent exposure while limiting damage to surrounding tissues. In order to accomplish this task without subsequent untoward complication incurrence, capability to convert the two-dimensional preoperative imaging information into 3D anatomical interpretation would be essential.

References

1. Heuer GJ. So-called hour-glass tumors of the spine. Arch Surg. 1929;18:935–61.
2. Asazuma T, Toyama Y, Maruiwa H, Fujimura Y, Hirabayashi K. Surgical strategy for cervical

dumbbell tumors based on a three-dimensional classification. Spine. 2004;29:E10–4.
3. Tomii M, Itoh Y, Numazawa S, Watanabe K. Surgical consideration of cervical dumbbell tumors. Acta Neurochir. 2013;155:1907–10.
4. Jinnai T, Koyama T. Clinical characteristics of spinal nerve sheath tumors: Analysis of 149 cases. Neurosurgery. 2005;56:510–5.
5. Ozawa H, Kokubun S, Aizawa T, Hoshikawa T, Kawahara C. Spinal dumbbell tumors: An analysis of a series of 118 cases. J Neurosurg Spine. 2007;7:587–93.
6. Lu DC, Dhall SS, Mummaneni PV. Mini-open removal of extradural foraminal tumors of the lumbar spine. J Neurosurg Spine. 2009;10:46–50.
7. El-Mahdy W, Kane PJ, Powell MP, Crockard HA. Spinal intradural tumours: part I—extramedullary. Br J Neurosurg. 1999;13:550–7.
8. Conti P, Pansini G, Mouchaty H, Capuano C, Conti R. Spinal neurinomas: Retrospective analysis and long-term outcome of 179 consecutively operated cases and review of the literature. Surg Neurol. 2004;61:34–43; discussion 44.
9. Safavi-Abbasi S, Senoglu M, Theodore N, Workman RK, Gharabaghi A, Feiz-Erfan I, et al. Microsurgical management of spinal schwannomas: Evaluation of 128 cases. J Neurosurg Spine. 2008;9:40–7.
10. Gelabert-Gonzalez M, Castro-Bouzas D, Serramito-Garcia R, Santin-Amo JM, Aran-Echabe E, Prieto-Gonzalez A, et al. Tumours of the nerve root sheath in the spine. Rev Neurol. 2011;53:390–6.
11. Seppala MT, Haltia MJ, Sankila RJ, Jaaskelainen JE, Heiskanen O. Long-term outcome after removal of spinal schwannoma: A clinicopathological study of 187 cases. J Neurosurg. 1995;83:621–6.
12. Hakuba A, Komiyama M, Tsujimoto T, Ahn MS, Nishimura S, Ohta T, et al. Transuncodiscal approach to dumbbell tumors of the cervical spinal canal. J Neurosurg. 1984;61:1100–6.
13. George B, Laurian C, Keravel Y, Cophignon J. Extradural and hourglass cervical neurinomas: The vertebral artery problem. Neurosurgery. 1985;16:591–4.
14. Eden K. The dumb-bell tumors of the spine. Br J Surg. 1941;28:549–70.
15. Costello F, Kardon RH, Wall M, Kirby P, Ryken T. Lee AG (2002) Papilledema as the presenting manifestation of spinal schwannoma. J Neuroophthalmol Off J N Am Neuroophthalmol Soc. 2002;22:199–203.
16. Kudo H, Tamaki N, Kim S, Shirataki K, Matsumoto S. Intraspinal tumors associated with hydrocephalus. Neurosurgery. 1987;21:726–31.
17. Sun H, Tian H. Intraspinal tumors accompanied by hydrocephalus: Case report, systematic review, and discussion of treatment strategy. Neurologist. 2011;17:342–5.
18. Parmar HA, Ibrahim M, Castillo M, Mukherji SK. Pictorial essay: Diverse imaging features of spinal schwannomas. J Comput Assist Tomogr. 2007;31:329–34.
19. Raysi Dehcordi S, Marzi S, Ricci A, Di Cola F, Galzio RJ. Less invasive approaches for the treatment of cervical schwannomas: Our experience. Eur Spine J. 2012;21:887–96.
20. Uede T, Kurokawa Y, Wanibuchi M, Ze PH, Ohtaki M, Hashi K. Surgical approach for cervical dumbbell type neurinoma: Posterior approach by partial hemilaminectomy with preservation of a facet joint. No Shinkei Geka Neurol Surg. 1996;24:675–9.
21. McCormick PC. Surgical management of dumbbell tumors of the cervical spine. Neurosurgery. 1996;38:294–300.
22. Lot G, George B. Cervical neuromas with extradural components: surgical management in a series of 57 patients. Neurosurgery. 1997;41:813–20; discussion 820–22.
23. George B, Bruneau M. Schwannomas of the cervical spine. in: erik van de kelft, editor. Surgery of the spine and spinal cord: A neurosurgical approach. Springer International Publishing AG Switzerland; 2016. p. 679–90.
24. Kiris T, Kilinçer C. Cervical spondylotic myelopathy treated by oblique corpectomy: A prospective study. Neurosurgery. 2008;674–82; discussion; 674–82.
25. Bruneau M, George B. Surgical technique for the resection of tumors in relation with the V3 and V4 segments of the vertebral artery. In: George B, Bruneau M, Spetzler R, editors. Pathology and surgery around the vertebral artery. Paris: Springer; 2011. p. 361–404.

How to Approach Anatomical Compartment; Extradural Intracanal Tumor

8

Jun Ho Lee and Chun Kee Chung

Abstract

Extradural tumors are within the spine but outside the sac (dura) are the largest group, accounting for up to 55% of the spinal tumors. The majority of extradural tumors represents metastases while the primary extradural spine tumors are rare, and there is little high-quality evidence outlining the optimal treatment for these lesions. Extradural intracanal portion of the spine tumors poses significant challenges to surgeons as the aim is to achieve satisfactory surgical outcomes with clean tumor margins while minimizing morbidity. Improvements in radiotherapy technology, advances in chemotherapy, novel molecular drug targets, and other multimodality protocols may increase survival rates.

Keywords

Extradural tumor · Intra-spinal canal · Metastases · Primary spinal bone tumors · Spondylectomy

8.1 Introduction

Extradural tumors are within the spine but outside the sac (dura) that holds the spinal cord, nerve roots, and spinal fluid. These are the largest group, accounting for up to 55% of the spinal tumors. They may arise from the cells covering the nerve roots, vertebral bodies (most extradural lesions), epidural structures or may invade the spinal canal secondarily from the nearby structures (Fig. 8.1) [1–2].

Extradural intracanal portion of the spine tumors pose significant challenges to surgeons as the aim is to achieve satisfactory surgical outcomes with clean tumor margins (e.g., thus avoid recurrence) while minimizing morbidity. Improvements in radiotherapy, chemotherapy, and novel molecular drugs may increase survival rates and improve overall outcomes. In this chapter, the author describes about the features

J. H. Lee
Department of Neurosurgery, Kyung Hee University Medical Centre, Seoul 02447, Republic of Korea
e-mail: moo9924@khu.ac.kr

C. K. Chung (✉)
Department of Neurosurgery, Seoul National University Hospital, Seoul National University College of Medicine, Seoul, Republic of Korea
e-mail: chungc@snu.ac.kr

Neuroscience Research Institute, Seoul National University Medical Research Center, Seoul, Republic of Korea

Clinical Research Institute, Seoul National University Hospital, Seoul, Republic of Korea

Department of Brain and Cognitive Sciences, Seoul National University College of Natural Sciences, Seoul, Republic of Korea

C. K. Chung (ed.), *Surgery of Spinal Cord Tumors Based on Anatomy*,
https://doi.org/10.1007/978-981-15-7771-0_8

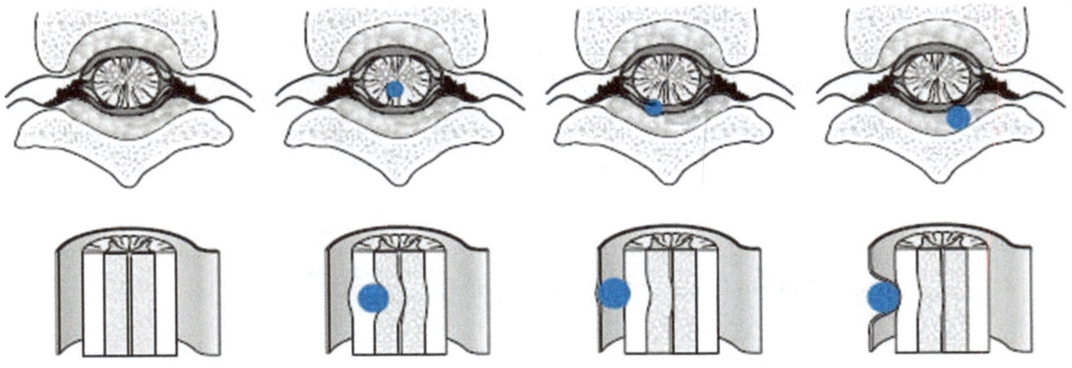

Fig. 8.1 Difference of the intracanal spinal tumors among the normal, intramedullary, intradural-extramedullary, and extradural in their origination

and their preceded considerations for these "extradural intracanal" tumors.

8.1.1 The Largest Group of Extradural—Intracanal Tumors: Metastasis

The majority of extradural tumors represent metastases, or cancerous tumors that have traveled from other parts of the body. Kidney, breast, prostate, and lung cancers will commonly travel to the bony spine. Metastatic spine tumors can cause pain (from bony destruction, fracture, or instability) or neurological dysfunction from compression of the spinal cord or nerve roots. Some of the well-verified features regarding these metastases are [1–2]

- Solitary vertebral lesions are less frequent than tumors with multiple locations.
- Metastases are most frequent in the thoracic spine followed by the lumbar spine.
- The most common primary tumors giving rise to metastatic spinal tumors are lung, breast, and prostate tumors.
- Most lesions are osteolytic (Fig. 8.2); osteoblastic metastases occur frequently with metastases from prostate and breast cancers.
- In elderly patients, the differential diagnosis with plasmocytoma/myeloma must be done.

Treatments for these tumors are aimed at preserving spinal stability, reducing/eliminating pain and maintaining neurological function. Common treatment modalities include surgery and radiation therapy. The typical goals of surgery are to confirm diagnosis, eliminate any compression of the spinal cord or nerve roots, and maintain stability by correcting deformity or restoring structural integrity (Fig. 8.3).

Complete surgical removal of tumors to the bony spine is rarely possible or practical. As such, radiation therapy is often used in conjunction with surgery to eliminate remaining tumor tissue or at least slow its progression. Such therapy can be delivered in multiple small doses over the course of several weeks (radiotherapy) or sometimes in much larger doses given just a few times or even once.

8.1.2 Primary Extradural—Intracanal Spinal Tumors: Bone Tumors

There are also primary tumors that affect the extradural bony spine. These are considerably less common than metastatic tumors and tend to be seen more commonly in children and young adults. Primary extradural tumors of the spine are rare and constitute approximately 4% of all spine tumors [3]. Despite their rarity, these tumors (Fig. 8.4) can pose significant surgical challenges as their aggressive nature makes achieving a clean tumor margin difficult; this may be particularly complicated by the critical surrounding anatomy (e.g., nerve roots/spinal cord) [4].

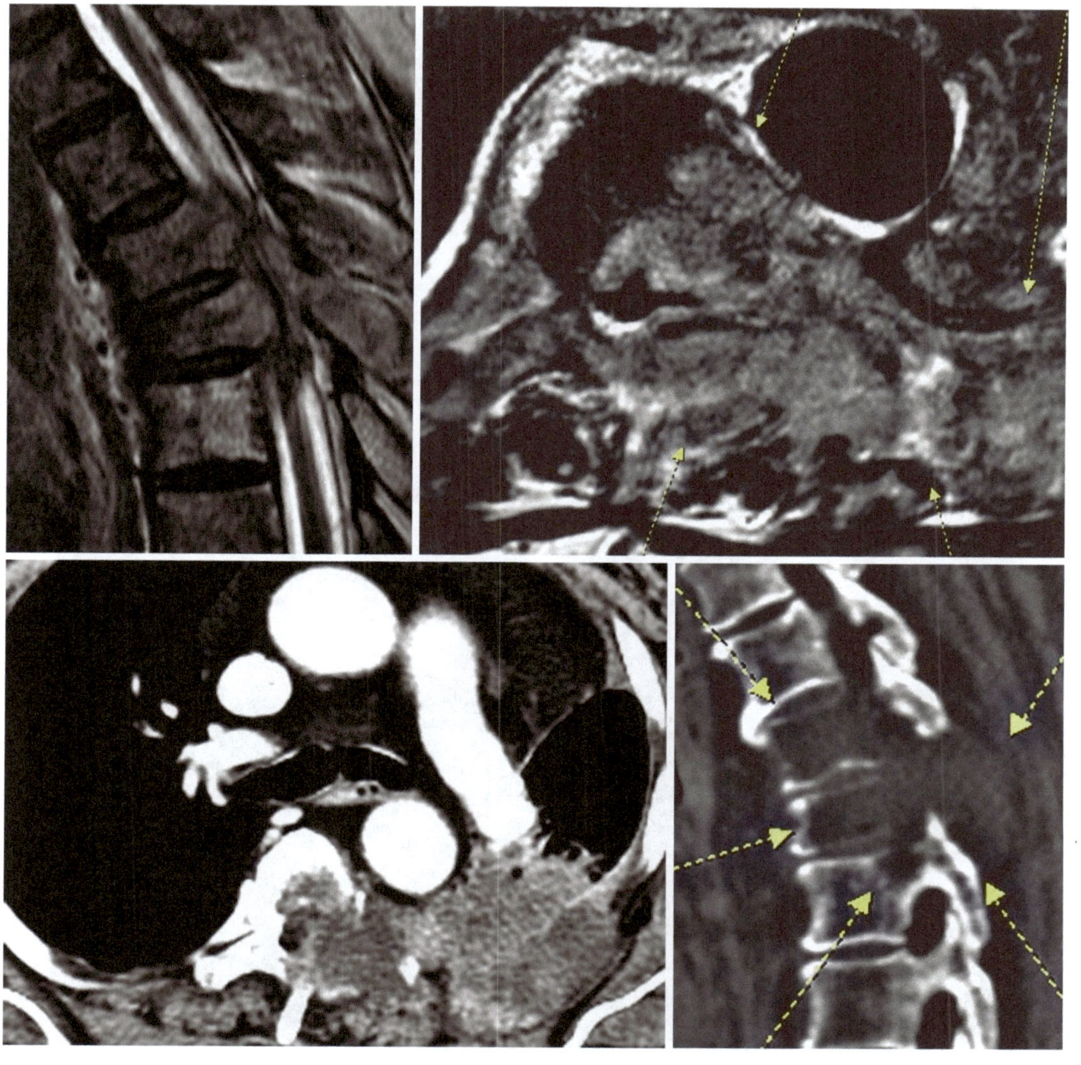

Fig. 8.2 Preoperative MRI (sagittal; upper left, axial; upper right) depiction of the extradural metastatic spinal tumor from the inherent lung cancer. Note the massive extension from the left retropleural cancer origin featured in the chest CT scan (lower left) to the left vertebral body, pedicle and dorsal lamina, spinous process, and multifidus muscles (arrow, upper right). The corresponding cancer incurred an osteolytic metastatic spinal tumor (lower right) on T6, 7 levels according to the sagittal CT scan

There are several types of these tumors that are benign but can cause problems by being locally destructive or invasive (e.g., hemangiomas, giant cell tumors and osteoblastomas). These are most often treated surgically to eliminate their destructive tendencies [5].

- Vertebral hemangioma is the most common benign spinal tumor (Fig. 8.5).
- Most occur in the vertebral body and about 10% extend into the posterior elements.
- The thoracic region is the most frequent.
- There are two different types: 1—asymptomatic; 2—aggressive, symptomatic types with intraspinal tumor extension and cord compression.
- Lesions with high T1 signal are considered benign. Low signal on both T1- and

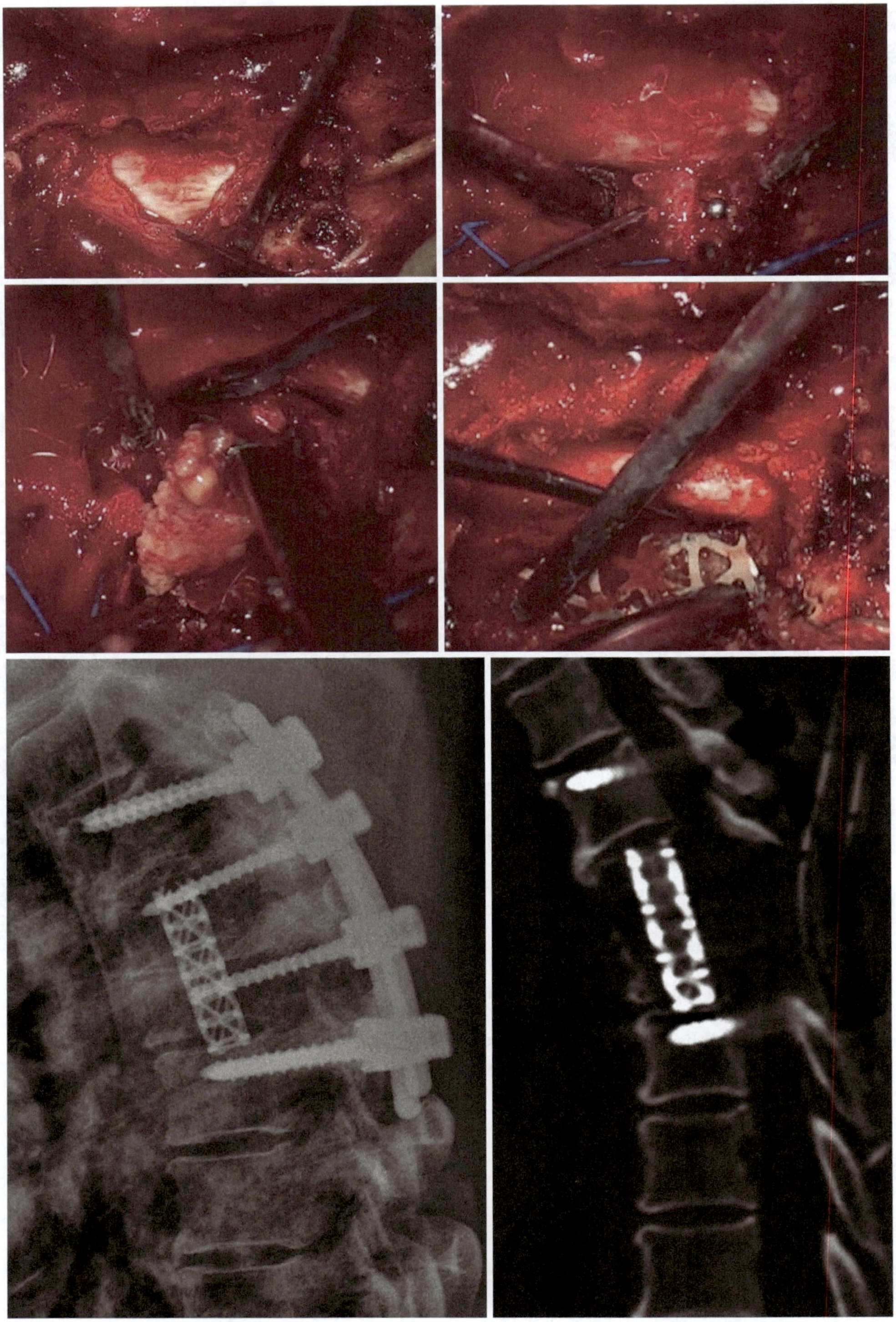

Fig. 8.3 Intraoperative process for the removal of an extradural metastatic spinal tumor. Dissection of the tumor portion from the dorsal cord sac (upper left), identification of the exiting nerve root from the corresponding spinal level (upper right), removal of the main, extradural portion of the tumor (lower left), and insertion of a mesh graft for the stabilization (lower right). The postoperative X-ray lateral view (left) & sagittal CT scan view (right) reveals well-reconstructed thoracic spinal levels from the metastasis with mesh graft inserted from below of superior endplate of T6 to above of upper endplate of T8

Variables	Benign	Malignant
Tumor	Aneurysmal bone cyst (*)	Chordoma
Location	Mainly posterior elements of the thoracolumbar spine, with extension into the vertebral body in 40% of cases	Over 50% of cases occur in the sacrum followed by the clivus (35%). One-sixth arise in the cervical, thoracic, and lumbar spine
Frequency	15% of all primary spine tumors	1-4% of primary bony tumors
Tumor	Giant cell tumor (*)	Chondrosarcoma
Location	Sacrum most common, then thoracic, cervical, and lumbar	Cervical (20%); thoracic (20%); lumbar (20%); sacral (20%)
Frequency	2-4% of all primary spine tumors	10% of all bone tumors but rarely in the spine
Tumor	Hemangioma	Ewing's sarcoma
Location	Most common in the thoracic and lumbar spine	Most commonly occurs at the sacrum
Frequency	Most common tumor of the spine, 12% incidence	Very rare to have primary spinal disease
Tumor	Osteoblastoma (*)	Lymphoma
Location	Most common in the cervical spine, then in the sacrum	Mostly involved the thoracic and lumbar spines
Frequency	1-3% of all primary bone tumors	Exceedingly rare, 1.7% of all primary bone lymphomas
Tumor	Osteochondroma	Osteosarcoma
Location	About 60% located in the lumbar spine, cervical (27%), thoracic (12%), sacrum (2%)	Mostly in the sacrum
Frequency	Most common benign bone tumor (30-40%), 1-4% occur in the spine	<5% of cases arise in the spine; comprise 3.6-14.5% of primary spinal tumors
Tumor	Osteiod osteoma	Plasmacytoma/multiple myeloma
Location	50% of cases occur in the cervical spine, followed by thoracic region	Lower thoracic and lumbar spine
Frequency	3% of all primary bone tumors, 10% occur in the spine	Most common primary tumor of the spine

(*): Aggressive benign tumors

Fig. 8.4 Summary of the primary extradural spinal tumors (courtesy from Lam FC et al. Surg Neurol Intl 2014)

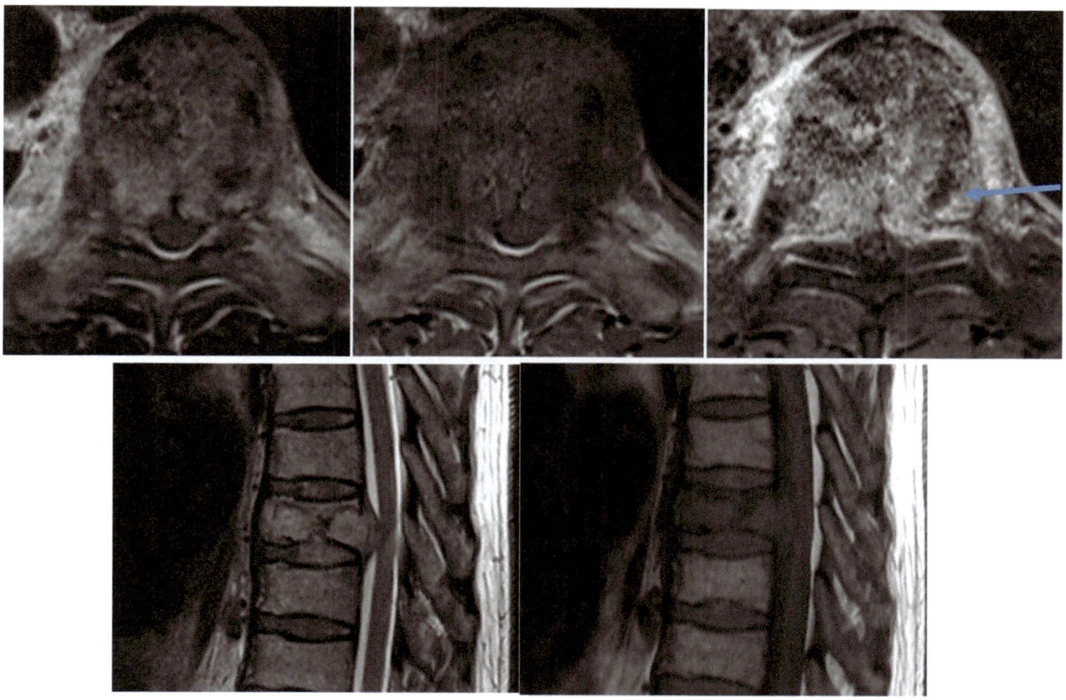

Fig. 8.5 An upper thoracic vertebral hemangioma featured through T2-, T1-, contrast-enhanced axial (upper 3 images in sequence), and sagittal (lower 2 images) MRI view. The lesion is associated with an intraspinal extradural component that is well enhanced with gadolinium (arrows)

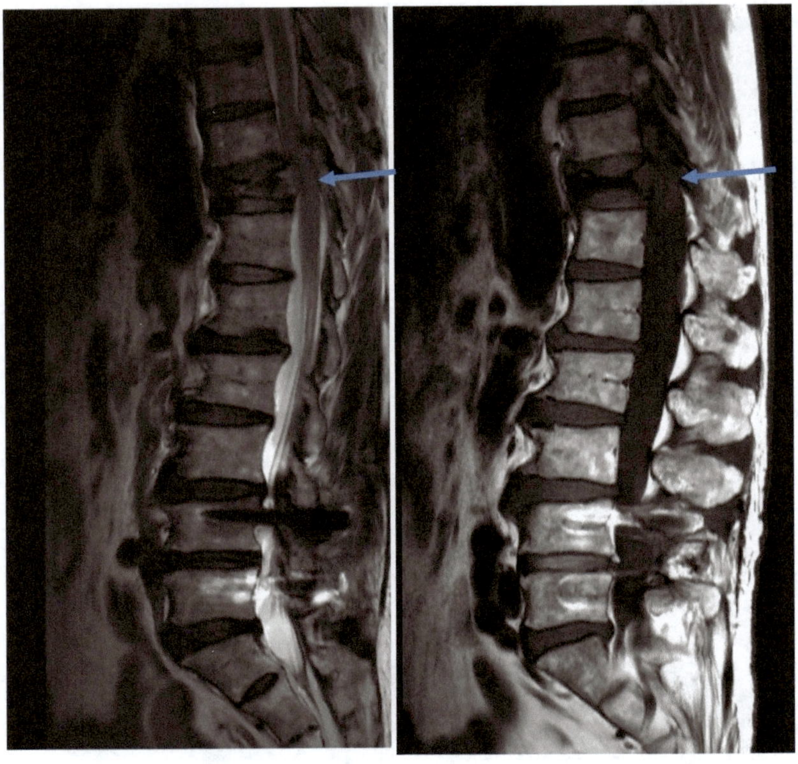

Fig. 8.6 Sagittal T2- (left) and T1- (right) weighted MRI images featuring solitary vertebral lesion, multiple myeloma. Note the dorsal cord and thecal sac compression (arrows)

T2-weighted sequences represents degenerative change/involution of the lesion. Low T1 signal together with high T2 signal may represent an atypical hemangioma.

Malignant tumor types (multiple myeloma, osteosarcomas, and Ewing's sarcoma), given their relative radioresistance and their typical malignant, invasive nature, surgery may be associated with fairly high morbidity and mortality rates [6]. Furthermore, it may be especially difficult to achieve gross total resections with tumor-free margins. These are often treated with multiple modalities including surgery, radiation, and chemotherapy [7].

- Myeloma is the most frequent primary malignant tumor of the spine (Fig. 8.6).
- The peak incidence is in the sixth to seventh decade.
- The spine and especially the vertebral bodies are the most common sites; epidural extension is common.

Useful information regarding the relative frequency of the various primary malignancies is available from large national registries and the cancer surveillance (SEER) programs [6]. Dorfman and Czerniak [8, 9] analyzed data on 2627 primary malignant tumors of bone collected in the SEER program during the period from 1973 to 1987. Osteosarcoma was the most frequently diagnosed sarcoma of bone (35.1%), followed by chondrosarcoma (25.8%), Ewing's sarcoma (16.0%), chordoma (8.4%), and malignant fibrous histiocytoma, including fibrosarcoma (5.6%). Important racial differences in the spectrum of tumors have been noted in several studies: osteosarcoma is more common in the Chinese and Japanese populations as compared with the White population, whereas chondrosarcoma is less common [10]. In the USA, chordomas and Ewing's sarcoma are seen almost exclusively in the White population.

In a more recent analysis, Damron and colleagues [11] looked at the survival and epidemiologic data from the National Cancer Database of the American College of Surgeons. Survival data were reported on cases with a minimum 5-year follow-up from 1985 to 1998. The relative 5-year survival rate was 53.9% for osteosarcoma, 75.2% for chondrosarcoma, and 50.6% for Ewing's sarcoma. In the Leeds tumor registry, which focuses on spine tumors, primary malignant tumors of the spine constituted only 4.6% of the cases registered between 1958 and 2000 [3]. The most common malignant spine tumors (based on clinical presentation) were multiple myeloma and plasmacytoma. The second most common tumor was chordoma, being most prevalent in the cervical and sacral regions. The third most common was osteosarcoma.

8.2 Surgery and Its Grading by the Extent of Resection

There are three major procedural methods for performing an en bloc excisions of the extradural intracanal spinal tumors; resection of the posterior arch and elements, sagittal resection along the lateral margin of the dura (spinal cord), and vertebrectomy (spondylectomy) [6]. These sequential surgical procedures are categorized by the tissue planes and manner of removal [12–13]. "Curettage" and "intralesional" are terms that describe the piecemeal removal of the tumor while "en bloc" indicates an attempt to remove the whole tumor in one piece, together with a layer of healthy tissue. Usually the specimen is then submitted for careful histological studies to further define the procedure as intralesional, marginal, or wide. The term "intralesional" is appropriate if the surgeon has elaborated within the tumor mass, "marginal" is appropriate if the surgeon has dissected along the pseudocapsule, which would be the layer of reactive tissue around the tumor, and "wide" is appropriate if the plane of surgical dissection is outside the pseudocapsule, thus removing the tumor with a continuous shell of healthy tissue. This wide en bloc procedure is usually called either excision or resection, which are the terms too widely used, confusing, and interchanged between them to be discriminated.

In order to avoid these confusions and to elucidate comparative results, it might be reasonable to differentiate this demanding, risky removal of the whole tumor in en bloc fashion from a simple intralesional (piecemeal removal from the whole extradural intracanal massive lesion) procedure. While this intralesional resection of malignant tumors may provide functional palliation and pain relief, it frequently results in a higher incidence of local recurrence.

8.3 Summary

The majority of extradural tumors represent metastases while the primary extradural spine tumors are rare, and there is little high quality evidence outlining the optimal treatment for these lesions. Trends in the literature support en bloc spondylectomy for low grade malignant tumors, but this aggressive approach proves technically challenging and may be associated with relatively high morbidity and mortality rates. Improvements in radiotherapy technology, advances in chemotherapy, novel molecular drug targets, and other multimodality protocols may increase survival rates.

References

1. Quiles AM, Gómez Roselló E, Laguillo G, García R, Caro JL. A comprehensive review of intraspinal tumors: Diagnostic, classification and radio-pathologic correlation. Presented at European Congress of Radiology (ECR) 2013 (poster number; C-2112). https://doi.org/10.1594/ecr2013/C-2112.
2. Abul-Kasim K, Thurnher MM, McKeever P, Sundgren PC. Intradural spinal tumors: Current classification and MRI features. Neuroradiology. 2008;50:301–14.

3. Kelley SP, Ashford RU, Rao AS, Dickson RA. Primary bone tumours of the spine: A 42-year survey from the leeds regional bone tumour registry. Eur Spine J. 2007;16:405–9.
4. Lam FC, Arle JE, Glazer PA, Kasper EM. Primary extradural tumors of the spine—Case review with evidence-guided management. Surg Neurol Int. 2014;28;5(Suppl 7):S373–5.
5. Harrop JS, Schmidt MH, Boriani S, Shaffrey CI. Aggressive "benign" primary spine neoplasms: Osteoblastoma, aneurysmal bone cyst, and giant cell tumor. Spine. 2009;34(22 Suppl):S39-47.
6. Sundaresan N, Rosen G, Boriani S. Primary malignant tumors of the spine. Orthop Clin North Am. 2009;40(21–36), v.
7. Kyle RA, Rajkumar SV. Multiple myeloma. N Engl J Med. 2004;351:1860–73.
8. Dorfman HD, Czerniak B. Bone cancers. Cancer. 1995;75:203–10.
9. Dorfman H, Czerniak B. Bone tumors. St. Louis (MO): Mosby; 1998.
10. Guo W, Xu W, Huvos AG, Healey JH, Feng C. Comparative frequency of bone sarcomas among different racial groups. Chin Med J. 1999;112:1101–4.
11. Damron TA, Ward WG, Stewart A. Osteosarcoma, chondrosarcoma, and Ewing's sarcoma: National Cancer Data Base Report. Clin Orthop Relat Res. 2007;459:40–7.
12. Sundaresan N, Digiacinto GV, Krol G, Hughes JE. Spondylectomy for malignant tumors of the spine. J Clin Oncol. 1989;7:1485–91.
13. Tomita K, Kawahara N, Baba H, Tsuchiya H, Fujita T, Toribatake Y. Total en bloc spondylectomy: A new surgical technique for primary malignant vertebral tumors. Spine. 1997;22:324–33.
14. Van Goethem JW, van den Hauwe L, Ozsarlak O, De Schepper AM, Parizel PM. Spinal tumors. Eur J Radiol. 2004;50:159–76.
15. Boriani S, Biagini R, De Iure F, Bertoni F, Malaguti MC, Di Fiore M et al. En bloc resections of bone tumors of the thoracolumbar spine. A preliminary report on 29 patients. Spine 1996;21:1927–31.

How to Approach Anatomical Compartment; Dural Tumor

9

Chi Heon Kim and Chun Kee Chung

Abstract

The representative tumor originated from dura is solitary fibrous tumor (SFT). SFT is a mesenchymal tumor of the fibroblastic type, presumably originating from soft tissue fibroblasts, and constitutes a heterogeneous group of rare spindle-cell tumors that include benign and malignant neoplasms. Most of the spinal SFTs are dense cellular tumors, mostly corresponding to the hemangiopericytoma phenotype, and are considered malignant (WHO grade II or III). The majority of patients (95%) was older than 21 years. Majority of patients complained of pain, hypoesthesia, paresis, urinary dysfunction, or combination of these as the initial presentation. Surgery is a mainstay treatment for spinal SFTs. As the tumor most likely originated from the spinal meninges, presumably meningeal fibroblasts, resection of the origin of tumor itself is essential to prevent recurrence even after gross total removal. Grade II or III tumors are considered malignant and treated with adjuvant therapy, typically radiotherapy.

Keywords

Solitary fibrous tumor · Spine · Surgery · Radiotherapy

C. H. Kim
Department of Neurosurgery, Seoul National University College of Medicine and Hospital, Seoul, South Korea
e-mail: chiheon1@snu.ac.kr

C. K. Chung (✉)
Department of Neurosurgery, Seoul National University Hospital, Seoul National University College of Medicine, Seoul, Republic of Korea
e-mail: chungc@snu.ac.kr

Neuroscience Research Institute, Seoul National University Medical Research Center, Seoul, Republic of Korea

Clinical Research Institute, Seoul National University Hospital, Seoul, Republic of Korea

Department of Brain and Cognitive Sciences, Seoul National University College of Natural Sciences, Seoul, Republic of Korea

9.1 Overview

The representative tumor originated from dura is solitary fibrous tumor (SFT). SFT is a mesenchymal tumor of the fibroblastic type, presumably originating from soft tissue fibroblasts, and constitutes a heterogeneous group of rare spindle-cell tumors that include benign and malignant neoplasms [1–3]. SFT is preferred by most pathologists to hemangiopericytoma, which includes a heterogeneous group of hemangiopericytoma like neoplasms [1, 3]. SFT was first described as a tumor originating from the pleura [4]. Surgery is the preferred choice of treatment with a 5-year

C. K. Chung (ed.), *Surgery of Spinal Cord Tumors Based on Anatomy*,
https://doi.org/10.1007/978-981-15-7771-0_9

survival rate of 100% when the benign SFT is completely removed. Most patients with malignant SFT don't survive more than 2 years due to progression or recurrence [4, 5]. The origin of spinal SFTs is variable, emerging from structures such as the dura mater, arachnoid, bone, periosteum, venous plexus, nerve root or spinal cord, and sometimes from structures with no correlation with the meninges [5–7]. So far, less than 100 spinal SFTs have been reported in the literature [7]. SFTs are rare (accounting for <1% of all primary CNS tumors) and usually occurs in the fourth to fifth decade of life [7, 8]. The tumors typically have a dural-based origin and is often located in supratentorial cranium, but about 10% are located in spine [8]. They comprise 0.08% of all primary bone tumors and 0.1% of primary malignant bone tumors [9, 10].

There are largely two morphological variants of SFT: the solitary fibrous tumor phenotype and the hemangiopericytoma phenotype [3, 8]. Detection of STAT6 nuclear expression or NAB2-STAT6 fusion is highly recommended to confirm the diagnosis [8]. In the central nervous system, a three-tiered histological WHO grading system is used [8]. A hypocellular, collagenized tumor with a classic solitary fibrous tumor phenotype is considered to correspond histologically to a WHO grade of I. Whereas, more dense cellular tumors, mostly corresponding to the hemangiopericytoma phenotype, are considered malignant (WHO grade II or III). The mitotic count is used to subclassify grade II (<5 mitosis/high power field [HPF]) and grade III (≥5 mitosis/HPF) [5, 8]. Grade I tumors are considered benign and is typically treated by surgical resection alone, but Grade II or III tumors are considered malignant and treated with adjuvant therapy, typically radiotherapy [8]. The majority of SFTs is benign and malignant SFTs compromise of 10% or less [2, 7].

9.2 Presentation

Albert GW et al. summarized 82 previous reports of spinal SFTs [7]. The ages ranged from 10 to 83 years (median 52 years) and the proportion of males was slightly higher (56% vs. 44%) [7]. The majority of patients (95%) was older than 21 years. SFTs were mostly located in thoracic spine (42%) followed by cervical spine (28%) and lumbar spine (13%), and were extradural in 27%, extradural and intradural extramedullary in 5%, intradural extramedullary in 35%, intradural extramedullary and intramedullary in 16%, and intramedurally in 15% [7, 11]. Majority of patients complained of pain, hypoesthesia, paresis, urinary dysfunction, or combination of those as the initial presentation [12–17]. An intramedullary SFT rarely causes a sudden paralysis [18, 19].

Spinal SFTs showed various morphologies with imaging; dumbbell-shaped or lobulated soft tissue mass, expansile intraosseous mass in the vertebral body, or posterior spinal element and long intraspinal canal mass (Fig. 9.1) [6, 12, 20]. Most SFTs were low or isointense on T1- and hypointense, mild hyperintense, or hyperintense on T2-weighted magnetic resonance imaging (MRI), which heterogeneously enhances when using contrast dye (Fig. 9.1) [7, 12, 13, 21, 22]. When SFTs are located in the intradural or extramedullary space, they mimic a meningioma or nerve sheath tumor (Fig. 9.1a, b) [7]. Malignant SFTs may present with multiple lesions as an initial presentation [2, 23].

9.3 Treatment and Outcomes

Surgery is a mainstay treatment for spinal SFTs. The extent of surgical removal determined clinical outcomes for patients with WHO grade I SFT, which compromised 93% of all reported cases of SFT [7, 9]. For WHO grade I SFT, no adjuvant treatment is recommended once gross total resection is achieved [6, 17, 24]. Gross total resection provided a recurrence-free rate of 90% at 1.2-year follow-up [7, 9]. Local recurrence was reported in less than 1% of patients after gross total removal and occurred over the long-term after surgery at 2 years, 8.5 years, and 14.5 years [7, 25–27]. Therefore, long-term clinical and radiological follow-ups are required [7, 28, 29]. As the tumor most likely originated from the spinal meninges, presumably meningeal fibroblasts, resection of the origin of tumor

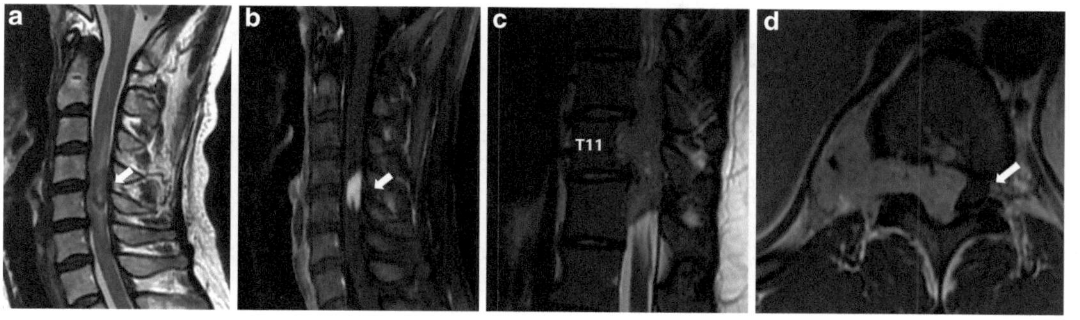

Fig. 9.1 Solitary fibrous tumor. A T2-weighted sagittal magnetic resonance image (MRI) showed a mixed low- and isosignal intensity intradural extramedullary (IDEM) mass (white arrow) in dorsal C4–5 spinal canal (**a**) and peritumoral edema extending from C3–6. The mass (white arrow) enhances intensely with gadolinium-enhanced T1-weighted MRI (**b**). A large isosignal extradural mass in T2-weighted sagittal MRI eroded T11 vertebra and extends from T10 to T12 spine (**c**). The spinal cord (white arrow) is deviated to the left by the well-enhanced compressing tumor in T1-weighed gadolinium-enhanced MRI (**d**)

itself is essential to prevent recurrence even after gross total removal [7, 24]. Gross total resection was achievable in 83% of patients with WHO grade I SFTs. Progression was detected in the majority of patients (5/6, 83%) with subtotal resection in a study follow-up period of 6 months to 21 years [7]. A malignant transformation was reported in only one case, 3.5 years after removal of the WHO grade I SFT [2].

Contrary to benign SFTs, a high rate of recurrence (about 25%) was reported in spite of adjuvant radiotherapy, for malignant SFTs (WHO grade II or III SFT) which comprises 7% of all spinal SFTs [6, 7]. Jia Q et al. analyzed 20 patients with WHO grade II or III SFT in spine [9]. The tumor was totally removed in 75% of patients. Mean recurrence/progression-free survival time was 37.6 months after gross total removal and 21 months after a subtotal resection [7]. The authors had a recurrence rate of 45% at median of 28 months (range, 12–73). Recurrence occurred in six out of nine patients (67%) with WHO grade III SFTs [9]. However, after a piece-meal manner removal, and when gross total removal was achieved, recurrence was reported in 60% of WHO grade III SFTs and 40% of grade II SFTs [7]. The recurrence rates after subtotal removal were 100% (3/3) with WHO grade III SFT and 50% (1/2) with WHO grade II SFTs [7].

Due to the rarity of the disease, treatment for metastasis from spinal SFT is rarely reported [13]. For example, Biawas et al. combined radiotherapy and chemotherapy (ifosfamide and epirubicin) for residual lesion and metastatic lung SFTs, but the treatment has not been standardized yet [13]. The most important prognostic factors for survival were found to be the extent of surgery for both benign and malignant SFTs, and standard therapy of both benign and malignant SFT. This may be an en block removal including the dural origin of tumor [9, 13, 17].

Case Series

From 2010 to 2017, seven patients underwent surgery for spinal SFTs in Seoul National University Hospital, South Korea (Table 9.1). Median age was 43 years (range 19–70) and five patients were male. All tumors were a solitary lesion and were located in the cervical spine in two patients, thoracic spine in two patients, occipital condyle in one patient, lumbar spine in one patient, and sacral spine in one patient. The SFTs were located in intradural extramedullary space in four patients, simultaneous intradural extramedullary and extradural space in two patients, and extradural space in one patient. Two patients also had neurofibromatosis type I. WHO grades were II/III in five patients and III/III in two patients. Weakness was the most common symptom

Table 9.1 Summary of patients

Patients No	Sex	Age at surgery	Symptom	Combined disease	Level	Location	Surgery extent	WHO grade	Adjuvant therapy	Recurrence	Time at recurrence (months)	Follow-up period (months)
1	M	43	Dysesthesia		Cervical	IDEM	GTR	II				61
2	M	21	Weakness, dysesthesia		Thoracic	ED	GTR, staged	II		Yes	9	45
3	F	49	Weakness, hypoesthe-sia		Cervical	IDEM	GTR	II				36
4	F	25	Pain		Sacral	IDEM	GTR	III		Yes	66	94
5	M	70	Weakness, hypoesthe-sia	NF-1	Thoracic	IDEM	NTR	II		Yes	58	85
6	M	51	Weakness		Occipital condyle	Both IDEM and ED	PR	III	Radiothe-rapy 60 Gy	Yes	49	70
7	M	19	Weakness, hypoesthe-sia	NF-1	Lumbar	Both IDEM and ED	PR	II		Yes	6	6

Abbreviations: *ED* extradural space; *GTR* gross total removal; *IDEM* intradural extramedullary space; *NF-1* neurofibromatosis type I; *NTR* near total removal (removal of 99%); *PR* partial removal (removal less than 90%)

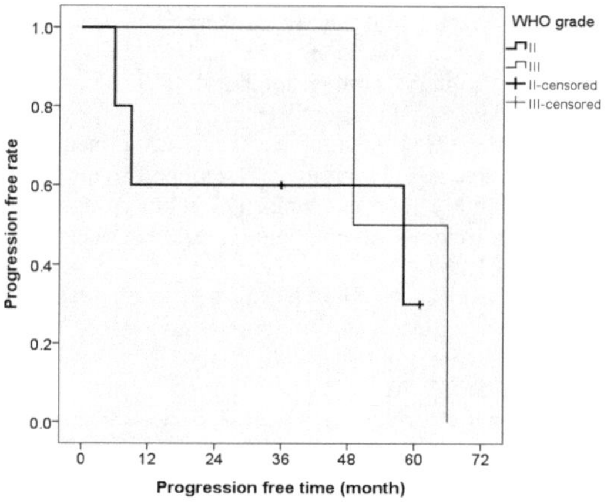

Fig. 9.2 Progression-free time. Mean progression-free times were 39 months (95% CI, 16–61) for WHO grade II solitary fibrous tumor and 58 months (95% CI, 9–41) for WHO grade III solitary fibrous tumor (log-rank test, p = 0.63)

presented in five patients, sensory symptoms such as hypoesthesia, or dysesthesia, or both, was the presenting symptom in five patients. Pain was the presenting symptom in one patient. The tumor was approached with a posterior midline approach and was totally removed in four patients, near totally removed in one patient, and partially removed in two patients but with an extradural tumor. Staged surgery was performed in patients with an extradural tumor that was located in both intraspinal and extraspinal spaces (Patient No 2, Fig. 9.1a, b), this was to preserve spinal stability in a 21-year-old man. Postoperative neurological status was uneventful in all patients. Radiotherapy was not performed in patients with WHO grade II SFTs. Radiotherapy was done for one patient with WHO grade III/III histology. Another 25-year-old female patient (Patient No 4) with a WHO grade III/III SFT in the sacral spine refused radiotherapy to preserve fertility. Recurrence/progression occurred in 3/5 WHO grade II SFT and 2/2 WHO grade III SFTs and mean progression-free times were 39 months (95% CI, 16–61) and 58 months (95% CI, 9–41) (log-rank test, p = 0.63), respectively (Fig. 9.2). Tumors that recurred were totally resected in four patients and further recurrence was not observed for 2–3 years thereafter. One patient (Patient No 7) presented with paraplegia (manual motor power grade 0/5) at recurrence and refused further surgery.

9.4 Conclusion

Although SFTs are rare and have various morphologies in imaging studies, it should be included in differential diagnoses. The presenting symptom is mostly pain or weakness that is recoverable with surgery. The mainstay of treatment is the gross total resection and postoperative radiotherapy is helpful to delay recurrence for WHO grade II or III tumors.

References

1. Penel N, Amela EY, Decanter G, Robin YM, Marec-Berard P. Solitary fibrous tumors and so-called hemangiopericytoma. Sarcoma. 2012;2012:690251.
2. Munoz E, Prat A, Adamo B, Peralta S, Ramon y Cajal S, Valverde C. A rare case of malignant solitary fibrous tumor of the spinal cord. Spine (Phila Pa 1976). 2008;33:E397–9.
3. Gengler C, Guillou L. Solitary fibrous tumour and haemangiopericytoma: Evolution of a concept. Histopathology. 2006;48:63–74.
4. Cardillo G, Lococo F, Carleo F, Martelli M. Solitary fibrous tumors of the pleura. Curr Opin Pulm Med. 2012;18:339–46.
5. Bisceglia M, Galliani C, Giannatempo G, et al. Solitary fibrous tumor of the central nervous system: A 15-year literature survey of 220 cases (August 1996-July 2011). Adv Anat Pathol. 2011;18:356–92.
6. Lang N, Zhang E, Xing X, Yuan H. Solitary fibrous tumour of the spine: Imaging features of a commonly misdiagnosed entity. Eur Radiol. 2018;28:3986–95.
7. Albert GW, Gokden M. Solitary fibrous tumors of the spine: A pediatric case report with a comprehensive review of the literature. J Neurosurg Pediatr. 2017;19:339–48.

8. Giannini C, Rushing EJ, Hainfellner JA, et al. Mesenchymal, non-meningothelial tumours. In: Louis DN, Ohgaki H, Wiestler OD, et al., editors. WHO classification of tumours of the central nervous system. Switzerland: WHO Press; 2016. p. 249–54.
9. Jia Q, Zhou Z, Zhang D, et al. Surgical management of spinal solitary fibrous tumor/hemangiopericytoma: A case series of 20 patients. Eur Spine J. 2018;27:891–901.
10. Tang JS, Gold RH, Mirra JM, Eckardt J. Hemangiopericytoma of bone. Cancer. 1988;62:848–59.
11. Ishii K, Nakamura M, Matsumoto M, Mukai M, Toyama Y, Chiba K. Intramedullary solitary fibrous tumor of the spinal cord. J Orthop Sci. 2009;14:450–4.
12. Yi X, Xiao D, He Y, et al. Spinal solitary fibrous tumor/hemangiopericytoma: A clinicopathologic and radiologic analysis of eleven cases. World Neurosurg. 2017;104:318–29.
13. Biswas R, Halder A, Ramteke PP, Pandey R. Malignant solitary fibrous tumor of thoracic spine with distant metastases: Second reported case and review of the literature. J Craniovertebr Junction Spine. 2017;8:79–81.
14. Walker CT, Amene CS, Pannell JS, et al. Hemorrhagic intramedullary solitary fibrous tumor of the conus medullaris: Case report. J Neurosurg Spine. 2015;23:438–43.
15. Basaran R, Kaksi M, Onoz M, Balkuv E, Sav A. Intradural solitary fibrous tumor of the lumbar spine: A distinctive case report. Case Rep Neurol Med. 2015;2015:708472.
16. Kakimaru H, Matsusaki M, Sanada H, Iwata A, Uchio Y. Dumbbell-type spinal solitary fibrous tumor with paraplegia. Orthopedics. 2009;32:213.
17. Jallo GI, Roonprapunt C, Kothbauer K, Freed D, Allen J, Epstein F. Spinal solitary fibrous tumors: A series of four patients: Case report. Neurosurgery. 2005;57:E195; discussion E195.
18. Bruder M, Tews D, Mittelbronn M, Capper D, Seifert V, Marquardt G. Intramedullary solitary fibrous tumor—A benign form of hemangiopericytoma? Case report and review of the literature. World Neurosurg. 2015;84:189, e187–9, e112.
19. Ogungbo B, Prakash S, Kulkarni G, Bradey N, Marks SM, Scoones D. Cervical intra-/extramedullary solitary fibrous tumour. Br J Neurosurg. 2005;19:254–7.
20. Lavrador JP, Oliveira E, Neto L, Pimentel J, Francisco AF, Livraghi S. Dumbbell-shaped spinal solitary fibrous tumor: Combined approach and a review of the literature. Neurochirurgie. 2015;61:287–91.
21. Mariniello G, Napoli M, Russo C, et al. MRI features of spinal solitary fibrous tumors. A report of two cases and literature review. Neuroradiol J. 2012;25:610–16.
22. Ogawa T, Moriyama E, Beck H, Sonobe H. Solitary fibrous tumor of the thoracic spinal cord. Neurol Med Chir (Tokyo). 2005;45:371–4.
23. Son S, Lee SG, Jeong DH, Yoo CJ. Malignant solitary fibrous tumor of tandem lesions in the skull and spine. J Korean Neurosurg Soc. 2013;54:246–9.
24. Martin AJ, Fisher C, Igbaseimokumo U, Jarosz JM, Dean AF. Solitary fibrous tumours of the meninges: Case series and literature review. J Neurooncol. 2001;54:57–69.
25. Mordani JP, Haq IU, Singh J. Solitary fibrous tumour of the spinal cord. Neuroradiology. 2000;42:679–81.
26. Fargen KM, Opalach KJ, Wakefield D, Jacob RP, Yachnis AT, Lister JR. The central nervous system solitary fibrous tumor: A review of clinical, imaging and pathologic findings among all reported cases from 1996 to 2010. Clin Neurol Neurosurg. 2011;113:703–10.
27. Caroli E, Salvati M, Orlando ER, Lenzi J, Santoro A, Giangaspero F. Solitary fibrous tumors of the meninges: Report of four cases and literature review. Neurosurg Rev. 2004;27:246–51.
28. Hashimoto K, Miyamoto K, Hosoe H, et al. Solitary fibrous tumor in the cervical spine with destructive vertebral involvement: A case report and review of the literature. Arch Orthop Trauma Surg. 2008;128:1111–6.
29. Kobayashi K, Imagama S, Ito Z, et al. Recurrence of solitary fibrous tumor of the cervical spinal cord. Nagoya J Med Sci. 2014;76:217–23.

How to Approach Anatomical Compartment: Intradural Extra-arachnoidal Tumor

10

Chang-Hyun Lee and Chun Kee Chung

Abstract

The most common tumor in the intradural extra-arachnoid space is meningioma. Meningiomas are thought to be derived from the arachnoid granulations or islands of arachnoid cells. In spine, the fenestration between cerebrospinal fluid (CSF) and blood may be on the inner surface of the dura mater at the entry zone of the nerve roots, where the spinal arteries penetrate. The surgical procedure depends on whether the spinal cord is pushed backward or forward. When the cord is pushed forward, the tumor can be removed via subdural epi-arachnoid approach without damages to arachnoid membrane and subarachnoid structure (particularly vascular structures). On the other hand, if the cord is pushed backward, an epi-arachnoid approach is sometimes impossible. The dura attached with meningioma need not be removed because the tumor did not originate from the dura. Dural curettage and coagulation results in as low a recurrence rate as aggressive excision of involved dura, and a substantially lower complication rate.

Keywords

Meningioma · Intradural extramedullary · Epi-arachnoid · Extra-arachnoid · Spinal cord tumor

10.1 Introduction

The intradural extra-arachnoid space is a potential one between dura and outer membrane of arachnoid. The most common tumor in this space is meningiomas, with dumbbell-shaped

---

Electronic supplementary material The online version of this chapter (https://doi.org/10.1007/978-981-15-7771-0_10) contains supplementary material, which is available to authorized users.

C.-H. Lee
Department of Neurosurgery, Seoul National University Hospital, Seoul, Republic of Korea
e-mail: imspinesurgeon@gmail.com

Department of Neurosurgery, Spine Center, Seoul National University Bundang Hospital, Seongnam, Republic of Korea

C. K. Chung (✉)
Department of Neurosurgery, Seoul National University Hospital, Seoul National University College of Medicine, Seoul, Republic of Korea
e-mail: chungc@snu.ac.kr

Neuroscience Research Institute, Seoul National University Medical Research Center, Seoul, Republic of Korea

Clinical Research Institute, Seoul National University Hospital, Seoul, Republic of Korea

Department of Brain and Cognitive Sciences, Seoul National University College of Natural Sciences, Seoul, Republic of Korea

C. K. Chung (ed.), *Surgery of Spinal Cord Tumors Based on Anatomy*,
https://doi.org/10.1007/978-981-15-7771-0_10

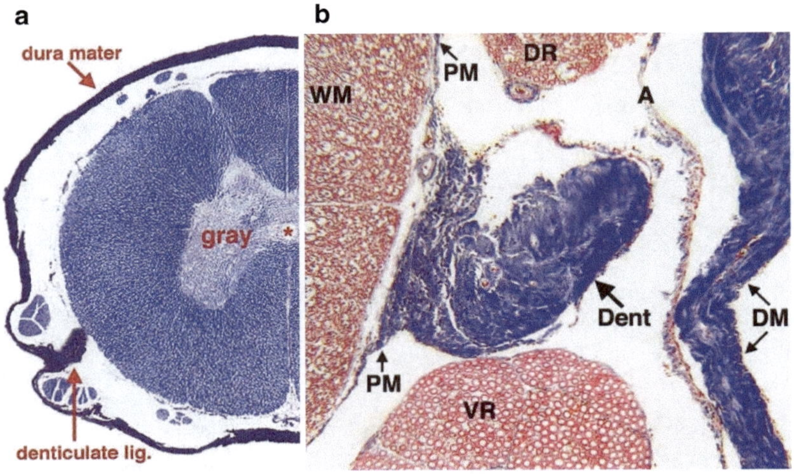

Fig. 10.1 **a** Cross-section of spinal cord (Luxol Blue stain). The central canal (asterisk) is surrounded by butterfly-shaped gray matter. The blue stained white matter is superficial to the gray matter. Pia mater is attached along the white matter surface. Dura mater is the most superficial menix. Arachnoid lines the dura mater. Bilaterally, a denticulate ligament extends from pia mater to dura mater. **b** High power view of the denticulate ligament (Dent) and neighboring structures (Triple stain). Pia mater (PM) is attached to the surface of spinal white matter (WM). The denticulate ligament is an expansion of pia mater collagen that periodically sends extensions toward the dura mater (DM). Arachnoid (A) and a dorsal root (DR) and a ventral root (VR) are also labelled. (Copyright by https://vanat.cvm.umn.edu/neurHistAtls/pages/men4.html)

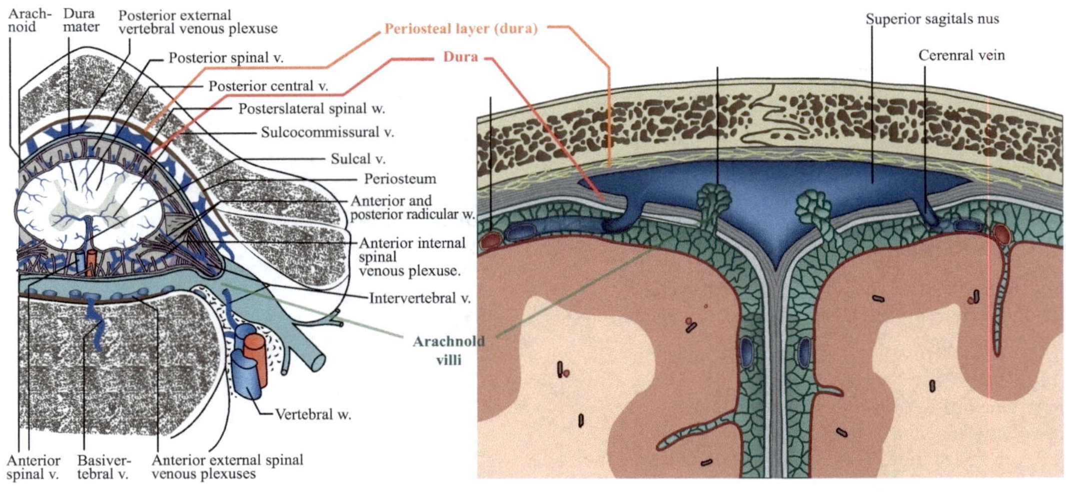

Fig. 10.2 Schematic drawing of the fenestration between CSF in the subarachnoid space and blood in the epidural space. Meningioma is known to be originated from the arachnoid cap cells and those cells lay on the inner surface of the dura mater at the entry zone of the nerve roots, where the spinal arteries penetrate

schwannomas and other tumors occurring rarely [1, 2]. During the surgeries of spinal cord, you can enter this space after incising dura. Dura is separated from arachnoid membrane without difficulty, but dentate ligament fixed dura and pia-arachnoid complex, as shown in Fig. 10.1. Below this space and bound with outer arachnoid, cerebrospinal fluid (CSF) circulates around the spinal cord and the spinal nerve roots project from it (Fig. 10.2). As these structures leave the spinal canal, arachnoid villi and arachnoid granulations form along the dura of the root sleeves and project into draining spinal veins [3]. The arachnoid membrane reflects back on the proximal portion of emerging nerve root and does not accompany it for any great length; this is known as the subarachnoid angle, where proliferations of arachnoid cells invade the dura and mark the limit of the subarachnoid space [4]. The base of these proliferations is continuous with the subarachnoid space and can penetrate the dura to varying degrees, allowing various amounts of CSF drainage among individuals [4]. It is fair to say that the relative contribution of these structures to net CSF reabsorption is poorly understood.

10.2 Pathogenesis

In 1831, Bright noticed the histologic similarities between meningioma cells and arachnoid villi cells. Cleland and Robin proposed for the first time that meningiomas derive from arachnoid cap cells. Thereafter, Schmidt observed obvious histologic similarities between meningioma cells and arachnoid cells at the ultrastructural level, with respect to cell adhesion mechanisms and the components of extracellular matrix [5].

Meningiomas are thought to be derived from the arachnoid granulations or islands of arachnoid cells. In the brain, the arachnoid cap cells are commonly observed at the superior sagittal sinus, which is an interface between CSF in the subarachnoid space and blood in the extradural region (Fig. 10.3). In spine, the fenestration between CSF and blood may be on the inner surface of the dura mater at the entry zone of the nerve roots, where the spinal arteries penetrate [5, 6]. For this reason, lateral tumors are more common than pure dorsal and ventral lesions [6, 7]. Previous investigators insisted that the spinal encapsulated meningiomas commonly develop into a small preserved subarachnoid space confined between the outer layer of arachnoid and the dura [8, 9]. Therefore, the tumor attached to the dura can be dissected from arachnoid membrane during intradural epi-arachnoid approach (Video 1, 2).

10.3 Epidemiology

Meningiomas of the spinal cord have a very low incidence in the first two decades of life, and arise most commonly in the fifth to seventh decades of life and have a striking female predominance, with only 20% occurring in males [10–12]. Meningiomas may be related to a putative hormonal influence on growth operating through progesterone receptors, and grow in pregnancy or breast carcinoma [13]. Gottfried et al. performed a meta-analysis including 566 cases from six published series, reaching the conclusion that most spinal meningiomas were located lateral to the spinal cord or had a component that extended laterally assuming a posterolateral or anterolateral location, of which they determined the posterolateral was

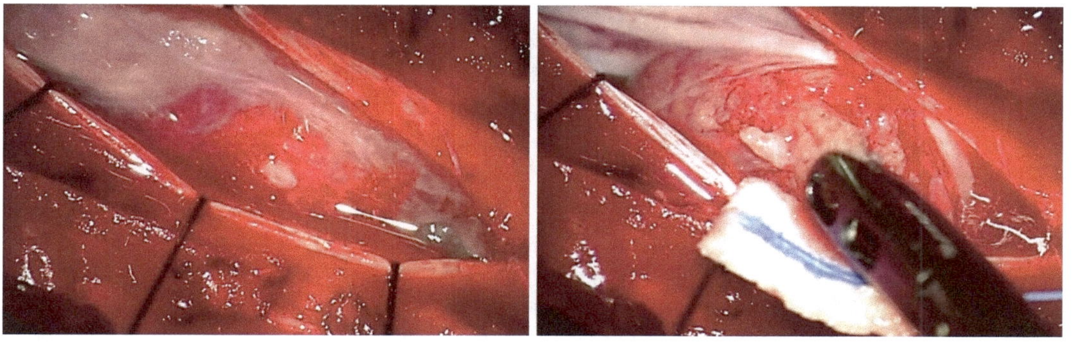

Fig. 10.3 The origin of meningioma. When dura was incised, an extra-arachnoidal tumor was shown. Because the tumor was attached to dorsal dura, a capsule of the tumor was opened. After dissecting covered the arachnoid membrane, the tumor was removed without incising arachnoid membrane

the more frequent [14]. Other authors reported that this tumor may be most commonly anterolateral above C7 and posterolateral below [15]. Traditionally, meningioma divided into ventral and dorsal meningioma and the standard for dividing is the dentate ligament. Clinically, it seems more reasonable to divide depending on pushing the spinal cord forward or backward because meningioma is located at lateral, ventral, and dorsal side.

Many previous researches reported the most common distribution of meningiomas along the spinal axis to be the thoracic segment (67%–84%), followed by the less frequent high cervical levels (14%–27%), and the extremely rare at lumbar levels (2%–14%) [7, 14, 16]. Even after accounting for the relative length of the thoracic spinal canal, a disproportionately high number of these lesions occur in the thoracic spine; meningiomas in the lumbar spine are unusual [17]. The propensity to involve the thoracic spine seems to be true only in females, as the relative involvement of the thoracic and cervical levels is approximately equal in males [17].

Although most of the spinal meningioma cases are intradural, few (5%–14%) occur at extradural or extraspinal locations [7, 14, 16, 18]. Most spinal meningiomas are globoid, but a few exceptions demonstrate *en plaque* configuration [19–22]. In pathologic subgroups of spinal meningioma, meningothelial and psammomatous meningiomas are the most common histologic subtypes of spinal meningioma [18, 23]. On the other hand, atypical (WHO grade II), the clear cell (WHO grade II), and malignant (WHO grade III) meningiomas are rare in the spinal meninges, with a combined incidence of 1.3% among all craniospinal meningiomas [14, 18, 24, 25].

10.4 Strategy of Surgical Treatment

Because spinal meningiomas are mostly benign tumors, their total surgical resection provides the best treatment option for a definitive cure for these patients. The surgical procedure depends on whether the spinal cord is pushed backward or pushed forward. When the cord is pushed forward, the dura is opened, the arachnoid is lifted (epi-arachnoid approach) and the tumor can be removed. Damages to subarachnoid structure (particularly vascular structures) can be avoided through an epi-arachnoid approach. On the other hand, if the cord is pushed backward, an epi-arachnoid approach is sometimes impossible [26]. In this case, surgeons can open the arachnoid first and enter the subarachnoid space; then, open the arachnoid again. In other words, the arachnoid is opened twice to enter the epi-arachnoid space [27, 28].

1. The dura should be opened longitudinally in the midline, but if the tumor is biased to one side, the perpendicular dura incision can be added at the same side of the tumor.
2. In prone position, the surgical site should be at the top. The head of the patient is located below the legs to avoid prevent blood and air (pneumocephalus) from entering the subarachnoid space (subarachnoid hemorrhage), which may result in arachnoiditis and air embolism complicating the postoperative period [19].
3. If the meningioma pushes the spinal cord forward, the surgeon does not need to incise outer layer of arachnoid membrane. Find the tumor along the interface between the dura and the outer layer of arachnoid membrane (intradural epi-arachnoid approach). Once the tumor is found, peel the outer arachnoid off from the tumor. Then, the tumor can be removed from the dura. The surgeon should continue dissection along this epi-arachnoid plane, applying force in the direction of the tumor avoiding pressure on the spinal cord, until the tumor is removed completely including the dural attachment.
4. If the meningioma is pushing the spinal cord backward, tumor removal via epi-arachnoid is usually but not always possible. If epi-arachnoid approach is possible, find and cut dentate ligaments along the interface between the dura and the arachnoid membrane (epi-arachnoid approach). If the outer layer of arachnoid membrane disturbs surgeon's vision, open the outer layer (dorsal

side) and go into the subarachnoid space. And then, open the outer layer (ventral side) and go out to the subdural space (extra-leptomeningeal route, Fig. 10.2).

5. Theoretically, the dura attached with meningioma need not be removed because the tumor is not originated from the dura. Because of the problem of arachnoid cap cells, removing the dura is an overshooting. It is enough to thoroughly curette the tightly adhered tumor from the inner dura [29]. Dural curettage and coagulation results in as low a recurrence rate as aggressive excision of involved dura, and a substantially lower complication rate [17].

Case Review

Case 1. Epi-arachnoid approach, spinal cord forward (Video 1).

A 59-year-old female patient complained of gait disturbance. The patient also complained of leg paresthesia. Her magnetic resonance (MR) images showed 1.7 × 1.2 × 1.1 cm-sized ovoid mass at the intradural extramedullary region in the T8-9 spinal canal (Fig. 10.4). The patient underwent spinal cord tumor removal. When dura was opened, the tumor was seen at epi-arachnoid space. The tumor was removed without incision of arachnoid membrane.

Case 2. Epi-arachnoid approach, spinal cord backward (Video 2).

A 68-year-old female patients complained of leg weakness for 3 months. She has felt tingling sense at both soles several years ago. The patient checked MR imaging, which demonstrated 1.2 × 1.1 × 1.3 cm mass at the T10 level

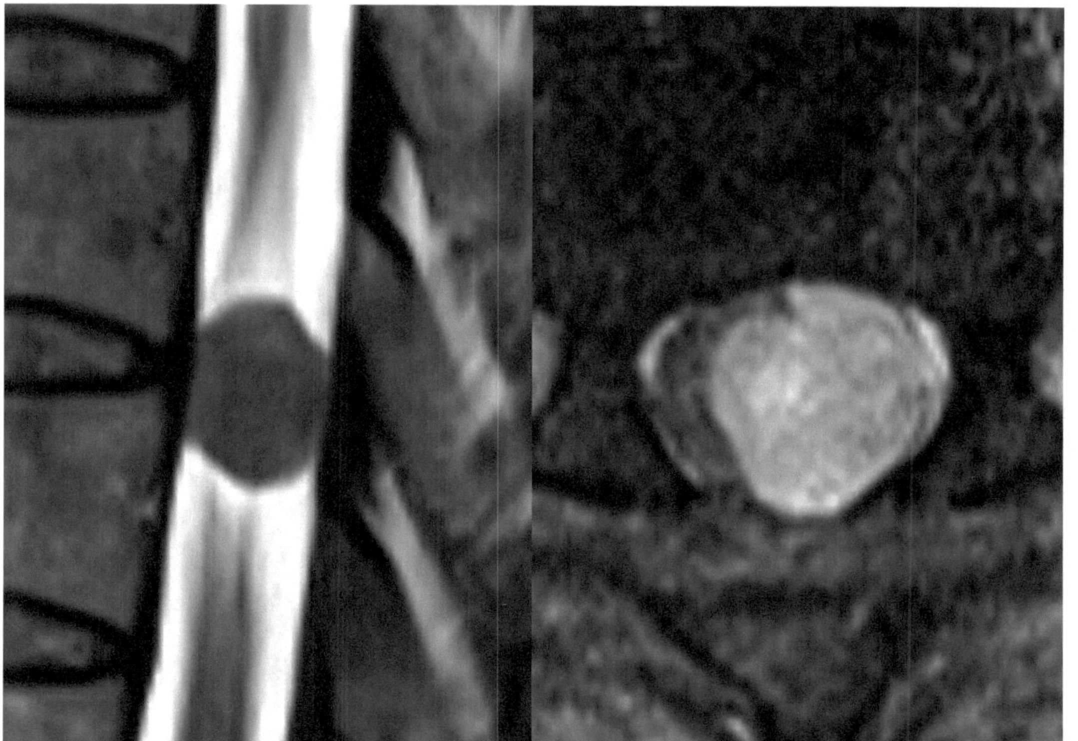

Fig. 10.4 Magnetic resonance images (MRI) of the thoracic spine revealed about 1.7 × 1.2 × 1.1 cm-sized ovoid mass at left side of T8-9 intradural extramedullary region. The tumor showed homogenous enhancement. The spinal cord displaced to the right

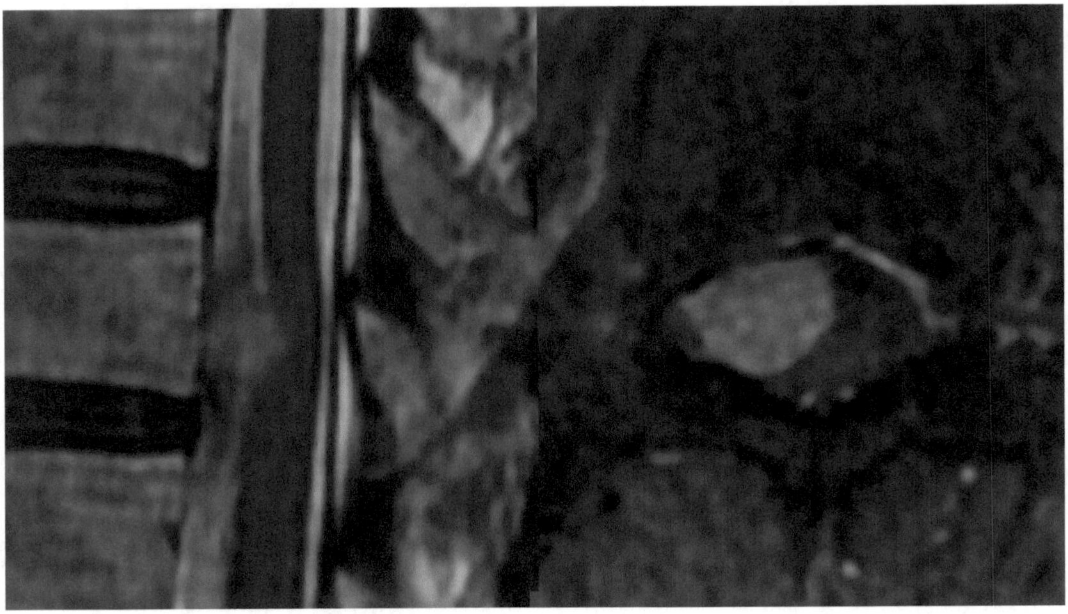

Fig. 10.5 Magnetic resonance images (MRI) of the thoracic spine revealed about 1.2 × 1.1 × 1.3 cm well enhancing mass at the right level T10. The tumor was located at intradural extramedullary region with suspicious focal dural enhancement. The spinal cord displaced to the backward

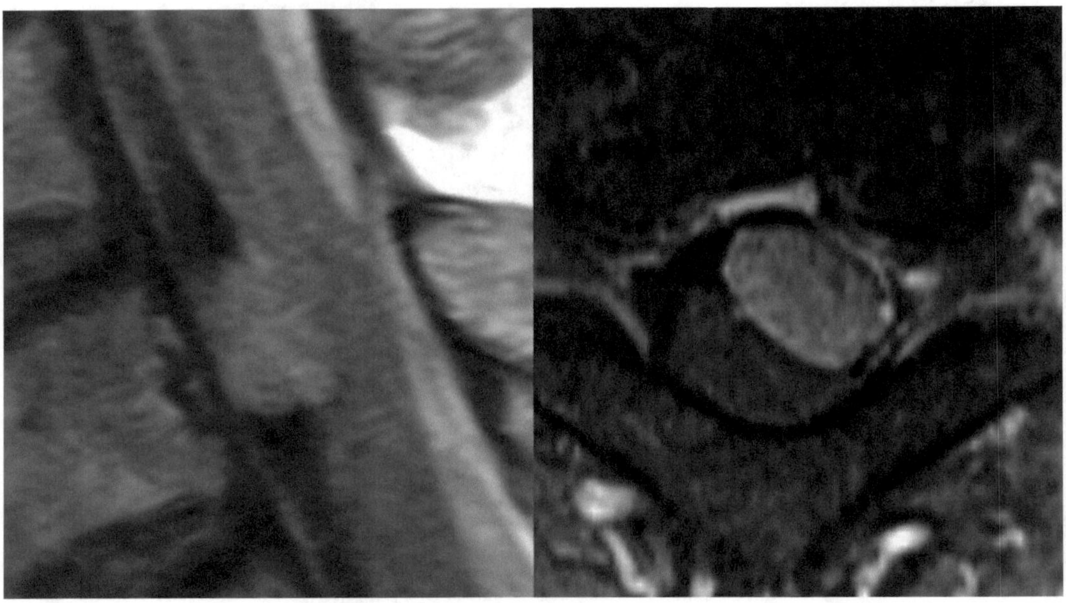

Fig. 10.6 Magnetic resonance images (MRI) of the thoracic spine demonstrated about 1.7 × 1.2 × 1.1 cm-sized ovoid mass at left side of T8-9 spinal canal, probable intradural extramedullary location. The spinal cord displaced to backward

(Fig. 10.5). Surgery for the patient was performed extra-leptomeningeal approach. After midline dura incision, the tumor was found via epi-arachnoid approach. The dentate ligament was cut to make the operation field. Arachnoid membrane was dissected from the tumor and the tumor was removed piecemeal pattern. Finally, dura of the tumor origin was coagulated with curettage.

Case 3. Extra-leptomeningeal approach, spinal cord backward (Video 3).

A 56-year-old woman presented with right shoulder pain. The pain was not relieved for 6 months, and the patient checked the MR imaging. The MR images showed $1.2 \times 0.7 \times 1.2$ cm-sized intradural extramedullary mass at T1 level (Fig. 10.6). The tumor was homogenously well enhanced with dural tail sign. Spinal cord was displaced to dorsal and right side. The patient underwent surgical removal of spinal cord tumor. When the dura opened, the surgeon tried to make operation field via epi-arachnoid approach. However, operation field was too narrow to remove the tumor safely. So, the dorsal layer of arachnoid membrane was opened, and the dentate ligament was cut. After then, the ventral layer of arachnoid membrane opened, and the tumor was removed successfully. Finally, dura of the tumor origin was scraped and then coagulated.

10.5 Conclusion

Intradural extra-arachnoidal tumor such as meningioma can be removed without incision of arachnoid membrane. It may be related with outcome and recurrence.

References

1. Barolat-Romana G, Benzel EC. Spinal intradural extraarachnoid metastasis. Surg Neurol. 1983;19(2):137–43.
2. Heran NS, Yong RL, Heran MS, Yip S, Fairholm D. Primary intradural extraarachnoid hodgkin lymphoma of the cervical. Spine. 2006;5(1):61.
3. Hartman AL. Normal anatomy of the cerebrospinal fluid compartment. In: Irani DN, editor. Cerebrospinal fluid in practice. Philadelphia: Saunders; 2009. p. 5–10.
4. Nicholas DS, Weller RO. The fine anatomy of the human spinal meninges. A light and scanning electron microscopy study. J Neurosurg. 1988;69(2):276–82.
5. Yamashima T. On arachnoid villi and meningiomas: Functional implication of ultrastructure, cell adhesion mechanisms, and extracellular matrix composition. Pathol Oncol Res. 1996;2(3):144–9.
6. Rasmussen TB, Kernohan JW, Adson AW. Pathologic classification, with surgical consideration, of intraspinal tumors. Ann Surg. 1940;111(4):513–30.
7. King AT, Sharr MM, Gullan RW, Bartlett JR. Spinal meningiomas: A 20-year review. Br J Neurosurg. 1998;12(6):521–6.
8. Caroli E, Acqui M, Roperto R, Ferrante L, D'Andrea G. Spinal en plaque meningiomas: A contemporary experience. Neurosurgery. 2004;55(6):1275–9; discussion 9.
9. Salpietro FM, Alafaci C, Lucerna S, Iacopino DG, Tomasello F. Do spinal meningiomas penetrate the pial layer? Correlation between magnetic resonance imaging and microsurgical findings and intracranial tumor interfaces. Neurosurgery. 1997;41(1):254–8.
10. Levy WJ Jr, Bay J, Dohn D. Spinal cord meningioma. J Neurosurg. 1982;57(6):804–12.
11. Sohn S, Kim J, Chung CK, Lee NR, Sohn MJ, Kim SH. A nation-wide epidemiological study of newly diagnosed primary spine tumor in the adult Korean population, 2009–2011. Journal of Korean Neurosurgical Society. 2017;60(2):195–204.
12. Gelabert-Gonzalez M, Garcia-Allut A, Martinez-Rumbo R. Spinal meningiomas. Neurocirugia (Asturias, Spain). 2006;17(2):125–31.
13. Roelvink NCA, Kamphorst W, Van Alphen HAM, Rao BR. Pregnancy-related primary brain and spinal tumors. Arch Neurol. 1987;44(2):209–15.
14. Gottfried ON, Gluf W, Quinones-Hinojosa A, Kan P, Schmidt MH. Spinal meningiomas: Surgical management and outcome. Neurosurg Focus. 2003;14(6):e2.
15. Levy WJ, Latchaw J, Hahn JF. Spinal neurofibromas: A report of 66 cases and a comparison with meningiomas. Neurosurgery. 1986;18(3):331–4.
16. Schaller B. Spinal meningioma: Relationship between histological subtypes and surgical outcome? J Neurooncol. 2005;75(2):157–61.
17. Hentschel SJ, McCutcheon IE. Intradural extramedullar spinal tumors. In: Dickman CA, Fehlings MG, Gokaslan ZI, editors. Spinal Cord and spinal column tumors. Newyork: Thieme Med. Publ; 2006. p. 335–48.

18. Gezen F, Kahraman S, Çanakci Z, Bedük A. Review of 36 cases of spinal cord meningioma. Spine. 2000;25(6):727–31.
19. Özgen S, Konya D. Spinal meningiomas. In: Pamir MN, Black PM, Fahlbusch R, editors. Meningiomas. Philadelphia: Saunders; 2010. p. 569–80.
20. Lee W, Chang KH, Choe G, et al. MR imaging features of clear-cell meningioma with diffuse leptomeningeal seeding. Am J Neuroradiol. 2000;21(1):130–2.
21. Im SH, Chung CK, Cho BK, Kim MK, Chi JG. Sclerosing meningioma: clinicopathological study of four cases. J Neurooncol. 2004;68(2):169–75.
22. Kim NR, Im SH, Chung CK, Suh YL, Choe G, Chi JG. Sclerosing meningioma: Immunohistochemical analysis of five cases. Neuropathol Appl Neurobiol. 2004;30(2):126–35.
23. Solero CL, Fornari M, Giombini S, et al. Spinal meningiomas: Review of 174 operated cases. Neurosurgery. 1989;25(2):153–60.
24. Peker S, Çerçl A, Özgen S, Isik N, Kalelioglu M, Pamir MN. Spinal meningiomas: Evaluation of 41 patients. J Neurosurg Sci. 2005;49(1):7–11.
25. Sade B, Chahlavi A, Krishnaney A, Nagel S, Choi E, Lee JH. World Health Organization Grades II and III meningiomas are rare in the cranial base and spine. Neurosurgery. 2007;61(6):1194–8; discussion 8.
26. Sohn S, Chung CK. Conventional posterior approach without far lateral approach for ventral foramen magnum meningiomas. Journal of Korean Neurosurgical Society. 2013;54(5):373–8.
27. Kim CH, Chung CK. Surgical outcome of a posterior approach for large ventral intradural extramedullary spinal cord tumors. Spine. 2011;36(8):E531–7.
28. Yoon SH, Chung CK, Jahng TA. Surgical outcome of spinal canal meningiomas. J Korean Neurosurg Soc. 2007;42(4):300–4.
29. Kim CH, Chung CK, Lee SH, et al. Long-term recurrence rates after the removal of spinal meningiomas in relation to Simpson grades. Eur Spine J: Official Publication of the European Spine Society, the European Spinal Deformity Society, and the European Section of the Cervical Spine Research Society. 2016;25(12):4025–32.

How to Approach Anatomical Compartment: Intradural Sub-arachnoidal Tumor

11

Sungjoon Lee and Chun Kee Chung

Abstract

Schwannoma is one of the most common pathologies that occur in the intradural sub-arachnoidal space. Spinal schwannomas present in various sizes, shape, and location. With proper adjustments, strategies and techniques used in spinal schwannoma surgeries could be applied to other tumors in the intradural sub-arachnoidal space. Spinal schwannomas can be classified into three categories, which are pre-ganglionic, ganglionic, and post-ganglionic type, according to their nerve root origin. Schwannomas arise from a Schwann cell and involves a single nerve fascicle. Thus theoretically, all of them could be removed without sacrificing the neighboring nerve fibers. In surgeries of ganglionic or post-ganglionic-type schwannomas, it is often not easy to isolate the tumor from other nerve tissues as in that of pre-ganglionic-type schwannomas. Suppose all schwannomas, regardless of their types, are actually located in the intradural sub-arachnoidal space, then it is quite helpful to find and secure the dissection plane between the tumor and the adjacent nerve fibers. With carefully planned surgical strategies and proper techniques, spinal schwannomas can be removed completely without causing neurologic deficits.

Keywords

Spinal cord neoplasms · Schwannoma · Operative surgical procedures

11.1 Introduction

The spinal cord is enveloped by three kinds of membranes. They are the pia, the arachnoid, and the dura matter from inside to outside, respectively. The intradural sub-arachnoid space is defined as the space between the arachnoid membrane and the pia matter. This space is

S. Lee
Department of Neurosurgery, Samsung Medical Center, Seoul, South Korea
e-mail: potata98@naver.com

C. K. Chung (✉)
Department of Neurosurgery, Seoul National University Hospital, Seoul National University College of Medicine, Seoul, Republic of Korea
e-mail: chungc@snu.ac.kr

Neuroscience Research Institute, Seoul National University Medical Research Center, Seoul, Republic of Korea

Clinical Research Institute, Seoul National University Hospital, Seoul, Republic of Korea

Department of Brain and Cognitive Sciences, Seoul National University College of Natural Sciences, Seoul, Republic of Korea

C. K. Chung (ed.), *Surgery of Spinal Cord Tumors Based on Anatomy*,
https://doi.org/10.1007/978-981-15-7771-0_11

filled with the cerebrospinal fluid (CSF) and it extends from the cranium to the S2 level of the spinal canal. Grossly, three kinds of structures are present in this space: the spinal nerve roots, ligaments such as the dentate ligaments and the filum terminale, and vessels such as the spinal arteries and veins. Common tumors that occur in the intradural sub-arachnoidal space are nerve sheath tumors such as schwannomas and neurofibromas, and ependymomas at the filum terminale [9]. Vascular origin tumors such as hemangioblastomas will not be discussed in this chapter, since the spinal arteries and veins run on the surface of the spinal cord, and the subject of the pial-extrapial lesions will be handled in Chap. 12.

For convenience, we are going to discuss surgical strategies and techniques of the intradural sub-arachnoidal pathologies focused on schwannomas. There are some reasons why we chose the schwannoma for the representative pathology. Most of all, a schwannoma is the most common pathology we encounter in daily practice. Second, due to their pathogenetic properties, most of them could be removed completely by proper surgical techniques, and with little adjustments, these techniques could be successfully applied to other intradural sub-arachnoidal pathologies. Third, schwannomas could also arise or extend beyond the spinal canal, and this usually complicates surgery plan. In comparison to other pathologies, schwannomas require more careful planning especially regarding surgical approaches. We thought that covering more complex subject with detailed explanation would be reasonable.

Some people might point out that the intradural sub-arachnoid space is limited within the spinal canal, and a pathology beyond the spinal canal should not be included in this chapter. However, the pathological concepts used in the schwannoma surgery are similar regardless of their location. An idea that suppose all schwannomas are actually located in the intradural sub-arachnoidal space is quite useful in planning the surgery. It is because this concept clearly guides us which and how many membranes should be opened, how to find a space or a plane for tumor dissection, and how to remove the tumor completely while saving the nearby nerve tissues. In this context, we think covering schwannomas of various locations is acceptable, and it would also help readers to understand and share our surgical strategies and techniques of spinal schwannomas.

In this chapter, we will give a brief overview of features of the spinal schwannoma at first, including epidemiology, pathogenesis, clinical features, and treatment outcomes. Then we will introduce our classification system and describe each surgical strategies and techniques according to the classification. General rules of the surgery will be described in the text, and specific examples of surgical cases will be presented in the figures.

11.2 Brief Overview of Epidemiology, Pathology, and Clinical Characteristics of Spinal Schwannoma

The annual incidence of spinal schwannoma has been estimated to be 0.3–0.5 per 100,000 [2, 22]. There is no sexual predilection, with a peak incidence in the fourth and fifth decade of life [2, 8]. It is uncommon in very young or old patients. However, it may become symptomatic at all ages [8, 22]. Along the longitudinal axis of the spine, they can occur anywhere. Location predilection differs between reports in the literature [21]. Most schwannomas occur sporadically. Only in about 3%–4% of cases, they occur in conjunction with a genetic disease such as neurofibromatosis type 2 or schwannomatosis [6, 14, 25].

Spinal schwannomas are benign neoplasms. They originate from Schwann cell progenitors [25]. Most of them are firm, encapsulated masses which arise from a single nerve axon, displacing other uninvolved nerve fibers as they grow [9]. The nerve fascicle of origin is usually non-functional [10]. Histologically, these lesions are characterized by compact, cellular Antoni A areas alternating with less cellular Antoni B areas [9, 22, 28]. Mitotic figures are sparse [22].

Common presentations of spinal schwannomas are local pain, either radiculopathy or axial pain, and focal neurologic deficits or signs, either attributable to functional loss of involved nerve root or compression of adjacent neural structures [9, 22, 25]. Myelopathy due to spinal cord compression or cauda equina syndrome by chronic compression is possible. Unusual manifestations such as subarachnoid hemorrhage, hydrocephalus, and syrinx formation have been reported in the literature [11, 17, 20].

Considering their benign nature and favorable prognosis, treatment decision should be made carefully. Usually symptomatic lesions are considered for treatment. In cases of non-symptomatic lesions, weighing risks and benefits of the treatment should be preceded before making treatment decision. The golden standard of schwannoma treatment has been gross total removal of the tumor with preserving adjacent neural structures as much as possible [22, 23, 25, 28]. Reported surgical outcomes have been mostly favorable [2, 4, 5, 8, 10, 16, 22, 23, 25, 28].

11.3 Strategy of Surgical Treatment

11.3.1 Classification

The clinico-radiologic features of spinal schwannomas are diverse. It is believed that most of intradural schwannomas arise from the Obersteiner-Redlich zone, where the transition from oligodendrocytes to Schwann cells happens [9]. These tumors, being located at the classic intradural sub-arachnoidal space, are usually small and round-shaped, and tend to be confined at the spinal canal when they are initially found. However, we quiet often meet patients with spinal schwannomas of various locations, sizes, and shapes. Many of them are not confined at the spinal canal. They extend to the paravertebral space. Anatomical barriers such as the dura matter or the neural foramen, or other bony structures often limit their growth, and often form the tumors into various dumbbell or hourglass shapes. Sometimes these slow-growing tumors penetrate and invade bony structures, presenting more varieties in sizes and shapes. Although it is out of scope of this chapter, schwannomas may be found at very unusual locations, such as the intramedullary spinal cord where no Schwann cells are known to be present [13].

Because of their diversity in presentation, clinicians had difficulties in treating these tumors in a considerable proportion of cases. Historically, efforts to classify spinal schwannomas had taken place to understand these complicated tumors better and to seek the standardized treatment. Before introducing our classification system, it would be helpful to briefly review the suggested classification systems of spinal schwannomas in the literature.

Eden's classification [3] might be the first widely used classification system for dumbbell-shaped tumors—mostly nerve sheath tumors—of the spine. By classifying the dumbbell-shaped spinal tumors, he tried to focus on understanding their main pathological types, and details of anatomical correlation related to clinical symptoms and surgical treatments. The ultimate goal of this classification system is to improve patient care, but an ideal classification system should provide an appropriate treatment guideline incorporated with its precise outcome. In this point of view, Eden's pioneering work was not satisfactory.

Earlier, advances in imaging modalities such as computed tomography (CT) and magnetic resonance imaging (MRI) and evaluating tumors of the spine were limited. Meaningful classification of spinal schwannomas which would guide a proper surgical strategy emerged after 1990s when MRI used in the diagnosis of spinal pathology was generalized. McCormick's classification [15], which was one of the early proposed system, was designed to guide surgical strategies for paraspinal and dumbbell-shaped spinal pathologies. It was simple and easy to follow. Limitations were also clear. It was based on various spinal pathologies, including not only primary but also metastatic tumors. Together with small number of patients included in the study, his classification failed to show the consistent and reliable prognosis between the groups.

In early 2000s, more detailed classifications were proposed according to size, shape, and extent of the tumor [1, 8, 24]. It seems that they tried to subclassify every possible shapes of nerve sheath tumors that could be found in spinal MRIs. As much as nine divided categories were observed [1]. Considering limited prognosis data of the nerve sheath tumors in accordance to their various sizes, locations, and shapes, it was reasonable to classify the tumors in very detailed way. However, the later proposed classifications simplified their categories again as accumulation of the treatment outcome data increased [18, 25]. The biggest change in these classification systems was that subcategorizing giant schwannomas and extending to extra-spinal spaces became less significant. It was because the reported surgical outcomes of these tumors had been generally good and differences between the groups were not significant [1, 7, 12, 19, 28]. We presume that this led to decrease in the needs for a highly sophisticated and detailed classification system.

In summary, spinal schwannomas present various clinico-radiologic and pathologic features. To discuss the surgical strategy, using of a suitable classification for this varied tumor would be helpful. The proposed classifications of spinal schwannomas were mostly based on anatomical locations. Therefore, terms such as intradural, epidural, foraminal, dumbbell, and extra-spinal were used. However, usefulness of subdividing the tumors into more detailed, specific categories according to the anatomical locations is under question. In the following section, we will divide spinal schwannomas into just three categories—pre-ganglionic, ganglionic, and post-ganglionic—according to their nerve root origin (Fig. 11.1). With this simple classification, we are going to discuss the anatomical considerations for schwannoma surgery, and the appropriate surgical planning and approach for each tumor category.

11.3.2 General Principles and Anatomical Considerations in Schwannoma Surgery

Schwannoma arises from a single Schwann cell. It involves one nerve axon, and it slowly grows pushing away other nerve fibers and fascicles near it. Theoretically, it is possible to remove only the tumor without sacrificing its neighboring nerve fibers. By meticulous microdissection between the tumor and other functional nerve fibers, we can minimize any neurologic deficits which a patient might experience after the

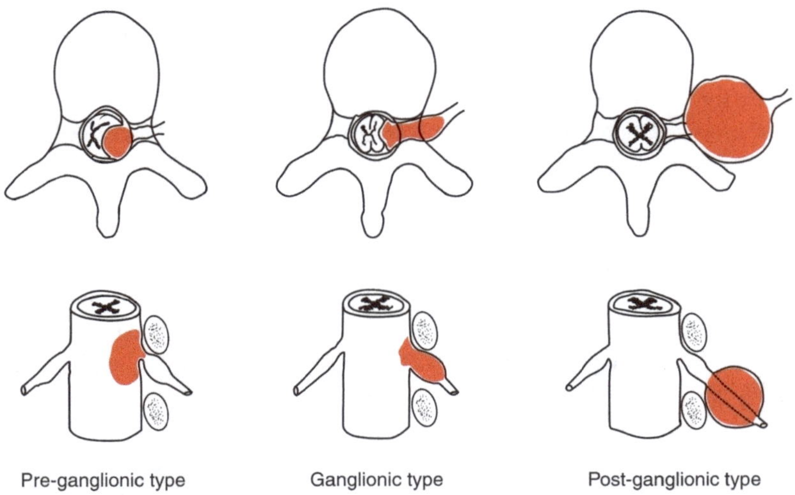

Fig. 11.1 Schematic drawing of schwannoma types in axial and coronal plane according to our classification system

operation. Therefore, the goal of schwannoma surgery should be focused on not only curative resection of the tumor, but also saving adjacent functional neural tissues as much as possible.

In cases of schwannomas located in the intradural sub-arachnoidal space (the pre-ganglionic type), the tumor mass and the involved nerve fascicle can be easily identified. Most of the tumors are found as a well-encapsulated mass hanging from its originated nerve root. Adhesion with other neural tissues such as the spinal cord is scarce and that en bloc resection can be achieved without much effort after freeing the tumor from its originated nerve root. On the other hand, schwannomas located at the spinal nerve roots (the ganglionic, post-ganglionic types) are not easy to readily discern from other neural tissues. When we initially encounter the tumor during the operation, what we see is only an enlarged nerve root containing the tumor inside. Mistakes such as removing the whole involved nerve root and not only the tumor but also functioning nerve fibers often happen.

Schwannomas of these two locations appear to be pathologically different from each other. However, they share common anatomical characteristics that could be applied to the surgery. In the spinal root, a nerve axon is enclosed with endoneurium. A group of axons form a fascicle, and it is covered by a coarse connective tissue which is called perineurium. A nerve root is comprised of several fascicles, and it is bound by a fibrous connective tissue, epineurium. In the intradural sub-arachnoidal space, a nerve root is formed by one or two more fascicles. Several roots from dorsal and ventral sides of the spinal cord bound together and form a spinal root as they exit the dura.

Extension of the spinal dura passing laterally around the spinal nerve roots forms dural root sleeves and continues with the epineurium of the spinal nerves [8]. Simply think that the endoneurium extends from the pia matter, and the perineurium extends from the arachnoid membrane. To remove a pre-ganglionic-type schwannoma, we have to open the dura and the arachnoid membrane consecutively to reach the tumor. Similarly, we should open the epineurium and the perineurium to directly access a ganglionic or post-ganglionic schwannoma and separate it from normally functioning nerve fibers. Histologically, the perineurium is a loose connective tissue, and it provides relatively clear dissection plane between the fascicles. In addition, it contains a small amount of CSF-like tissue fluid. Although it is a potential space which is much different from the CSF-filled sub-arachnoid space, this provides an excellent surgical plane to dissect the tumor.

Surgical techniques to remove spinal schwannomas should be similar regardless of their types. How to approach the tumor should be the most concerning problem. Anatomical relationships of the spine or the vital structures such as great vessels, heart, or other solid organs, often limit proper access to and exposure of the tumor. If necessary, multiple route and/or staged operation should be considered. In cases of giant spinal schwannomas, intentional partial resection can be a reasonable option if total removal of the tumor is not possible.

11.3.3 Surgical Strategies

11.3.3.1 Pre-ganglionic Type

This is the most common type of the three [8, 25]. As we described in the previous section, this type of tumor is small and is usually confined in the intradural sub-arachnoidal space when initially found. As most of slow-growing, benign tumors do, schwannomas tend to grow in direction to less crowded space where no anatomical barriers resist. Because of laterally located barriers such as dura and spinal bony structures like pedicles and facets, they grow rather in the sagittal or medial direction than the lateral. The spinal cord or the cauda equina is compressed and the patient becomes symptomatic much earlier than other two types.

In some cases, epidural extension over the spinal dura mater may present. Compared to the main mass, this extension is usually small in volume. Additional approach from outside of

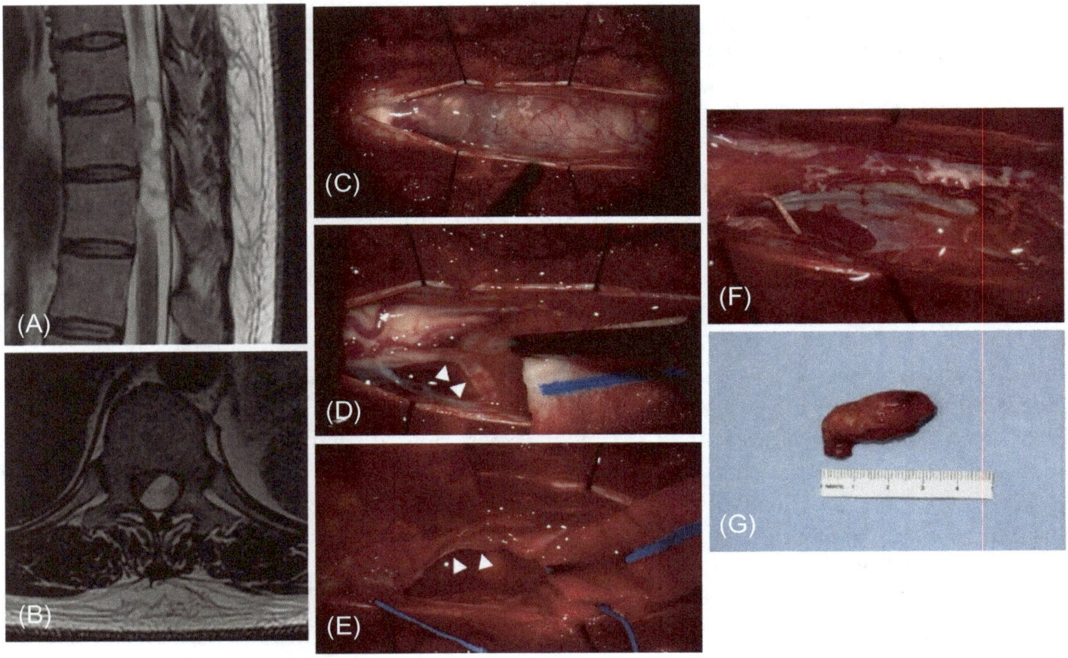

Fig. 11.2 A pre-ganglionic-type schwannoma. **a**, **b** MRI shows an intradural extramedullary tumor of heterogeneous signal on T2 weighted images. Its extent is near two vertebral segments on sagittal plane, but it is confined in the spinal canal. **c** After opening the dura, the tumor is seen under the arachnoid membrane. **d** Attached nerve roots (white arrowheads) should be carefully dissected away from the tumor. Unless their fascicles are involved by the tumor, this procedure should not be a trouble. **e** Identify the tumor origin, and disconnecting the tumor from its originated nerve root would end the surgery. **f** Intraoperative photo and **g** gross pathology photo of the removed tumor mass are shown

the dura is mostly unnecessary. If a volume of the epidural extension is similar or even larger than the intradural mass, it may not be the pre-ganglionic type but the ganglionic type. In this case, the approach should be started extradurally first. What looks like the intradural mass on MRI might be actually located at the epidural space, pushing the dura and the spinal cord medially.

Posterior midline approach with laminotomy would suffice for the pre-ganglionic-type schwannoma. Descriptions below are our surgical routine in this type of tumor. Some authors reported good surgical outcomes by minimally invasive surgery (MIS) techniques [26]. However, we think MIS techniques in the spinal tumor surgery should be tailored to individual cases, not recommended in general.

Figure 11.2 illustrates a typical pre-ganglionic-type schwannoma surgery.

(a) The patient is placed in prone position. Make sure that the surgical site is on the top, and the patient's abdomen is not compressed anywhere by the positioning. Intraoperative neurophysiologic monitoring is so helpful that we recommend its routine use in the spinal schwannoma surgery.
(b) Midline skin incision is made. Back muscles meticulously dissected from the spine. Do laminotomies. The bony opening should be large enough to expose the tumor entirely.
(c) Open the dura in midline longitudinally. For easier exposure, a paramedian incision toward the tumor can be adopted. Open the arachnoid membrane, and tag it to the dura.

Repairing it after the tumor removal might decrease the chance of postoperative complications such as arachnoiditis.

(d) Find the tumor, and its originating nerve root. Dissect every root adhering to the tumor. Other than the originating root, dissection should not be difficult. Dissect every nerve fascicles which could be saved from the originating root. Stimulate the remaining fascicles to check whether it is functional or not. As described in the previous section, the involved nerve root is mostly non-functional. Cut the last remaining fascicles, and remove the tumor with them.

(e) If the size of the tumor is large then it cannot be removed by en bloc fashion, so decrease the tumor volume first by internal debulking using an ultrasonic aspirator, and then take it out. During the tumor removal, always be cautious not to insult the spinal cord.

(f) Repair the arachnoid membrane, and close the dura watertightly. The removed lamina bones are reattached with lamina screws [27]. Close the wound layer-by-layer. Drains are usually not required.

11.3.3.2 Ganglionic Type

This type of schwannoma is located at the neural foramen. Surrounding bony structures limit the growth such that it grows in either one or both the directions toward the spinal canal and the extra-foraminal space. Dumbbell or hour-glass shapes are common in this type. Extension to inside of the spinal dura is also commonly found [1, 8, 18]. However, we recommend to approach the tumor outside of the spinal dura

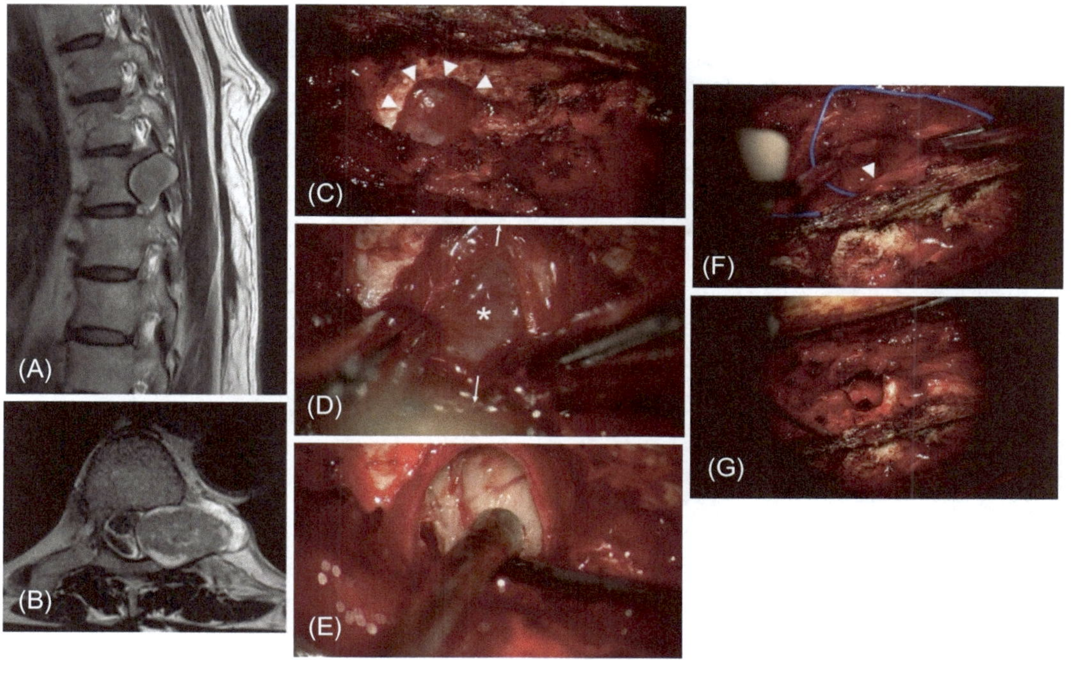

Fig. 11.3 A ganglionic-type schwannoma. **a**, **b** T2-weighted MRI shows a heterogeneous extradural mass located at a left neural foramen of the thoracic spine. Widening of the foramen is observed. **c** Lamina bone was partially removed to expose the tumor (white arrow heads). Full extent of exposure is not always necessary. In consideration of the spinal stability, bony removal of the spine should be carefully planned. **d** After making incision on the epineurium along the root (direction by white arrows), glassy tumor mass appears (white asterisk). Clear tissue fluid between the perineurium and the tumor helps to find the dissection plane. **e** By following the proper dissection plane, the tumor could be dissected from other nerve tissues without much difficulty. **f** The tumor origin (white arrowhead) is identified. **g** Intraoperative photo after the tumor removal is shown

first. Tumors at the extradural location are most frequent [18]. Also the intradural portion of the tumor could be removed from the outside of the spinal dura in many times. Consider the intradural exploration when the size of the intradural portion is too big or concerns of damage to the spinal cord are present.

To properly expose the tumor, violation of the facet joint is often inevitable. If the bony removal makes the spine unstable, instrumentation should be considered. However, in some cases like shown in Fig. 11.3, the tumor could be removed not causing the spinal instability. Therefore, careful surgical planning before the operation is mandatory.

Posterior approach usually suffices. However, a combined approach should be considered when a tumor grows beyond the anterior vertebral body and/or far laterally. Resecting the whole involved nerve root should be avoided. After opening the epineurium, finding the dissection plane which is located under the perineurium of the involved nerve fascicle is the most important step for successful surgery. An easy and successful strategy to find this plane is approaching the most bulged spot, where the distance between the epineurium and the tumor is the shortest. It is also a safe way since there are minimal chances for normal functioning nerve fibers present on this short way to the tumor.

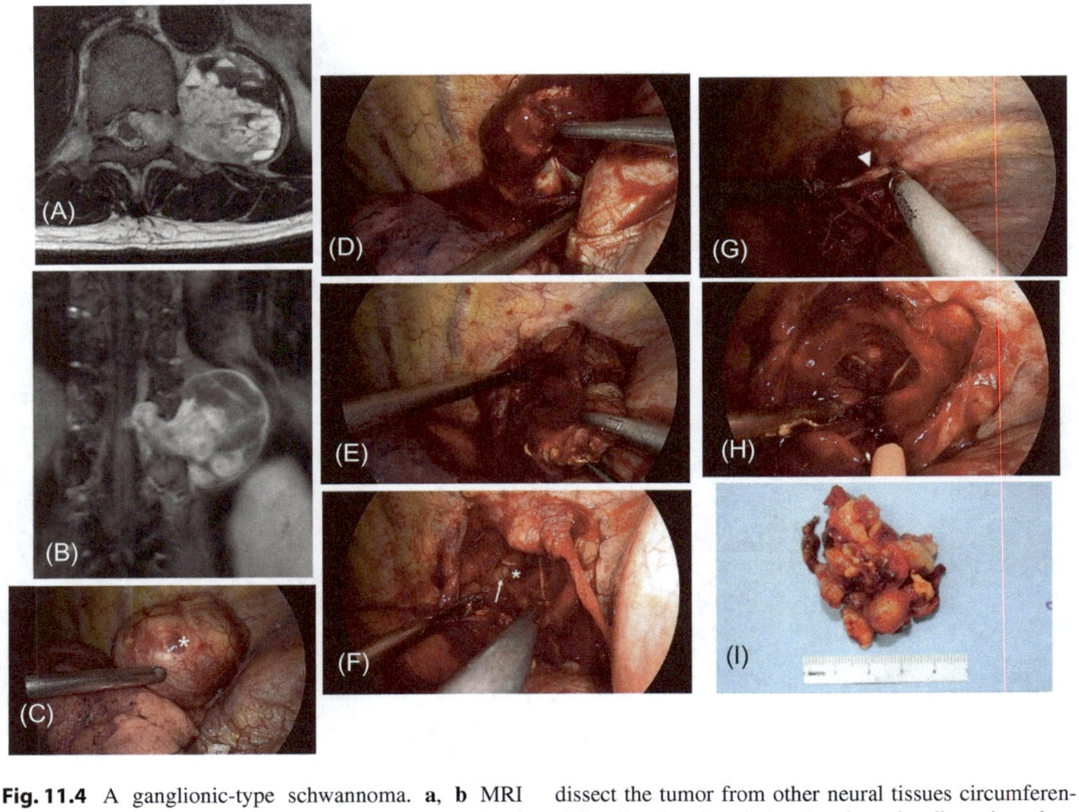

Fig. 11.4 A ganglionic-type schwannoma. **a, b** MRI shows a heterogeneous, contrast-enhanced extradural mass extending from the neural foramen to the extra-spinal pleural cavity. Thinking a combined approach in mind, we decided to perform the extra-spinal approach using thoracoscopy. **c** Entering the pleural cavity, the protruded tumor mass (white asterisk) is observed. Lung at the left lower corner, and diaphragm at the right lower corner is also seen. **d, e** After incising the epineurium, dissect the tumor from other neural tissues circumferentially. Keeping in mind not to lose the dissection plane formed between the perineurium and the tumor, tumor is removed in piecemeal fashion. **f** The proximal tumor origin (white arrow) is revealed after mass removal of the extra-spinal tumor. The white asterisk is marked at the neural foramen. **g** The distal origin (white arrow) is identified and removed. **h** Intraoperative photo and **i** gross pathology photo after the tumor removal are shown

Figures 11.3 and 11.4 illustrate our surgical procedures for the ganglionic-type schwannomas. Compared to the pre-ganglionic type, the ganglionic types present more wide range of anatomical and morphological variations. Therefore, surgeons should adjust the surgical procedures properly to suit their individual cases.

(a) Patient position and preoperative preparations are similar to those of the pre-ganglionic type. With very few exceptional cases, select posterior approach at first.
(b) After muscle dissection, remove the posterior spinal bone enough to expose the involved nerve root. A schwannoma grows along the involved nerve fascicle. But basically they expand, pushing away neighboring neural tissues. Even if the surgical window is relatively small, complete removal can be achieved by pulling the tumor in conjunction with sharp dissection following the proper surgical plane. Therefore, the extent of bony removal should be carefully planned beforehand. If the spinal stability after this exposing procedure is in question, spinal instrumentations should be considered.
(c) Identify the root involved by the tumor. Make incision on the epineurium along the root. Choosing the most bulged area, the tumor encapsulated with endoneurium would readily show itself. If any nerve roots appear to run at the incision site, it is better to find other site to bypass them. However, if it is not possible to avoid, then use stimulator to check whether they have any motor functions. Based on this stimulation result, decision should be made whether to try a completely different approach or to sacrifice them and proceed.
(d) The tumor surface is glassy, similar to the pre-ganglionic type of schwannoma (Fig. 11.3d). A small amount of CSF-like fluid is usually present on its surface. The tumor and the surrounding neural tissues should be easily dissected. This dissecting plane is the space between the perineurium covering the involved fascicle and the endoneurium encapsulating the tumor. The surgical window is small for en bloc resection in most of cases. Piecemeal resection is acceptable unless not losing the dissection plane.
(e) After the complete removal, look for the origin sites, and make sure there are no remaining tumor. If the tumor was removed in piecemeal fashion, bleeding might be profuse, but usually controllable. Meticulous bleeding control after the tumor removal is mandatory.
(f) If necessary, do the intradural exploration. Surgical techniques in this procedure would be the same as that of the pre-ganglionic types.
(g) Repair the epineurium and/or the dura. Complete spinal instrumentations if the spine is unstable after the surgery. If the extra-spinal portion is left, consider a combined approach.

11.3.3.3 Post-ganglionic Type

Schwannomas of this type are similar in pathologic form to those which arise from peripheral nerves of other body parts. However, surgeries of this type of spinal schwannomas are quite challenging. It is mainly because this type of tumors is deeply seated in the body such as the pleural or the retroperitoneal space, and vital structures and organs are often block the surgical corridor. Therefore, how to approach the tumor is the most important factor for a successful surgery in the post-ganglionic schwannomas.

Approaches should be decided on where the most extraspinal portion of the tumor is located. Because the neural foramen works as the anatomical barrier, most of post-ganglionic origin schwannomas outgrow to the extra-spinal space (Figs. 11.5 and 11.6). Normally, the spinal nerves are located juxta to the spine. In addition, the spine locates at the center of the body. This means that approaching to the tumor out-to-in direction naturally leads us to the safe spot where no functioning normal nerve fibers are present. Exploring the spinal canal is mostly unnecessary. Posterior approach is only

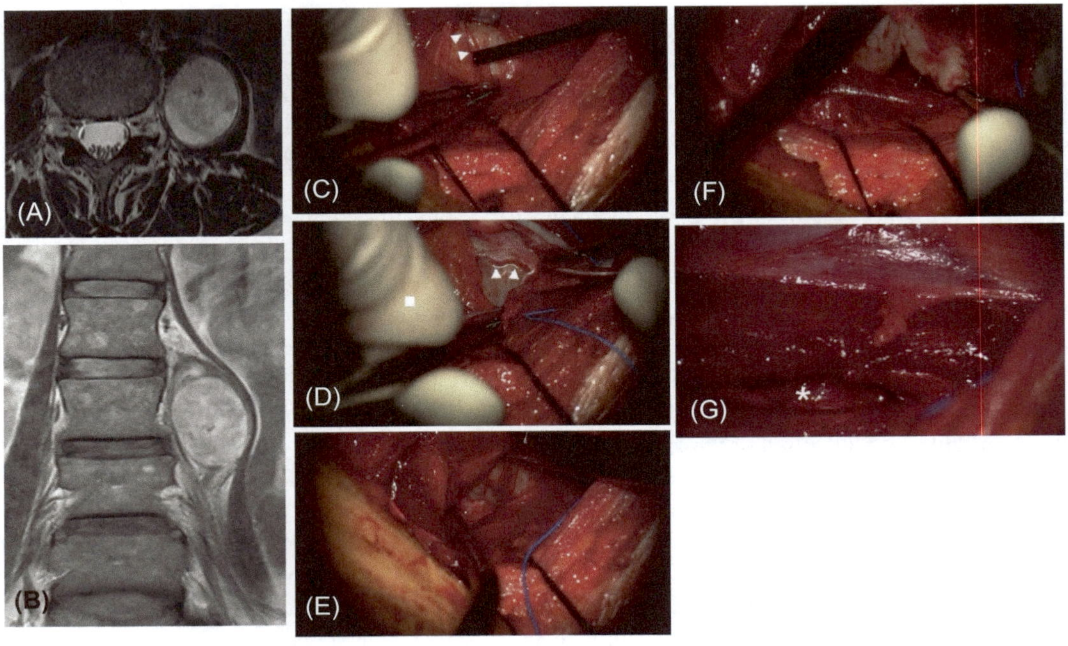

Fig. 11.5 A post-ganglionic-type schwannoma. **a, b** MRI shows a round shape extra-spinal mass which has a heterogenous T2 weighted signal intensity. It is located inside of the left psoas muscle. **c** Strip the psoas muscle away and expose the tumor. By using a nerve stimulator, identify any functioning nerve root (white arrowheads) at risk of injury. **d** Incise the epineurium and find the dissection plane (white arrowheads). Be careful not to damage any identified functional roots beforehand. **e, f** Circumferential dissection following the plane is performed and remove the tumor totally. **g** Intraoperative photo after the tumor removal (white asterisk—the site of tumor removal) is shown

considered when the extra-spinal tumor grows to dorsal direction. (Fig. 11.6).

Any surgical instruments can be adopted if they are feasible for the surgery. Tumors in pleural space can be removed under thoracoscope (Fig. 11.4). Laparoscopic or robotic devices could also be used in tumors in the abdominal and pelvic cavities. Once approaching to the tumor is done, surgical technique to isolate and remove the tumor is similar to those of the ganglionic type of schwannomas.

(a) Patient position should be tailored to the surgical plan made preoperatively. As previously mentioned, any surgical instrument can be used. Other preoperative preparations are similar to those of the surgeries of pre-ganglionic and ganglionic schwannomas.
(b) Encountering the tumor, make incision on the epineurium. In most cases, the rendezvous location is where the most bulged spot of the nerve root is involved. Without much efforts, the tumor mass covered by the endoneurium should be exposed. Keeping the dissection plane, the tumor can be removed minimizing the damage to adjacent normal functioning nerve fibers. Identify the nerve fascicle of tumor origin, and the proximal and the distal ends should be identified and cut.
(c) After the removal, look for any remaining tumor mass at the nerve origin. Do meticulous bleeding control. Unlike other two types, repairing the opened epineurium is often not necessary due to very low risk of CSF leakage. Repair the wound layer-by-layer in reverse order.

11.4 Conclusion

Several pathologies may arise in the intradural sub-arachnoidal space. The most common neoplasm in this space is nerve-sheath tumors, especially schwannomas. Schwannomas can

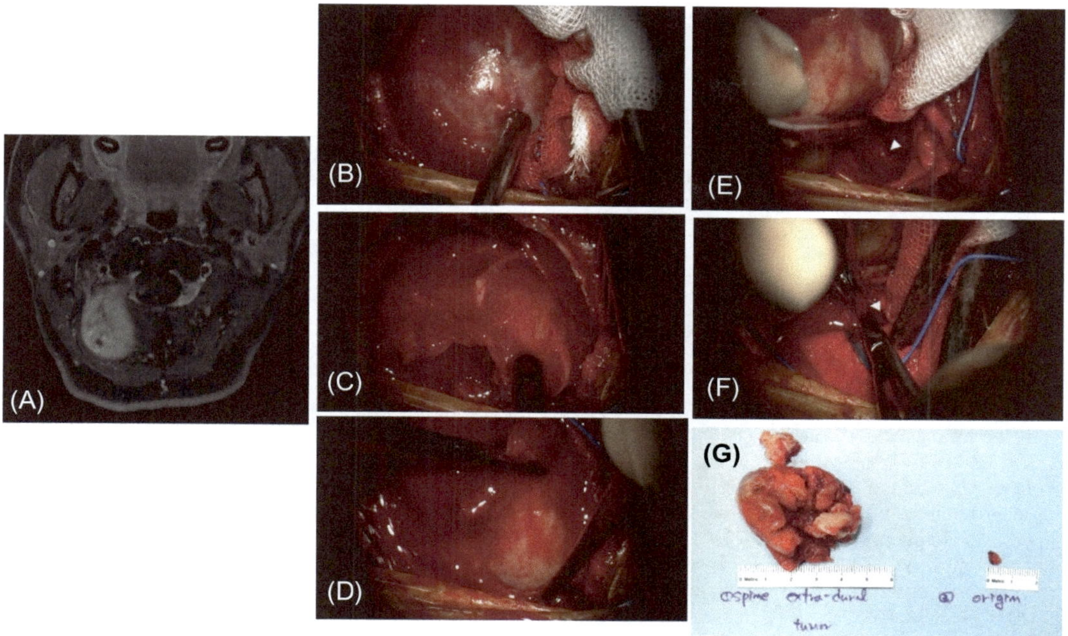

Fig. 11.6 A post-ganglionic-type schwannoma. **a** MRI shows a well-enhancing extradural mass which is extended to dorsal direction. **b** A posterior paramedian approach, directly targeting the extra-spinal mass portion is performed. The tumor is seen after stripping away dorsally covered posterior neck muscles. **c**, **d** After making vertical incision on the epineurium, circumferential dissection of the tumor is performed maintaining the dissection plane. **e** As dissection progresses to the ventral side of the tumor, distal portion of the origin root is identified (white arrowhead). It is coagulated and cut. **f** By following the dissection plane upward, proximal portion of the origin root is also identified (white arrowhead). After disconnecting the tumor from the proximal origin, it is then taken out. **g** The gross pathology photo is shown

be classified into three types: pre-ganglionic, ganglionic, and post-ganglionic types. Only the pre-ganglionic type is located in the intradural sub-arachnoidal space according to its classic definition. However, by understanding the similarity of pathologic and anatomical relationships among these three types, we can learn how to perform successful surgeries in treating the spinal schwannomas.

References

1. Asazuma T, Toyama Y, Maruiwa H, Fujimura Y, Hirabayashi K. Surgical strategy for cervical dumbbell tumors based on a three-dimensional classification. Spine (Phila Pa 1976). 2004;29:E10–14.
2. Conti P, Pansini G, Mouchaty H, Capuano C, Conti R. Spinal neurinomas: Retrospective analysis and long-term outcome of 179 consecutively operated cases and review of the literature. Surg Neurol. 2004;61:34–43; discussion 44.
3. Eden K. The dumb-bell tumours of the spine. BJS. 1941;28:549–70.
4. Fehlings MG, Nater A, Zamorano JJ et al. Risk factors for recurrence of surgically treated conventional spinal schwannomas: Analysis of 169 patients from a multicenter international database. Spine (Phila Pa 1976). 2016;41:390–8.
5. Halvorsen CM, Ronning P, Hald J, et al. The long-term outcome after resection of intraspinal nerve sheath tumors: Report of 131 consecutive cases. Neurosurgery. 2015;77:585–2; discussion 592–583.
6. Holland K, Kaye AH. Spinal tumors in neurofibromatosis-2: management considerations—A review. J Clin Neurosci: Off J Neurosurg Soc Australa. 2009;16:169–77.
7. Jiang L, Lv Y, Liu XG et al. Results of surgical treatment of cervical dumbbell tumors: Surgical approach and development of an anatomic

classification system. Spine (Phila Pa 1976). 2009;34:1307–14.
8. Jinnai T, Koyama T. Clinical characteristics of spinal nerve sheath tumors: Analysis of 149 cases. Neurosurgery. 2005;56:510–15; discussion 510–15.
10. Kim P, Ebersold MJ, Onofrio BM, Quast LM. Surgery of spinal nerve schwannoma. Risk of neurological deficit after resection of involved root. J Neurosurg. 1989;71:810–4.
11. Kudo H, Tamaki N, Kim S, Shirataki K, Matsumoto S. Intraspinal tumors associated with hydrocephalus. Neurosurgery. 1987;21:726–31.
12. Lee CH, Chung CK, Hyun SJ, Kim CH, Kim KJ, Jahng TA. A longitudinal study to assess the volumetric growth rate of spinal intradural extramedullary tumour diagnosed with schwannoma by magnetic resonance imaging. Eur Spine J. 2015;24:2126–32.
13. Lee SE, Chung CK, Kim HJ. Intramedullary schwannomas: Long-term outcomes of ten operated cases. J Neurooncol. 2013;113:75–81.
14. MacCollin M, Chiocca EA, Evans DG, et al. Diagnostic criteria for schwannomatosis. Neurology. 2005;64:1838–45.
15. McCormick PC. Surgical management of dumbbell and paraspinal tumors of the thoracic and lumbar spine. Neurosurgery. 1996;38:67–74; discussion 74–65.
16. McCormick PC. Surgical management of dumbbell tumors of the cervical spine. Neurosurgery. 1996;38:294–300.
17. Mills B, Marks PV, Nixon JM. Spinal subarachnoid haemorrhage from an "ancient" schwannoma of the cervical spine. Br J Neurosurg. 1993;7:557–9.
18. Ozawa H, Kokubun S, Aizawa T, Hoshikawa T, Kawahara C. Spinal dumbbell tumors: An analysis of a series of 118 cases. J Neurosurg Spines. 2007;7:587–93.
19. Pongsthorn C, Ozawa H, Aizawa T, Kusakabe T, Nakamura T, Itoi E. Giant sacral schwannoma: A report of six cases. Ups J Med Sci. 2010;115:146–52.
20. Quencer RM, el Gammal T, Cohen G. Syringomyelia associated with intradural extramedullary masses of the spinal canal. AJNR Am J Neuroradiol. 1986;7:143–8.
21. Safavi-Abbasi S, Senoglu M, Theodore N, et al. Microsurgical management of spinal schwannomas: Evaluation of 128 cases. J Neurosurg Spine. 2008;9:40–7.
9. Sellin JN, Tatsui CE, Rhines LD. Assessment and treatment of benign intradural extramedullary tumors. Elsevier; 2016.
22. Seppala MT, Haltia MJ, Sankila RJ, Jaaskelainen JE, Heiskanen O. Long-term outcome after removal of spinal schwannoma: A clinicopathological study of 187 cases. J Neurosurg. 1995;83:621–6.
23. Sohn S, Chung CK, Park SH, Kim ES, Kim KJ, Kim CH. The fate of spinal schwannomas following subtotal resection: A retrospective multicenter study by the Korea spinal oncology research group. J Neurooncol. 2013;114:345–51.
24. Sridhar K, Ramamurthi R, Vasudevan MC, Ramamurthi B. Giant invasive spinal schwannomas: Definition and surgical management. J Neurosurg. 2001;94:210–5.
25. Sun I, Pamir MN. Non-syndromic spinal schwannomas: A novel classification. Front Neurol. 2017;8:318.
26. Turel MK, D'Souza WP, Rajshekhar V. Hemilaminectomy approach for intradural extramedullary spinal tumors: An analysis of 164 patients. Neurosurg Focus. 2015;39:E9.
27. Yang SH, Kim CH, Chung CK, Park SB, Sohn S, Lee S. Bone fusion rate in the thoracic and lumbar spine after laminoplasty with laminar screws. Spine (Phila Pa 1976). 2014;39:E1325–30.
28. Yu NH, Lee SE, Jahng TA, Chung CK. Giant invasive spinal schwannoma: Its clinical features and surgical management. Neurosurgery. 2012;71:58–66.

How to Approach Anatomical Compartment: Intradural Pial-Extrapial Tumor

12

Sung Hwan Hwang, Hyun Joo Park and Chun Kee Chung

Abstract

Spinal cord hemangioblastomas are benign, high vascular tumors and are considered intramedullary spinal tumors, but they are anatomically located in the pial-extra parenchymal and are considered exactly juxtamedullary tumors. The focus of the surgical procedure on this tumor is to perform a complete resection while preserving the surrounding normal neural tissue. Most authors believe that surgical procedures require circumferential coagulation around the tumor that has been advocated to control intraoperative bleeding. However, circumferential coagulation (CC) could not avoid the collateral damage to the spinal cord tissue itself. Hence, instead of circumferential coagulation, circumferential dissection with minimal use of coagulation (CD) has been applied to prevent unwanted damage to the spinal cord from coagulation. The efficacy and limitations of digital subtraction angiography and embolization as a preoperative procedure should be considered. Efficacy of intraoperative indocyanine green fluorescence angiography is sufficient to replace digital subtraction angiography. Intraoperative neuromonitoring is also necessary because the neurological changes during surgery can be identified immediately.

Keywords

Hemangioblastoma · Pial-extrapial · Spinal cord tumor · Intraoperative indocyanine green fluorescence angiography · Intraoperative neuromonitoring · Circumferential dissection

Electronic supplementary material The online version of this chapter (https://doi.org/10.1007/978-981-15-7771-0_12) contains supplementary material, which is available to authorized users.

S. H. Hwang
Department of Neurosurgery, The Armed Forces Capital Hospital of Korea, Seong-nam, South Korea
e-mail: ssabys@hanmail.net

H. J. Park
Department of Neurosurgery, Seoul National University Hospital, Seoul, South Korea
e-mail: hjp624@gmail.com

C. K. Chung (✉)
Department of Neurosurgery, Seoul National University Hospital, Seoul National University College of Medicine, Seoul, Republic of Korea
e-mail: chungc@snu.ac.kr

Neuroscience Research Institute, Seoul National University Medical Research Center, Seoul, Republic of Korea

Clinical Research Institute, Seoul National University Hospital, Seoul, Republic of Korea

Department of Brain and Cognitive Sciences, Seoul National University College of Natural Sciences, Seoul, Republic of Korea

C. K. Chung (ed.), *Surgery of Spinal Cord Tumors Based on Anatomy*,
https://doi.org/10.1007/978-981-15-7771-0_12

12.1 Introduction

The spinal pia mater closely follows and encloses the curves of the spinal cord, and is attached to it through a connection to the anterior fissure. The membrane in this area is thicker, more compact, and less vascular than the cranial pia mater, separated from the glia limitans by a subpial layer of collagen that continues with the collagen core of the dentate ligaments [1] (Fig. 12.1). The superficial vascular layer, or epipial tissue, consists of a dense network of collagenous fibers run by superficial blood vessels. The deep avascular layer is a thin meshwork of reticular and elastic fibers adhering to the glia limitans [2]. Between the two layers are spaces which exchange information with the subarachnoid cavity as well as blood vessels. In most current accounts the function of the pia mater is described as that of a scaffold for the vasculature of spinal cord parenchyma such as the anterior and posterior spinal arteries [3, 4]. Most of the spinal cord hemangioblastomas are located under the pia mater of the spinal cord and are on the posterior part of the spinal cord, with a few cases on the ventral part of the spinal cord [5–7]. Spinal cord hemangioblastomas are more accurately considered juxtamedullary tumors because they arise from the pia in the vast majority of cases [8]. The surface presentation and pial origin of spinal cord tumors provide the fundamental basis of the surgical resection strategy and technique.

12.2 Pathogenesis

Hemangioblastomas can occur sporadically or in conjunction with Von Hippel Lindau (VHL). In both types, the pathogenesis is due to inactivation of the VHL tumor suppressor gene located on chromosome 3p [9]. The typical spinal cord hemangioblastoma usually enlarges the cord, is well demarcated, and consists of a highly vascular nodule with an associated cyst; leptomeningeal vessels are prominent. Histologically, these tumors are composed of an intricate vascular network of irregular and often dilated capillaries with intervening stromal cells. These stromal cells can produce erythropoietin, resulting in erythrocytosis. Erythropoietin and vascular endothelial growth factor have also been shown to be upregulated and may

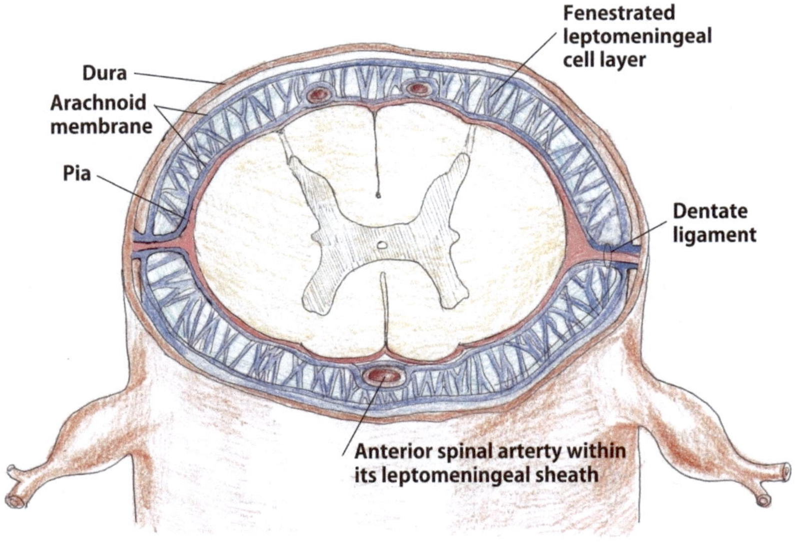

Fig. 12.1 Ultrastructure of spinal leptomeninges. A fenestrated leptomeningeal cell layer is interposed between the arachnoid and the pia. The ligamentum denticulatum is made of a collagen core continuous with the dura mater at its points of attachment and lined by a pial layer. Penetrating vessels dive into the parenchyma encased with their leptomeningeal sheath [1]

contribute to the pathogenesis of hemangioblastomas [10]. Additional comparative genomic hybridization has shown loss of chromosome 6, 9, 18q and a gain of chromosome 19 [11–13].

12.3 Epidemiology

Spinal cord hemangioblastomas (SCH) are uncommon highly vascular neoplasm with a benign nature, and it constitutes 1.6%–6.4% of all spinal cord tumors [14, 15]. It is known to predominate in males and the mean age of symptom onset is the 4th decade of life [16–19]. Most hemangioblastomas appear sporadically. However, in approximately 25% of cases, they are associated with Von Hippel Lindau (VHL) disease. Surgery is curative in sporadic cases [17–19]. Imagama et al. reported that 84.6% of hemangioblastomas were intramedullary, 11.5% were intramedullary + extramedullary, and 3.8% were extramedullary [20]. The thoracic spinal cord is the most frequently affected site, and the intramedullary location is the most common [16, 21–23]. In Lee DK et al. series, SCH represented 2% of all spinal cord tumors, 6.8% of all intramedullary tumors, and 13.6% of all CNS hemangioblastomas. These incidences are similar to those previously published. Males predominated (male:female = 11:3) and the mean age was also in the expected range (37.2 years). The intramedullary location was the most common (intramedullary:intradural-extramedullary:extradural = 13:0:1). The predominance of the cervical location (cervical:thoracic:multiple = 7:4:3) was different as compared to the previous literature [15]. SCH typically follow an indolent course, and patients later present with neurological symptoms due to a slowly progressive mass effect [24]. The most commonly reported clinical manifestations of SCH are pain (50%–80%), sensory changes (39%–69%), and motor deficits (7%–40%) [17, 19, 25–27]. And the earliest manifestation of sensory change is usually the impairment of proprioception because the intramedullary tumor is almost always located in dorsal area of the spinal cord [17, 18]. Several cases presenting with subarachnoid hemorrhage have been reported, although asymptomatic cases have been found [28–30].

12.4 Strategy of Surgical Treatment

Excessive intraoperative bleeding is the main reason to hinder complete resection of SCH, because it obscures the operative field leading to damage to surrounding tissues [23, 31]. Therefore, the minimization of intraoperative bleeding is critical in surgical resection and for the subsequent achievement of total resection. Complete removal of the tumor is the goal for treatment, and is strongly associated with improved functional outcomes [8, 15, 32–34].

Most of the authors recommend a digital subtraction angiography (DSA) prior to the operation and emphasized the need for a precise angiographic study to delineate the feeding arteries and draining veins associated with the hemangioblastomas [35]. Several authors have reported upon the preoperative embolization of hemangioblastoma [23, 36–38]. However, a risk of post-procedural edema or new neurological deficit should be taken into consideration. In some cases, the preoperative embolization may complicate the following surgical procedure because of the stiffness of the embolization material, which may render the dissection more difficult [39]. Furthermore, a few complications associated with the procedure such as an intradural hemorrhage and an aggravation of hydrocephalus were also reported [36].

Some authors believe that intraoperative ultrasound (IOUS) is a sensitive intraoperative tool to guide the surgical approach and to give adequate information about the extent of the tumor as well as its morphology [40]. However, our experiences showed that while the surgical site was narrow, the ultrasound device was large and had problems with its use. There was also a problem that the sensitivity was not high.

In the surgery of spinal hemangioblastoma, several reports describe the usefulness of intraoperative indocyanine green (ICG) fluorescence angiography [41–43]. This technique provides real-time information about the precise location of the tumor lesion and the feeding arteries and draining veins, as well as additional feeding arteries that were not revealed by preoperative spinal angiography. Additionally, post-resection ICG videoangiography can be used to identify tumor removal in the slowing of blood vessel filling and identification of residual pathological blood vessels or tumors in most patients [41].

Neurophysiological monitoring is mandatory and the electrodes should be placed depending on the location of the lesion. Motor (MEP) and somatosensory evoked potentials (SSEP) are recorded throughout the surgery to provide feedback to the surgeon during spinal cord manipulation. The baseline recording preoperative period should be performed to have a reference during surgical manipulation of the spinal cord.

Most authors have reported that tumoral capsule is coagulated using a fine bipolar forceps with low intensities, respecting the venous drainage and attempting to avoid any bleeding [34]. This circumferential coagulation technique around the tumor has been advocated in order to control the intraoperative bleeding. SCH can be removed with circumferential dissection of the tumor–pial interface to devascularize and detach the tumor. Circumferential coagulation (CC) could not avoid the collateral damage to the spinal cord tissue itself. Hence, instead of circumferential coagulation, circumferential dissection with minimal use of coagulation (CD) has been applied to prevent unwanted damage to the spinal cord from coagulation. Pial vessels that cross the margin of the tumor at its junction with the pia mater are sharply divided to clearly expose the margin of the tumor at the pial surface. The plane of dissection is developed in a circumferential manner using microscissors, microforceps, and small cottonoid strips. If the collateral damage to the spinal cord tissue itself can be reduced by this plane of dissection method, the sensory abnormality in patients after surgery may be reduced. Currently, after surgery in this way, there was no problem in removing the tumor with en bloc and improvement in functional deterioration.

Case review

Case 1. C2-3 level posterior approach, spinal cord backward (Video 1).

A 22-year-old male patient complained of right hand grasp power weakness and right shoulder pain. His magnetic resonance (MR) images showed 3.4 cm-sized hypervascular avid enhancing mass at the intramedullary region in the C2-3 level (Fig. 12.2). The patient underwent spinal cord tumor removal. Tumor was removed by circumferential dissection with minimal use of coagulation method.

Case 2. Cervicomedullary junction posterior approach, spinal cord backward (Video 2).

A 55-year-old female patient complained of right arm weakness and right hand tingling sensation. Her magnetic resonance (MR) images showed that 1 cm-sized hypervascular tumor staining at right side cervicomedullary junction (Fig. 12.3). Tumor was removed by circumferential dissection with minimal use of coagulation method.

Case 3. C4-5 level posterior approach, spinal cord backward (Video 3).

A 37-year-old male patient complained of right hand fine motor impairment and tingling sensation. His magnetic resonance (MR) images showed 1.1 cm-sized hypervascular avid enhancing mass at the intramedullary region in the C4-5 level (Fig. 12.4). Tumor was removed by circumferential dissection with minimal use of coagulation method.

Case 4. L1-2 level posterior approach, spinal cord backward.

A 44-year-old female patient complained of both leg tingling sensation. Her magnetic resonance (MR) images showed that 1.4 cm-sized hypervascular avid enhancing mass at the intramedullary region in the L1-2 level (Fig. 12.5). Tumor was removed by circumferential dissection with minimal use of coagulation method.

12.5 Conclusion

Preoperative embolization and intraoperative ultrasound are not necessary for SCH surgery, and intraoperative indocyanine green

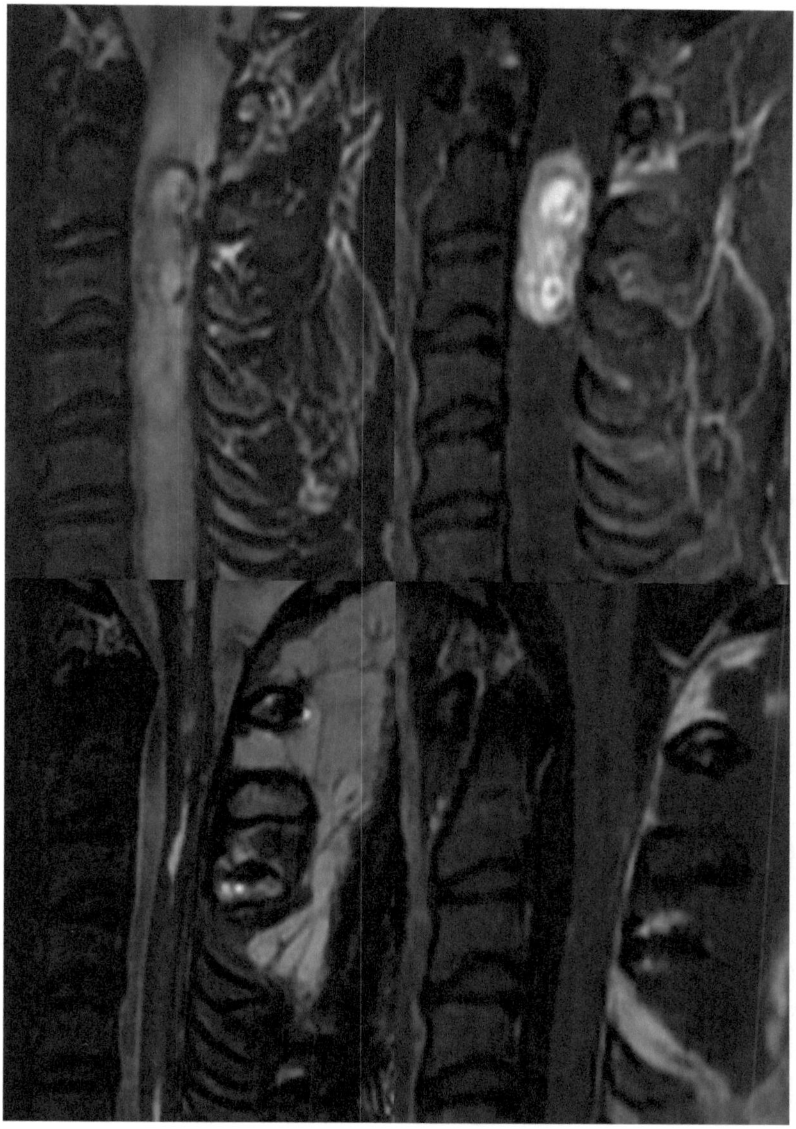

Fig. 12.2 Preoperative magnetic resonance images (MRI) of the cervical spine revealed about 3.4 cm-sized hypervascular avid enhancing mass at the intramedullary region in the C2-3 level. Postoperative MRI showed that all the advanced tumors were removed and syrinx also improved

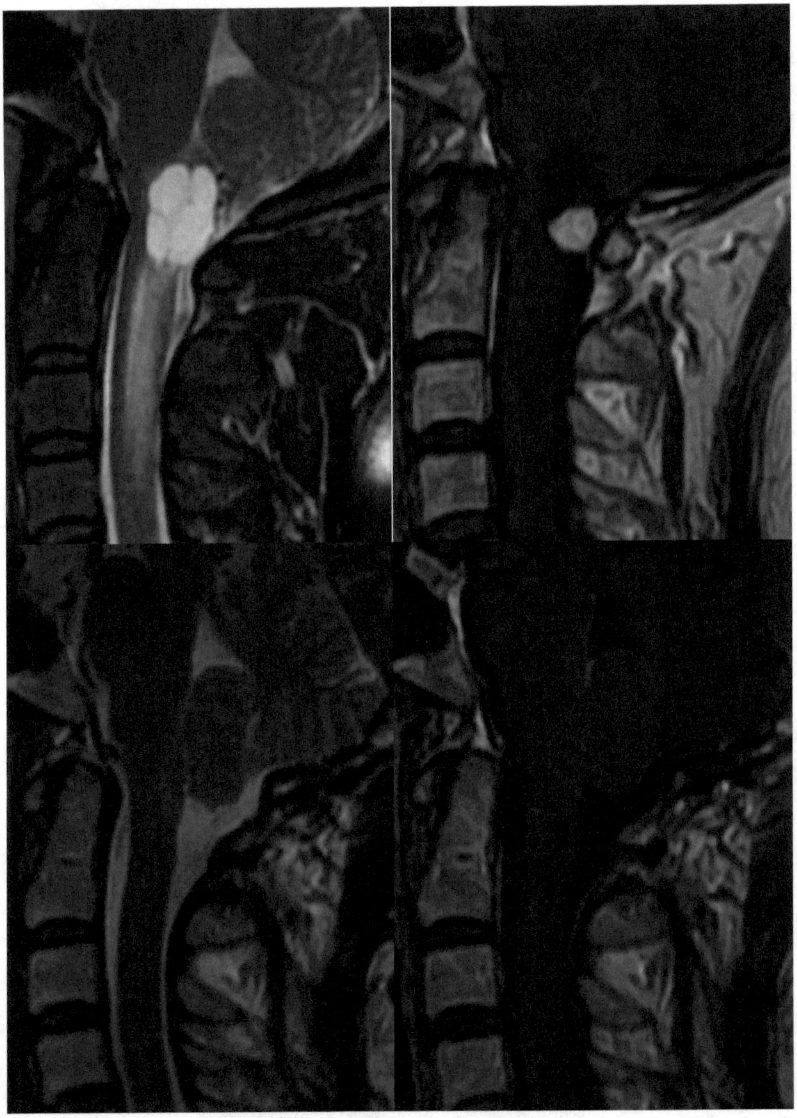

Fig. 12.3 Preoperative magnetic resonance images (MRI) of the cervical spine revealed about 1 cm-sized hypervascular tumor staining at the right side of cervicomedullary junction. Postoperative MRI showed that all the advanced tumors were removed and syrinx also improved

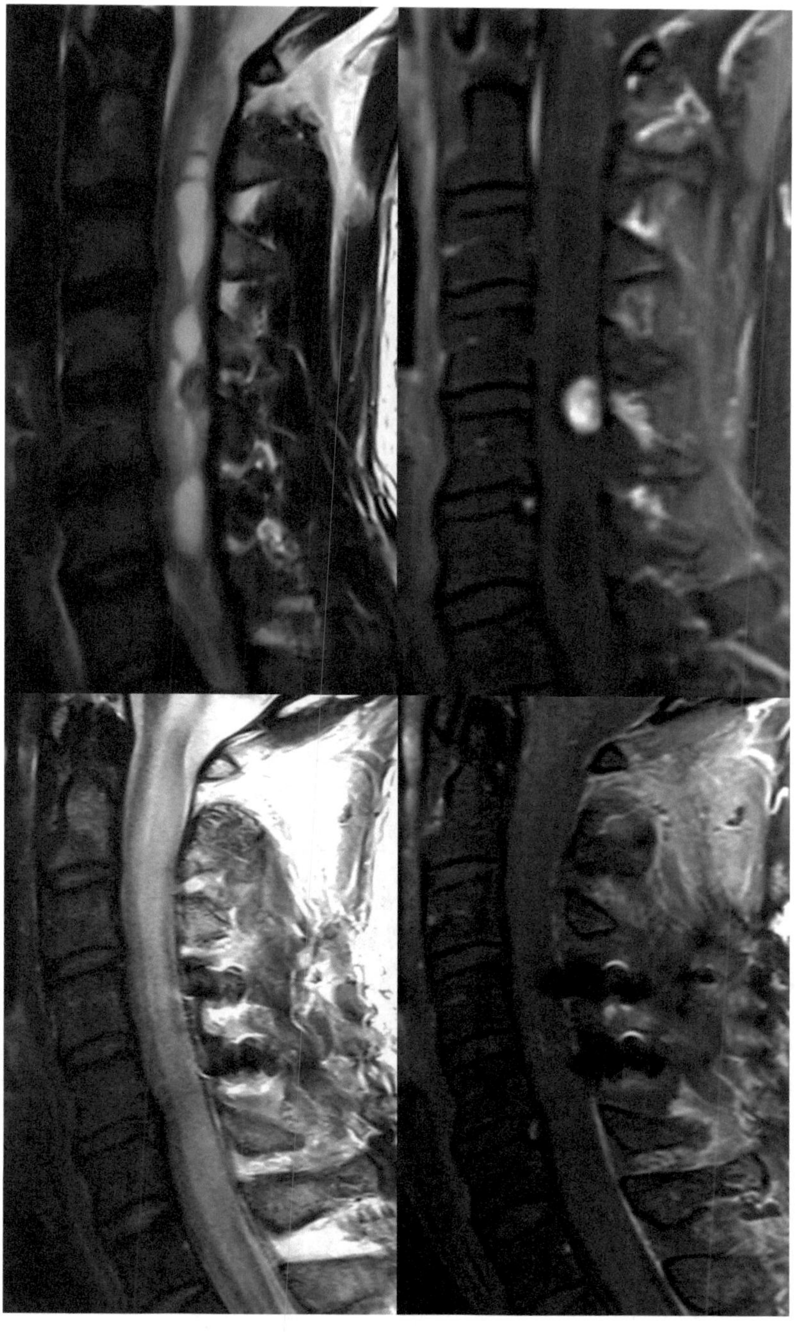

Fig. 12.4 Preoperative magnetic resonance images (MRI) of the cervical spine revealed about 1.1 cm-sized hypervascular avid enhancing mass at the intramedullary region in the C4-5 level. Postoperative MRI showed that all the advanced tumors were removed

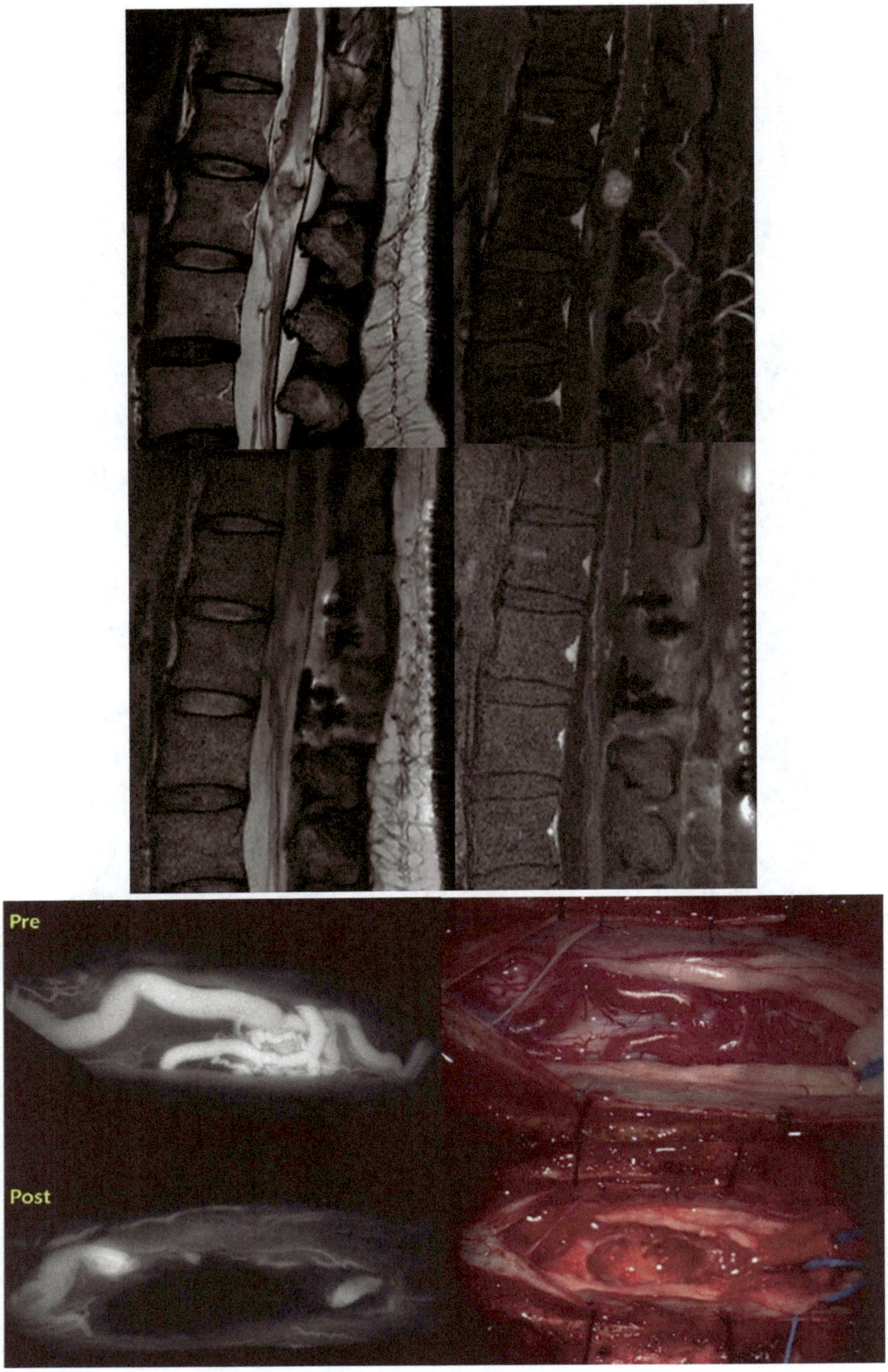

Fig. 12.5 Preoperative magnetic resonance images (MRI) of the lumbar spine revealed about 1.4 cm-sized hypervascular avid enhancing mass at the intramedullary region in the L1-2 level. Postoperative MRI showed that all the advanced tumors were removed. Preoperative and postoperative intraoperative fluorescence angiography provides real-time information about the precise location of the tumor lesion and the feeding arteries and draining veins

fluorescence angiography and intraoperative neuromonitoring are helpful.

Circumferential dissection with minimal use of coagulation is helpful for developing tumor–cord interface clearly and for providing a better functional outcome.

References

1. Nicholas DS, Weller RO. The fine anatomy of the human spinal meninges: a light and scanning electron microscopy study. J Neurosurg. 1988;69(2):276–82.
2. Alcolado R, Weller R, Parrish E, Garrod D. The cranial arachnoid and pia mater in man: anatomical and ultrastructural observations. Neuropathol Appl Neurobiol. 1988;14(1):1–17.
3. Millen J, Woollam D. On the nature of the pia mater. Brain. 1961;84(3):514–20.
4. White A. Physical properties and functional biomechanics of the spine. In: Clinical biomechanics of the spine. 1990;22.
5. Iwasaki Y, Koyanagi I, Hida K, Abe H. Anterior approach to intramedullary hemangioblastoma: case report. Neurosurgery. 1999;44(3):655–7.
6. Pluta RM, Iuliano B, Devroom HL, Nguyen T, Oldfield EH. Comparison of anterior and posterior surgical approaches in the treatment of ventral spinal hemangioblastomas in patients with von Hippel—Lindau disease. J Neurosurg. 2003;98(1):117–24.
7. Nakashima H, Tokunaga K, Tamiya T, Matsumoto K, Ohmoto T, Furuta T. Analysis of spinal cord hemangioblastoma in von Hippel-Lindau disease. no Shinkei Geka Neurological Surgery. 1999;27(6):533–40.
8. Mandigo CE, Ogden AT, Angevine PD, McCormick PC. Operative management of spinal hemangioblastoma. Neurosurgery. 2009;65(6):1166–77.
9. Zadnik PL, Gokaslan ZL, Burger PC, Bettegowda C. Spinal cord tumours: advances in genetics and their implications for treatment. Nat Rev Neurol. 2013;9(5):257.
10. Krieg M, Marti HH, Plate KH. Coexpression of erythropoietin and vascular endothelial growth factor in nervous system tumors associated with von Hippel-Lindau tumor suppressor gene loss of function. Blood. 1998;92(9):3388–93.
11. Gijtenbeek JM, Jacobs B, Sprenger SH, et al. Analysis of von Hippel—Lindau mutations with comparative genomic hybridization in sporadic and hereditary hemangioblastomas: possible genetic heterogeneity. J Neurosurg. 2002;97(4):977–82.
12. Weil RJ, Vortmeyer AO, Zhuang Z, et al. Clinical and molecular analysis of disseminated hemangioblastomatosis of the central nervous system in patients without von Hippel—Lindau disease: Report of four cases. J Neurosurg. 2002;96(4):775–87.
13. Sprenger SH, Gijtenbeek JM, Wesseling P, et al. Characteristic chromosomal aberrations in sporadic cerebellar hemangioblastomas revealed by comparative genomic hybridization. J Neurooncol. 2001;52(3):241–7.
14. Biondi A, Ricciardi GK, Faillot T, Capelle L, Van Effenterre R, Chiras J. Hemangioblastomas of the lower spinal region: report of four cases with preoperative embolization and review of the literature. Am J Neuroradiol. 2005;26(4):936–45.
15. Lee DK, Choe WJ, Chung CK, Kim HJ. Spinal cord hemangioblastoma: surgical strategy and clinical outcome. J Neurooncol. 2003;61(1):27–34.
16. Browne TR, Adams RD, Roberson GH. Hemangioblastoma of the spinal cord: review and report of five cases. Arch Neurol. 1976;33(6):435–41.
17. Murota T, Symon L. Surgical management of hemangioblastoma of the spinal cord: a report of 18 cases. Neurosurgery. 1989;25(5):699–708.
18. Yasargil M, Antic J, Laciga R, Fideler R, Boone S. The microsurgical removal of intramedullary spinal hemangioblastomas. Report of twelve cases and a review of the literature. Surg Neurol. 1976;(3):141–48.
19. Roonprapunt C, Silvera VM, Setton A, Freed D, Epstein FJ, Jallo GI. Surgical management of isolated hemangioblastomas of the spinal cord. Neurosurgery. 2001;49(2):321–8.
20. Imagama S, Ito Z, Wakao N, et al. Differentiation of localization of spinal hemangioblastomas based on imaging and pathological findings. Eur Spine J. 2011;20(8):1377.
21. Xu Q-W, Bao W-M, Mao R-L, Yang G-Y. Magnetic resonance imaging and microsurgical treatment of intramedullary hemangioblastoma of the spinal cord. Neurosurgery. 1994;35(4):671–6.
22. Corr P, Dicker T, Wright M. Exophytic intramedullary hemangioblastoma presenting as an extramedullary mass on myelography. Am J Neuroradiol. 1995;16(4):883–4.
23. Tampieri D, Leblanc R, TerBrugge K. Preoperative embolization of brain and spinal hemangioblastomas. Neurosurgery. 1993;33(3):502–5.
24. Liu A, Jain A, Sankey EW, Jallo GI, Bettegowda C. Sporadic intramedullary hemangioblastoma of the spine: a single institutional review of 21 cases. Neurol Res. 2016;38(3):205–9.
25. Cristante L, Herrmann H-D. Surgical management of intramedullary hemangioblastoma of the spinal cord. Acta Neurochir. 1999;141(4):333–40.
26. Deng X, Wang K, Wu L, et al. Intraspinal hemangioblastomas: analysis of 92 cases in a single institution. J Neurosurg: Spine. 2014;21(2):260–9.

27. Lonser RR, Butman JA, Huntoon K, et al. Prospective natural history study of central nervous system hemangioblastomas in von Hippel-Lindau disease. J Neurosurg. 2014;120(5):1055–62.
28. Rawe SE, Van JG, Rothman S. Radiographic diagnostic evaluation and surgical treatment of multiple cerebellar, brain stem, and spinal cord hemangioblastomas. Surg Neurol. 1978;9(6):337–41.
29. Yu JS, Short MP, Schumacher J, Chapman PH. Intramedullary hemorrhage in spinal cord hemangioblastoma. Report of two cases. J Neurosurg. 1994;81(6):937–40.
30. Cerejo A, Vaz R, Feyo PB, Cruz C. Spinal cord hemangioblastoma with subarachnoid hemorrhage. Neurosurgery. 1990;27(6):991–3.
31. Horton JA, Eelkema E, Albright AL. Preoperative embolization of a hemangioblastoma. Am J Neuroradiol. 1989;10(1):203–203.
32. Wang Z, Liu A. Differential diagnosis and operative timing of intramedullary spinal cord tumors. Zhongguo Yi Xue Ke Xue Yuan Xue Bao Acta Academiae Medicinae Sinicae. 1999;21(2):88–93.
33. Wang C, Zhang J, Liu A, Sun B. Surgical management of medullary hemangioblastoma: report of 47 cases. Surg Neurol. 2001;56(4):218–26.
34. Messerer M, Cossu G, Pralong E, Daniel R. Intramedullary hemangioblastoma: Microsurgical resection technique. Neurochirurgie. 2017;63(5):376–80.
35. Malis LI. Atraumatic bloodless removal of intramedullary hemangioblastomas of the spinal cord. J Neurosurg: Spine. 2002;97(1):1–6.
36. Eskridge JM, McAuliffe W, Harris B, Kim D, Scott J, Winn H. Preoperative endovascular embolization of craniospinal hemangioblastomas. Am J Neuroradiol. 1996;17(3):525–31.
37. Vazquez-Anon V, Botella C, Beltran A, Solera M, Piquer J. Preoperative embolization of solid cervicomedullary junction hemangioblastomas: report of two cases. Neuroradiology. 1997;39(2):86–9.
38. Standard SC, Ahuja A, Livingston K, Guterman LR, Hopkins LN. Endovascular embolization and surgical excision for the treatment of cerebellar and brain stem hemangioblastomas. Surg Neurol. 1994;41(5):405–10.
39. David P, Messerer M, Aghakhani N, et al. Les hémangioblastomes intramédullaires. Neurochirurgie. 2017;63(5):366–71.
40. Regelsberger J, Fritzsche E, Langer N, Westphal M. Intraoperative sonography of intra-and extramedullary tumors. Ultrasound Med Biol. 2005;31(5):593–8.
41. Hao S, Li D, Ma G, Yang J, Wang G. Application of intraoperative indocyanine green videoangiography for resection of spinal cord hemangioblastoma: advantages and limitations. J Clin Neurosci. 2013;20(9):1269–75.
42. Hwang SW, Malek AM, Schapiro R, Wu JK. Intraoperative use of indocyanine green fluorescence videography for resection of a spinal cord hemangioblastoma. Neurosurgery. 2010;67(3 Suppl Operative):300–3; discussion 303.
43. Murakami T, Koyanagi I, Kaneko T, Iihoshi S, Houkin K. Intraoperative indocyanine green videoangiography for spinal vascular lesions: case report. Oper Neurosurg 2011;68(suppl_1): E241–E245.

How to Approach Anatomical Compartment; Intrapial Intra-axial Tumor

13

Woo Jin Choe and Chun Kee Chung

Abstract

Intramedullary spinal cord tumors can be surgically removed through exact understanding of the anatomical location and an appropriate microsurgical technique. Proper myelotomy procedures are necessary for the safe and successful approach to the intra-axial tumors like astrocytoma. In the chapter, the authors describe several requisite guidelines to access intra-axial intramedullary lesion, while preserving neurological functions of the spinal cord.

W. J. Choe
Department of Neurosurgery, Konkuk University Hospital, 120-1, Neungdong-ro, Hwayang, Seoul 05030, Gwangjin, South Korea
e-mail: 20050100@kuh.ac.kr

C. K. Chung (✉)
Department of Neurosurgery, Seoul National University Hospital, Seoul National University College of Medicine, Seoul, Republic of Korea
e-mail: chungc@snu.ac.kr

Neuroscience Research Institute, Seoul National University Medical Research Center, Seoul, Republic of Korea

Clinical Research Institute, Seoul National University Hospital, Seoul, Republic of Korea

Department of Brain and Cognitive Sciences, Seoul National University College of Natural Sciences, Seoul, Republic of Korea

Keywords

Intramedullary · Intra-axial · Myelotomy · Astrocytoma

13.1 Introduction

In the first half of the twentieth century, surgical treatment of intramedullary spinal cord tumor produced devastating outcomes. Since the introduction of microsurgical techniques and with the aid of bipolar cautery/ultrasonic tissue aspirator, the more aggressive tumor resection could be possible without inflicting injury to adjacent neural tissue. Technical advances have resulted in improved clinical outcome, while the morbidity and mortality are reduced. Near-complete or complete surgical resection has been reported to have great results in case of tumors with clear cleavage margin [1–3]. In highly invasive tumors, radical resection is usually limited to minimize the neural damage in the spinal cord. However, several studies have demonstrated a better clinical outcome of surgical resection over minimal biopsy even in invasive lesions [4–6].

Therefore, we will discuss fundamental principles to remove the lesion, while minimizing spinal cord injury in the surgical treatment of intramedullary tumors.

C. K. Chung (ed.), *Surgery of Spinal Cord Tumors Based on Anatomy*,
https://doi.org/10.1007/978-981-15-7771-0_13

13.2 Strategy of Surgical Treatment

13.2.1 General Considerations

The two main goals of the surgical interventions are: (1) tumor removal while preserving or improving neurological status and (2) get a pathological diagnosis [1].

Laminectomy is usually limited to one spinal level above and below the tumor. Ultrasound can be helpful in delineating tumor margin. Intramedullary tumors are usually hyperechoic in the solid portion and hypoechoic in the cystic or necrotic portion [7, 8]. When there is a risk of postoperative kyphotic deformity or instability, osteoplastic laminotomy (laminoplasty) or posterior instrumentation could be considered [2, 9].

Atraumatic myelotomy with minimal damage to the spinal cord can provide an appropriate corridor to a successful surgery [1–3]. The axial tumor location and plane according to intramedullary tumor pathology should be understood and inspected for adequate myelotomy (Fig. 13.1).

The traditional approach to intramedullary cord tumor is through a posterior midline sulcus, and the posterolateral approach using dorsal root entry zone (DREZ) is followed [10–13]. Direct transpial approach can be considered especially in vascular tumors such as hemangioblastoma or cavernous hemangioma [14, 15]. The exact axial location of tumor is the most important factor defining the myelotomy site and should be figured out by thorough interpretation of MR images and careful inspection in the operating field [1].

In case of tumors without prominent cleavage margins, it is better to stay in the tumor and dissection should be performed within the tumor margin to minimize damage to the spinal cord. Identifying the cephalic-caudal pole may be helpful in resecting as much tumors as possible [1–3].

13.2.2 Posterior Midline Myelotomy

Posterior midline myelotomy is a surgical approach to access the tumor via the dorsal (posterior) median sulcus, which is preferred for most gliomas. The sulcus is located in the middle of the posterior lateral sulci on both sides. The vessels branching from the midline dorsal medullary vein may be helpful in identifying the sulcus [2, 16]. However, distortion and transformation of the normal anatomical structures can make the recognition of the midline difficult. In a large tumor, the spinal cord usually enlarged and rotated, and dorsal medial sulcus is hard to identify. Careful inspection of the arrangement of central veins on the surface of the posterior column helps to identify the surgical orientation. Checking the midpoint of bilateral DREZ is also useful in confirming the dorsal midline [2, 6, 10, 17].

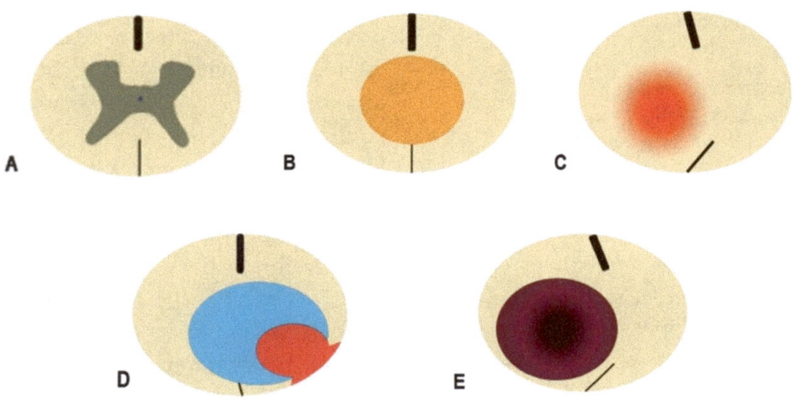

Fig. 13.1 Schematic diagram of the axial locations and appearances of intramedullary spinal cord tumors. **a** Normal **b** Ependymoma **c** Astrocytoma **d** Hemangioblastoma **e** intramedullary metastasis

The posterior spinal veins do not need to be saved unless they are judged to play a critical role in the venous circulation. Indocyanine green videoangiography (iCg-Va) can be applied in identifying collateral venous circulation [18]. Small blood vessels crossing the midline on the dorsal surface of the spinal cord can be carefully coagulated using bipolar cautery [2]. The incision of posterior median septum is made with a diamond arachnoid knife or microscissors, and then myelotomy is extended rostral or caudal over the length of the solid tumor. Pial strut sutures using #6–0 suture material may be made to facilitate for securing the operating field [1]. However, controversy arises because this suture may increase the tension of the spinal cord and can cause damage to the functioning neural tissue [19].

The incision can be deepened until the tumor is identified. After the tumor is encountered, it is important to delineate the cleavage plane between the tumor and spinal cord using a microdissector. If tumor has cystic portion, drainage of the cyst at its poles is quite useful in both decompression of the spinal cord and identifying the tumor margin [1]. At tumor margin, coagulation is performed on the surface of the tumor and tissue is obtained for frozen biopsy. Further dissecting procedures are dependent on the presence of the cleavage margin and tumor size [19, 20]. If the tumor has an apparent dissection plane, fibrous and vascular attachments between the parenchyma and the tumor are meticulously divided using cautery from the dorsal to lateral portion of the tumor. In invasive tumors, tumor is removed from center to periphery of the tumor margins (inside-out techniques). If gliosis-associated or hemosiderin-deposited tissue is encountered, it may be thought as a borderline between normal tissue and tumor and it is better to preserve those tissue [10, 20]. Larger tumors may require internal debulking with ultrasonic aspirator for better visualization of the lateral and ventral tumor margins.

After confirmation of the lateral margin, dissection can be carefully progressed to the ventral side. In large tumors, it is important to preserve ventral pia and not to damage the perforating arteries of the anterior spinal artery in the ventral portion, and indocyanine green videoangiography (iCg-Va) can also be useful [18].

In dorsal midline approach with a large eccentrically located tumor, it must be kept in mind that dorsal median sulcus may be leant oblique, and is not perpendicular to dorsal surface of the spinal cord (Fig. 13.1). Even though dorsal midline sulcus is correctly identified at cord surface, there are lots of possibilities damaging dorsal columns and commissural fibers during the deepening procedure. Commissural circuits of interneurons of the spinal cord provide the coordination of both sides of the body, and ensure proper alternation or synchrony of muscle activities during the locomotion. They also transmit proprioceptive information to the cerebellum via spinocerebellar and cuneocerebellar tracts [21, 22]. Therefore, despite careful dissection of dorsal midline sulcus, patients may complain of imbalance or discoordination after midline myelotomy.

13.2.3 Posterolateral Myelotomy

Posterolateral sulcus approach is the so-called dorsal root entry zone (DREZ) myelotomy [13, 23, 24]. This approach may be indicated for tumors eccentrically located in spinal cord [17]. The basic procedure is the same as posterior midline approach. The incision is made using an arachnoid diamond knife or a microscissor along the ipsilateral posterolateral sulcus. The myelotomy site is just medial to the DREZ, while paying attention to the injury of the posterior spinal artery on the same side. The posterolateral sulcus naturally leads to the posterolateral tract of Lissauer. After myelotomy is extended rostro-caudally, a careful microsurgical dissection is employed to establish the plane between the tumor and spinal cord. Internal debulking of the tumor with ultrasonic surgical aspirator and bipolar coagulation are often used to facilitate mobilization of the tumor and recognizing tumor margins [16, 25].

The advantage of this approach is to reduce the neurological symptoms associated with the damage to the dorsal column, but the risk of neurological symptoms owing to lateral column injury may increase [13].

13.2.4 Direct Transpial Approach

This approach utilizes a direct incisional corridor at the site where lesion is identified in the surgical field. Vascular diseases such as hemangioblastoma or cavernous malformation are the main indications of this approach [14, 15]. Most hemangioblastomas arise from the dorsal spinal cord with apparent pial attachment. Also, glioma can grow exophytically to subarachnoid space through pial membrane. Various malignant neoplasm can infiltrate and replace surface spinal cord tissue and grow out to subarachnoid space.

In these instances, myelotomy may not be necessary and pial incision through the tumor-spinal cord juncture can make tumor margin clear [3]. The pial attachment site can be used as a corridor with circumferential pial incision.

13.2.5 Closure

When the main procedure is completed, the pial strut sutures are removed after meticulous hemostasis. The pial edges are sutured so that they can be approximated with each other. Exceptionally in direct transpial approach, pial sutures usually are not mandatory. The arachnoid membrane may be closed with the dura mater using watertight suture. It is preferred to repair pia mater, arachnoid membrane, and dura mater separately in layer-by-layer pattern, if possible. Occasionally, expansile duroplasty is necessary if significant residual tumor was left [1, 2, 16].

13.2.6 Surgical Treatment of Astrocytoma

Astrocytomas are the most common intramedullary tumors in children, and second common intramedullary tumor following ependymoma in adult. The vast majority of spinal cord astrocytomas are of low-grade and the cervical spinal cord is the most frequently affected site [1, 3].

Spinal cord astrocytomas are infiltrating in nature and cleavage margin to normal functioning spinal cord is obscure. Astrocytomas tend to be physically heterogeneous with variable tumor color and consistency, and intra-tumoral cysts are commonly observed [2–4, 26]. They are usually eccentrically located from the center of the spinal cord, and their asymmetrical location can cause the rotation/distortion of cord and make the recognition of the dorsal median sulcus confusing. Pilocytic astrocytomas in children can be clearly distinguished from surrounding tissue, while fibrillary astrocytomas are similar in consistency and appearance to functioning spinal cord at the boundary [26, 27]. The tumor resection should proceed from the center to the periphery until the tumor demarcation becomes unclear or when changes of evoked potentials are noted [2].

In low-grade astrocytomas, the efficacy of radical resection is not confirmed and controversial. Before surgery, the goal and the extent of the resection should be carefully planned [28]. Diffusion tensor MR imaging and fiber tractography is helpful in planning of (1) myelotomy site and approaching route and (2) extent of tumor removal. Also, this study is useful in predicting neurological prognosis after surgical procedure. Attempting total resection in fibrillary astrocytoma is deemed to be impossible due to its microscopically infiltrating characteristics, and may be harmful [11]. There is no evidence that the radical resection can result in cure in low-grade tumors and change the natural history of intramedullary astrocytoma [1, 29, 30]. But, McCormick et al. described that many low-grade gliomas have boundary and amenable to resection [31].

The rare high-grade astrocytoma or glioblastoma has very poor prognosis and is not affected by the extent of the surgical intervention [1, 3]. They tend to recur early after resection, and other treatment options like radiotherapy/chemotherapy should be considered after conservative surgery. Kim et al. reported that extent of resection did not influence the survival and the histological grade was the most significant predictor of prognosis in patients with astrocytoma of the spinal cord [32].

13.3 Case Illustrations

13.3.1 Case 1. Approach Through Posterior Midline Sulcus

A 17-year-old male patient presented with gait disturbance and paresthesia in the chest. Weakness in the right leg and voiding problem were noted. Magnetic resonance (MR) images showed an expansile swelling and diffuse enhancing mass in the intramedullary spinal cord in upper thoracic spine (T3-5, Fig. 13.2). Posterior midline myelotomy was used to approach the mass. The tumor being infiltrative and the demarcation unclear, subtotal removal of the tumor and decompression of spinal cord with duroplasty were performed (Fig. 13.3). The pathological diagnosis was high-grade glioma consistent with anaplastic astrocytoma. After surgery, the tumor volume was slightly decreased, and the neurological status was unchanged (Fig. 13.4). The patient received additional radiotherapy and chemotherapy.

13.3.2 Case 2. Approach Through Right Dorsal Root Entry Zone

A 36-year-old female patient having a history of breast cancer presented with a Brown-Séquard syndrome. She had been receiving chemotherapy for two years, but suffered from multiple systemic metastasis including brain. She complained of weakness in the right hand and leg. Magnetic resonance (MR) images showed a $2.3 \times 1.3 \times 1.0$ cm-sized ovoid-shaped enhancing mass inside the spinal cord at the level of C5-6 vertebrae (Fig. 13.5). A myelotomy on dorsal root entry zone was made as it was the shortest route to the mass. Tumor demarcation was partially unclear at the border and near total removal of the mass with decompression of the spinal cord was performed (Fig. 13.6). A metastatic adenocarcinoma was confirmed on histological study. After surgery, motor weakness in the right hand and leg was improved and she could ambulate by herself. Postoperative MR showed marked decrease of tumor volume and peritumoral edema (Fig. 13.7). The

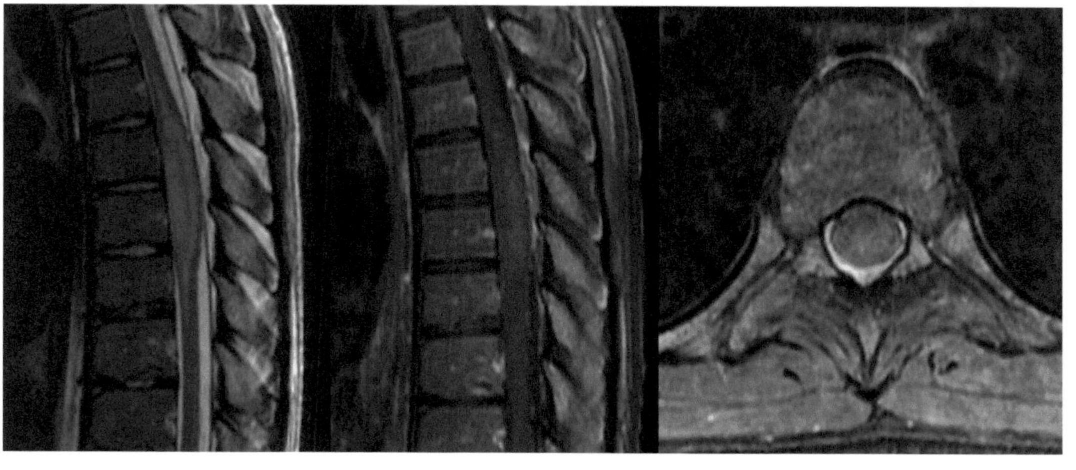

Fig. 13.2 Case 1: Magnetic resonance (MR) images of the upper thoracic spine showed enlargement of the spinal cord and diffuse enhancing intramedullary tumor. The tumor demarcation was not clear

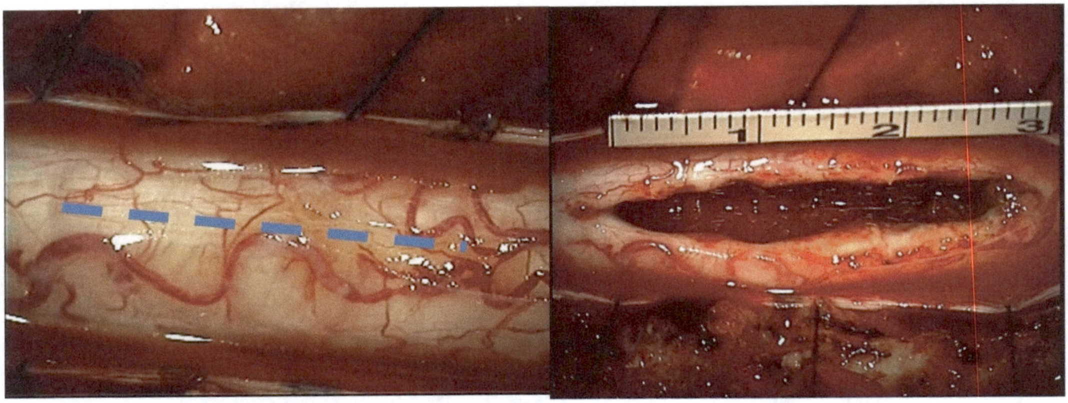

Fig. 13.3 Case 1: Surgical approach was done through dorsal median sulcus (dotted line) on the swollen spinal cord. Midline was confirmed by checking both dorsal root entry zone (DREZ) and dorsal venous vasculature. Subtotal removal and decompression of spinal cord were performed using tumor forceps and Cavitron Ultrasonic Surgical Aspirator (CUSA)

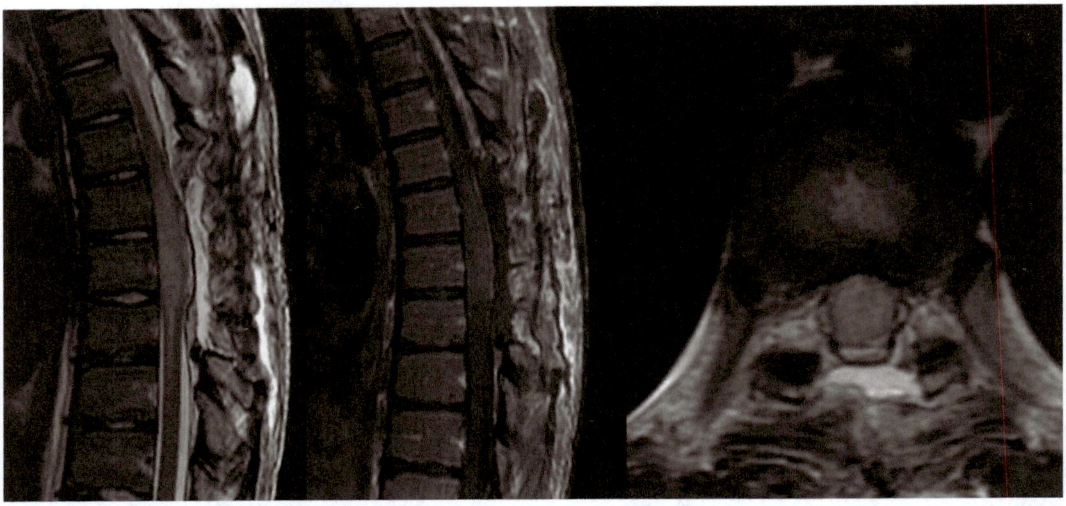

Fig. 13.4 Case 1: A postoperative MRI showed slightly decreased tumor volume and decompression of the spinal cord with duroplasty. The neurological status of the patient was not changed after surgery, and he received additional radiotherapy and chemotherapy

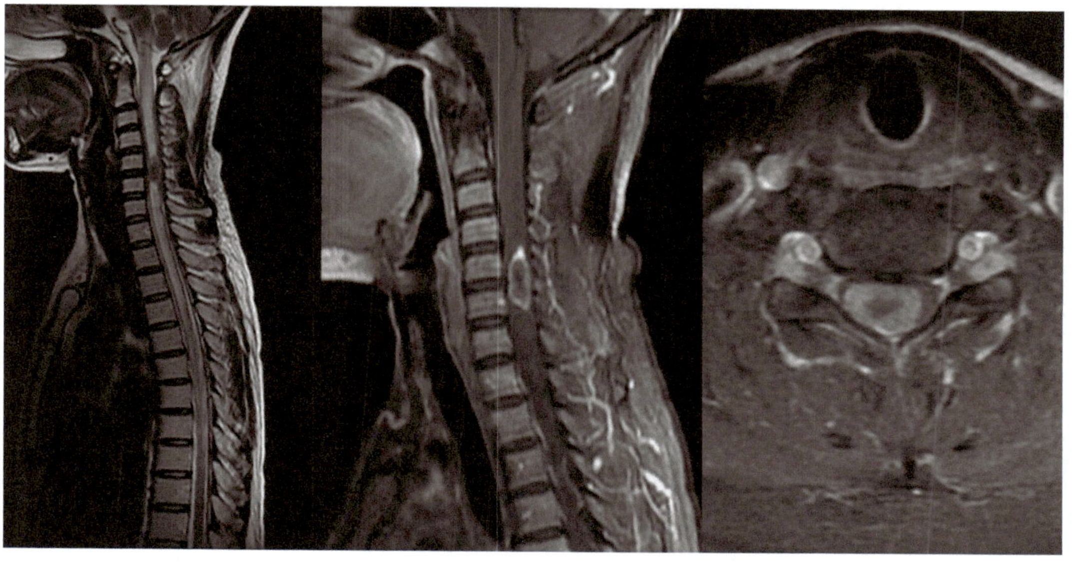

Fig. 13.5 Case 2: A well-enhancing ovoid-shaped intramedullary mass was found by a cervical magnetic resonance (MR) study. The tumor was compressing the normal spinal cord and seems to have cleavage margin to neural tissue. Extensive peritumoral edema was observed from medulla to midthoracic spinal cord

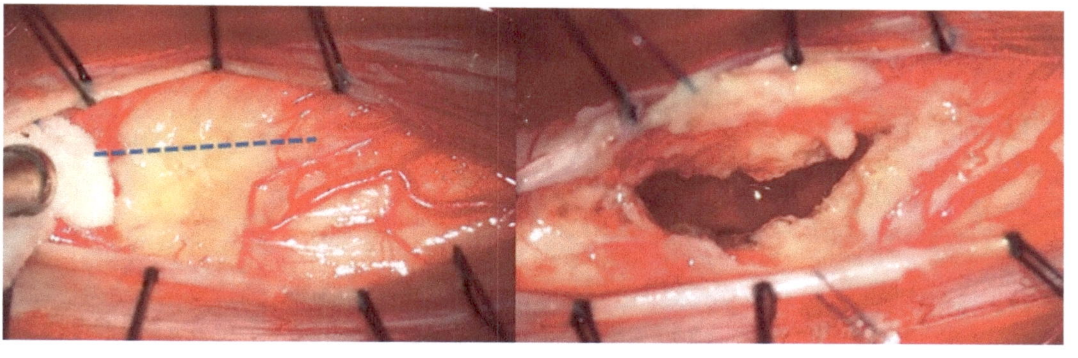

Fig. 13.6 Case 2: A myelotomy was mad through dorsal root entry zone (dotted line) in the right side. The tumor was firm and yellowish and the cleavage line was partially unclear at the ventral and medial side. Near total removal of the tumor was performed

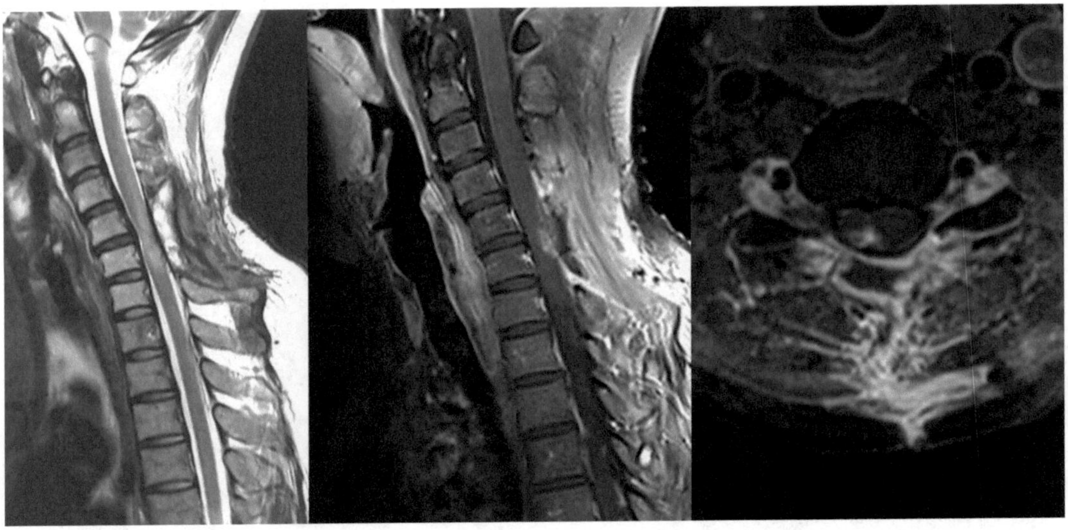

Fig. 13.7 Case 2: After surgery, the motor power in the hand and the lower extremities was improved and the patient could walk with the aid of walking frame. Postoperative MR showed that a large portion of the mass was removed and peritumoral edema was markedly decreased

patient received additional chemotherapy with a changed regimen.

References

1. Cooper PR, Hida K. Intramedullary spinal cord tumors. In: Dickman CA, Fehlings MG, Gokaslan ZI, editors. Spinal cord and spinal column tumors. New York: Thieme Medical Publishers; 2006. p. 315–34.
2. McCormick PC, Anson JA. Intramedullary spinal cord lesions. In: Benzel EC, editor. Spine surgery. Philaderphia: Elsevier Sauders. Pub; 2012. p. 983–90.
3. Epstein FJ, Farmer J, Freed D. Adult intramedullary astrocytomas of the spinal cord. J Neurosurg. 1992;77(3):355–9.
4. Rodriguez GB, Waldron JN, Wong CS, Laperriere NJ. A retrospective analysis of 52 cases of spinal cord glioma managed with radiation therapy. Int J Radiat Oncol Biol Phys. 2002;48(3):836–42.
5. Kahn J, Loeffler JS, Niemierko A, Chiooca EA, Batchelor T, Chakravarti A. Long-term outcomes of patients with spinal cord gliomas treated by modern conformal radiation techniques. Int J Radiat Oncol Biol Phys. 2011;81(1):232–8.
6. McGirt MJ, Goldstein IM, Chaichana KL, Tobias ME, KothbauerKF, JAllo GI. . Extent of surgical resection of malignant astrocytomas of the spinal cord: outcome analysis of 35 patients. Neurosurgery. 2008;63(1):55–60.
7. Epstein FJ, Farmer JP, Schneider SJ. Intraoperative ultrasonography: an important surgical adjunct for intramedullary tumors. J Neurosurg. 1991;74:729–33.
8. Maiuri F, Iaconetta G, Gallicchio B, Stella L. Intraoperative sonography for spinal tumors. Correlations with MR findings and surgery. J Neurosurg Sci. 2000;44:115–22.
9. Goh KY, Velasquez L, Epstein FJ. Pediatric intramedullary spinal cord tumors: is surgery alone enough? Pediatr Neurosurg. 1997;27:34–9.
10. McCormick PC. Intramedullary tumors of the spinal cord. In: Menezes AH, Sonntag VKH, editors. Principles of spinal surgery. Mcgraw-Hill;1996. pp. 1355–70.
11. Brotchi J. Intrinsic spinal cord tumor resection. Neurosurgery. 2002;50:1059–63.
12. Ohata K, Takami T, Gotou T, El-Bahy K, Morino M, Maeda M, Inoue Y, Hakuba A. Surgical outcome of intramedullary spinal cord ependymoma. Acta Neurochir (Wien). 1999;141:341–6; discussion 346–7.
13. Takami T, Yamagata T, Ohata K. Posterolateral sulcus approach for spinal intramedullary tumor of lateral location: technical note. Neurol Med Chir (Tokyo). 2013;53:920–7.
14. Malis L. Atraumatic bloodless removal of intramedullary hemangioblastomas of the spinal cord. J Neurosurg. 2002;97(1 Suppl):1–6.
15. Mitha AP, Turner JD, Spetzler RF. Surgical approaches to intramedullary cavernous malformations of the spinal cord. Neurosurgery 2011;68(2 Suppl operative):317–24; discussion 324.

16. Manzano G, Green BA, Vanni S, Levi AD. Contemporary management of adult intramedullary spinal tumors—pathology and neurological outcomes related to surgical resection. Spinal Cord. 2008;46:540–6.
17. Raco A, Esposito V, Lenzi J, Piccirilli M, Delfini R, Cantore G. Long-term follow-up of intramedullary spinal cord tumors: a series of 202 cases. Neurosurgery. 2005;56(5):972–81.
18. Takami T, Yamagata T, Naito K, Arima H, Ohata K. Intraoperative assessment of spinal vascular flow in the surgery of spinal intramedullary tumors using indocyanine green videoangiography. Surg Neurol Int. 2013;4:135.
19. Kucia EJ, Bambakidis NC, Chang SW, Spetzler RF. Surgical technique and outcomes in the treatment of spinal cord ependymomas, part 1: intramedullary ependymomas. Neurosurgery 2011;68(1 Suppl operative):57–63; discussion 63.
20. Toshihiro T. Surgical management of spinal intramedullary tumors: radical and safe strategy for benign tumors. Neurol Med Chir (Tokyo). 2015;55:317–27.
21. Chédotal A. Roles of axon guidance molecules in neuronal wiring in the developing spinal cord. Nat Rev Neurosci. 2019;20:380–96.
22. Castellani V. Building spinal and brain commissures: axon guidance at the midline. ISRN Cell Biol. 2013;2013:21, Article ID 315387.
23. Nashold BS, Ostdahl RH. Dorsal root entry zone lesions for pain relief. J Neurosurg. 1979;51:59–69.
24. Sindou M, Mifsud JJ, Boisson D, Goutelle A. Selective posterior rhizotomy in the dorsal root entry zone for treatment of hyperspasticity and pain in the hemiplegic upper limb. Neurosurgery. 1986;18:587–95.
25. Klekamp J. Treatment of intramedullary tumors: analysis of surgical morbidity and long-term results. J Neurosurg Spine. 2013;19:12–26.
26. Cooper PR. Outcome after operative treatment of intramedullary spinal cord tumors in adults. Intermediate and long-term results in 51 patients. Neurosurgery 1989;25:855–85.
27. Fischer G, Brotchi J, Chignier A, et al. Epidemiology. In: Fischer G, Brotchi J, editors., et al., Intramedullary spinal cord tumors. Stuttgart: Thieme; 1996. p. 9–10.
28. Brotchi J, Dewitte O, Levivier M, et al. A survey of 65 tumors within the spinal cord: surgical results and the importance of pre- Operative magnetic resonance imaging. Neurosurgery. 1991;29:651–7.
29. Sandler HM, Papadopoulos SM, Thornton AF Jr, Ross DA. Spinal cord astrocytomas: results of therapy. Neurosurgery. 1992;30:490–3.
30. Guidetti B, Mercuri S, Vagnozzi R. Long-term results of the surgical treatment of 129 intramedullary spinal gliomas. J Neurosurg. 1981;54:323–30.
31. McCormick PC, Stein BM. Intramedullary tumors in adults. Neurosurg Clin North Am. 1990;1:687–700.
32. Kim MS, Chung CK, Choe G, Kim IH, Kim HJ. Intramedullary spinal cord astrocytoma in adults: postoperative outcome. J Neurooncol. 2001;52(1):85–94.

How to Approach Anatomical Compartment; Intrapial Intra-Ependymal Tumor

14

Seung Heon Yang and Chun Kee Chung

Abstract

Treatment of spinal ependymoma is still challenging because of a concern of postoperative neurological deficit, which derived from its intramedullary location. Despite recent progression of adjuvant therapy, surgical resection is still a mainstay of the treatment, which can lead to an actual cure. To achieve successful surgical outcome minimizing the neurological deficits, the development and keeping the dissection plane throughout the tumor removal is the most important. Therefore, it is imperative to understand the anatomical relationship between the tumor and the surrounding tissues based on tumor origin. In this chapter, the authors suggest the concept of the intra-ependymal tumor, instead of the traditional intramedullary tumor for ependymoma based on the tumor origin and anatomical features. This concept may facilitate the development of the dissection plane and leads to the safe and effective removal of spinal ependymoma.

Keywords

Ependymoma · Intramedullary tumor · Ependymal layer · Central canal · Spinal cord · Tumor

Electronic supplementary material The online version of this chapter (https://doi.org/10.1007/978-981-15-7771-0_14) contains supplementary material, which is available to authorized users.

S. H. Yang
Department of Neurosurgery, Seoul National University Hospital, Seoul, South Korea
e-mail: nsdocyang@daum.net; nsdocyang@hanmail.net

C. K. Chung (✉)
Department of Neurosurgery, Seoul National University Hospital, Seoul National University College of Medicine, Seoul, Republic of Korea
e-mail: chungc@snu.ac.kr

Neuroscience Research Institute, Seoul National University Medical Research Center, Seoul, Republic of Korea

Clinical Research Institute, Seoul National University Hospital, Seoul, Republic of Korea

Department of Brain and Cognitive Sciences, Seoul National University College of Natural Sciences, Seoul, Republic of Korea

14.1 Introduction

Ependymoma (WHO grade II) and anaplastic ependymoma (WHO grade III) are grouped together with myxopaillary ependymoma (WHO grade I) and subependymoma (WHO grade I) representing ependymal neoplasm in the central nervous system because of their unique histological appearance in common [1]. However, these grade I ependymomas have distinct clinical behavior, tumor biology, and genetic features

C. K. Chung (ed.), *Surgery of Spinal Cord Tumors Based on Anatomy*,
https://doi.org/10.1007/978-981-15-7771-0_14

compared to grade II or III ependymomas [2, 3]. Myxopapillary ependymoma occurs almost exclusively in the region of conus medullaris, cauda equina, and filum terminale, which belongs to sub-arachnoid epi-pial space according to the authors' concept. Subependymoma is a rare CNS tumor which is usually found in the floor of the fourth ventricles and on the lateral ventricle walls although it occurs in any compartment of central nervous system [4, 5]. In this regard, most of this chapter will focus on classical ependymoma (WHO grades II and III) of the spinal cord.

Ependymoma is the most common intramedullary glial tumor which arises in the spinal cord in adults. However, unlike other intramedullary tumors, ependymoma is differentiated in that it has a more central location lined by ependymal layer, and it is well demarcated from its surrounding neural tissues which allow the development of a dissection plane of ependymal layer, which often lead to a complete resection without significant neurological problem (Fig. 14.1).

The origin of ependymoma has not been clearly specified yet. Traditionally, one of the primitive ependymal or subependymal cell around the ventricle or central canal has been thought to be a possible candidate. More recently, the radial glial cell has been suggested as the most potent candidate of tumor origin based on its similarity in immunophenotype

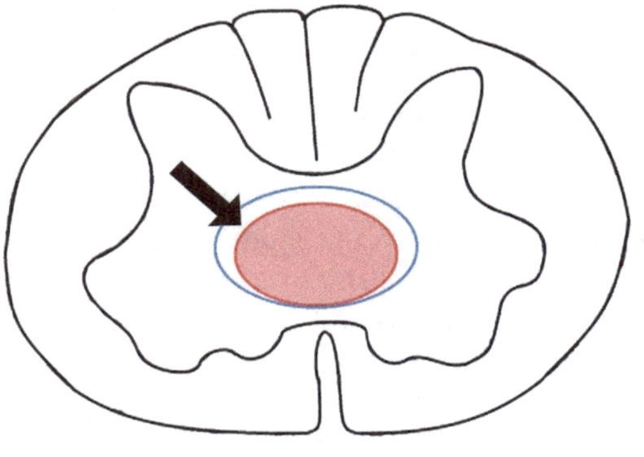

Fig. 14.1 Schematic drawing depicting subependymal space and cleavage plane between the cord and the ependymoma

with a self-renewing multipotent cancer cell [6, 7]. Interestingly, many of signature genes of ependymoma are significantly correlated with normally expressed genes in the developing central nervous system at embryonic period [6]. Furthermore, ependymoma in each compartment (supratentorial, infratentoral, and spinal) exhibits its distinct subset of gene expression, and these differences of gene expression are often found at accordant region during normal development of the central nervous system; all the signature genes of spinal ependymoma were expressed in the wall of the developing spinal canal and the "ventrolateral" spinal cord [6]. This might explain why ependymoma is commonly fed by branches of anterior spinal artery and a cleavage plane often become obscure or adherent to anterior median septum at the ventral surface of tumor.

The authors suggest that the ependymomas need to be considered separately from other intramedullary tumors and re-categorized into "intradural intraependymal" tumor from the aforementioned developmental and anatomical perspectives.

14.1.1 Presentation

Including all the subtypes, ependymoma is the third most common spinal cord tumor following schwannoma and meningioma accounting for 7.6%–23% of all spinal cord tumors. However, its annual incidence rate is known to be only 0.09–1 per 100,000 person, which shows the rarity of the tumor [8–10]. According to the national SEER (Surveillance Epidemiology and End Results) database, grades II and III ependymomas comprise up to 75% and 11% of all adult spinal ependymoma cases, respectively [11].

It is known to occur in any age group, but more than 50% of newly diagnosed ependymomas occur in middle age group (40–59 years). There seems no significant sexual difference in incidence for both grades II and III ependymomas [11].

Ependymoma occurs more frequently in the cervical or cervicothoracic region, up to 50%, despite the relatively small proportion of the segment [12–14]. Cyst or syringomyelia is often associated with ependymoma, and found in around two-thirds of cases [13, 15, 16]. Hemorrhage is also often found with ependymoma, in more than 20% of cases and it could be located at either tumor poles or inside the tumor [13, 17].

Ependymoma has an indolent course in symptomatic progression, so that symptom duration before the diagnosis is usually prolonged, ranging from 2 to 4 years [14, 18, 19]. Symptoms could be variable according to the location and size of the tumor. The most common symptom is sensory change, particularly hypesthesia and dysethesia below the affected level, and it could develop early in disease progression [16, 18, 19]. Localized aching pain at the level of the tumor may occur in early period either [19]. Thoracic ependymoma is known to cause more significant neurological deficits than cervical ependymoma [16]. Gait ataxia, motor weakness, and sphincter dysfunction are more likely to happen with thoracic ependymoma. Although its central, intramedullary location of the ependymomas, classic central cord syndrome is not common, and the weakness usually develops asymmetrically in advanced state of the tumor [19, 20].

14.2 Treatment and Outcomes

Surgery is the mainstay of treatment for spinal ependymoma. Along with histological grade, the extent of surgical removal is known to be associated with prolonged progression-free survival (PFS) and overall survival (OS). The role of adjuvant treatments for the management of spinal ependymoma has not been well established in association with its rarity of the tumors.

Unlike infratentorial ependymoma in children, in which its efficacy has been established [21], there have been conflicting results regarding the role of radiotherapy for spinal ependymomas [8, 22]. Although many investigators support the use of adjuvant radiotherapy for incompletely resected tumors, a recent study conducted by Oh et al. showed that the adjuvant radiation therapy for incompletely resected tumor did not make the difference in the overall survival [23]. Therefore, adjuvant radiotherapy is usually reserved and cautiously adopted in special circumstances; after the resection of "anaplastic" ependymoma, for a case of "unresectable" remnant tumor after a "revision" surgery, and for disseminated disease. We support a watchful waiting strategy for incompletely resected grade II ependymoma. Revision surgery is usually tried if the remnant tumor progress.

The role of systemic therapy in the management of ependymoma has not been well defined either. A single study reported a positive result with etoposide for the recurrent spinal ependymoma once, but supporting evidence is lacking [24, 25]. Targeted agents like Imatinib, everolimus, and bevacizumab has been tested for spinal ependymomas, and some of them showed potential to be a therapeutic agent, especially for NF2-related ependymoma [26–28]. However, more evidence is required for the clinical application.

A recent analysis using national SEER database reported that the 5-year and 10-year overall survivals were 94.7 and 85.1%, for the patients with grade II ependymoma and 58.2 and 46.4% for those with grade III disease [29]. The reported progression-free survival rates were 87%–97.5% at 5 years and 80%–92.6% at 10 years [14, 16, 23, 30]. Oh et al. executed a meta-analysis pooling grades II and III ependymomas and reported significantly better outcome in gross total resection (GTR) group; The 5-year PFS and OS were 97.9 and 98.8% for GTR group, 65.3 and 79.3% for subtotal resection with radiotherapy group, and 45.1 and 73.7% for subtotal resection without radiotherapy group [23]. In addition to GTR, histologic grade and patient's age were often suggested as significant prognostic factors. The reported rate of GTR spans wide range (20%–86%), and the rate of GTR seems to be increasing over time due to development of microsurgical technique and intraoperative neuromonitoring [14, 16, 29–32]. Although GTR is a primary target of surgical treatment currently, however, general consensus is that aggressive removal may not be attempted when serious neurological deficit is likely to occur. This policy is worth to consider, given that ependymoma is a slowly growing tumor.

There is a concern of postoperative neurological deficit because a myelotomy and manipulation of spinal cord are essential for surgical treatment. At immediate postoperative period, only about 6% of patients exhibited improved neurological function or symptoms [14]. Approximately 40%–60% of patients experienced deterioration of neurological function or neuropathic pain in some degree at immediate postoperative period. However, these neurological decline tended to improve during follow-up, and finally approximately 70%–75% of surgically treated patient remained stable or improved at follow-up [14, 16]. Permanent neurological decline was observed in 20%–27% of patients. Unfavorable functional outcome seems to be associated with preoperative functional status, longstanding symptom, and location in the thoracic level regardless of surgical extent. Delayed neurological deterioration is related with tumor recurrence or progression of remnant tumor [14, 16].

There is little known about the natural history of ependymoma yet. Behmanesh et al. analyzed the outcomes of 12 patients with intramedullary ependymoma who rejected treatment and suggested that wait and see strategy might be a viable option for intramedullary ependymomas [33]. However, given that preoperative neurological function is closely related to postoperative functional outcome, the authors recommend not to delay surgical treatment, especially when any neurological deficit is accompanied at presentation [14].

14.3 Surgical Approach

1. A Mayfield skull clamp is utilized for cervical and upper thoracic lesions. Neck flexion and head elevation (i.e., military prone) reduces the spinal curvature at these levels [19]. Abdomen should fall freely to keep abdominal pressure low, so that excessive epidural bleeding can be prevented.
2. During laminectomy, be cautious not to violate facet joints. Wide laminectomy does not necessary for ependymoma surgery because midline myelotomy is executed in most cases. Before the dura is opened, muscular and epidural bleeding should be meticulously controlled to prevent contamination of the surgical field with blood. The dura is opened in the midline and tented laterally. The arachnoid is opened and also tented by suturing to the dural edges.
3. Once the spinal cord is exposed, dorsal cord surface should be carefully inspected to delineate dorsal midline septum for proper myelotomy to minimize dorsal column injury. As is well known, several anatomical landmarks are primarily utilized to estimate the posterior midline septum: (1) the course and location of the posterior spinal vein and its perforating branches exiting from the cord; (2) the midpoints between the right and left posterior spinal artery; and (3) the midpoint of dorsal root entry zones at both sides. The spinal cord at the index level could be rotated or thinned with diminished anatomical characteristics, which may hinder the localization of the midline septum with anatomical landmarks [19]. In that case, dorsal column mapping might be helpful [34]. Nevertheless, the importance of anatomical approaches is not diminished.
4. A standard midline myelotomy is performed through the posterior median septum. For pial incision, a sharp blade is recommended. The author prefers an ophthalmic knife with pointed tip. The myelotomy site is deepened with micro-dissector until the tumor is exposed. The ependymoma is seen in purple-gray color and easily distinguishable from the normal cord tissue. Once the tumor is encountered, ependymal layer ought to be identified, since we should extend myelotomy under this layer in cranial and caudal direction with micro-dissector or micro-forceps. The myelotomy should be extended over entire length of tumor. If cyst

is present at either proximal or distal end, it is opened and drained at this step. This cystic space may facilitate identification of ependymal layer, providing a clear interface between the cord and the tumor.

5. Once the dorsal surface of tumor is exposed over the entire length, gentle dissection should be carried out. Not like intra-axial tumor, ependymoma exhibits quite clear dissection margin of ependymal layer despite the tumor is not encapsulated. Pial tenting could be applied at this point to enhance the dissection by applying retraction to the cord. However, this maneuver is not recommended as a routine procedure due to concerns that it may cause dorsal column dysfuction [35]. If dissection plane is not as clear as expected, intraoperative biopsy should be considered to rule out other intramedullary malignant neoplasms, which may necessitate to change the surgical objectives [19].
6. The basic technique of dissection is to apply traction force on the tumor against the cord tissue [19]. Micro-forceps, dissector, and suction tip are used depending on the circumstances. On applying counter traction on the spinal cord, the use of cottonoid can prevent cord damage and facilitate the dissection. During the dissection, small vessels bridging into the tumor surface may be encountered. Those vessels need to be cauterized and cut, and dissection continues to the ventral side. Once either tumor pole is dissected and freed from the spinal cord, ventral dissection plane could be developed relatively easily by applying traction force to the tumor pole perpendicular to the long axis of the spinal cord [19]. Feeding vessels from the anterior spinal artery could be isolated and cauterized. Excessive traction may cause avulsion injury of anterior spinal artery which can cause anterior spinal cord syndrome.
7. During the dissection, motor-evoked potential (MEP) should be frequently checked while somatosensory evoked potential is continuously recorded. While MEP decline more than 50% is generally accepted as a warning sign, the authors prefer all-or-none criteria [36]. Therefore, dissection is usually continued as long as the parenchyma of the cord is not violated and the dissection plane is secured even when the MEP is decreased more than 50%. Also, there may be tonic EMG responses when we dissect around the anterior horn. It is a sign that we are in the anterior horn; hence utmost care should be taken to save the anterior horn left behind to the remaining normal cord tissue.
8. After removal of the tumor, closure of the myelotomy is performed using 8–0 nylon by suturing pia matter to prevent cord tethering which may be a potential cause of morbidity in the postoperative period. (In case that only partial resection was achieved and cord swelling is present, closure of myelotomy site with pial suture might not be feasible. For those cases, care should be taken not to give too much pressure by pial suture.) Arachnoid membrane is also approximated, not very densely, with 8–0 nylon. For closure of durotomy, continuous, water-tight suture is preferred with 6–0 prolene. Patch graft is not required in most cases. Just before completing the dural closure, the dural sac is filled and inflated with normal saline injection to prevent epidural bleeding and intracranial hypotension.
9. Lamionoplasty is done for all spinal cord tumor cases. If spinal cord compression is a concern due to cord swelling, a lifted laminoplasty with miniplate is a viable option. A few investigator previously advocated that laminoplasty is not mandatory and it might not affect spinal kyphotic deformation in adults [19]. However, laminoplasty has several advantages other than preventing kyphotic deformity. First, it can provide anatomical barrier between muscular layer and dura. Unexpected cord compression by swollen muscles can be prevented with laminoplasty. Second, it can facilitate safe and effective approach in case a revision surgery is required. More importantly, we believe that the risk of CSF leakage could be decreased with laminoplasty. Open wound is closed

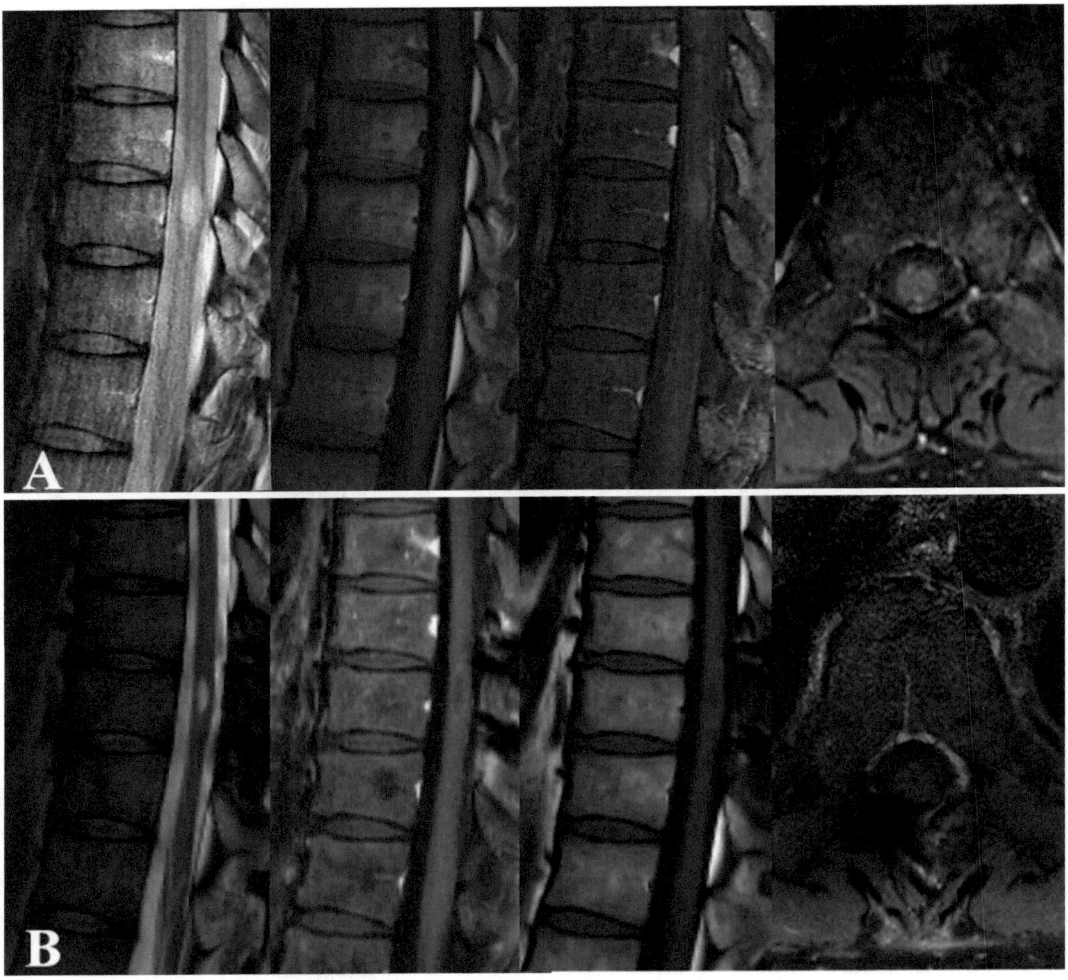

Fig. 14.2 **a** Preoperative magnetic resonance (MR) images of a 45-year-old patient presenting with paresthesia in lower extremities. A 1.5 cm-sized, well-circumscribed mass lesion is seen at T10 level. **b** Postoperative 1-year follow-up MR images

layer by layer without any suction drainage insertion [37].

14.4 Case Review

14.4.1 Case 1. (Video 1)

A 45-year-old male patient visited outpatient clinic complaining of paresthesia in both lower extremities. The symptom started 18 months ago, and aggravated 6 months prior to the visit. Her magnetic resonance (MRI) images revealed $1.5 \times 0.8 \times 0.8$ cm-sized intramedullary lesion at T10 level (Fig. 14.2). There was no hemorrhage or syrinx found. The patient underwent surgical resection and en-bloc tumor removal could be achieved. The paresthesia symptom did not change, though any additional deterioration did not occur after the surgery. The tumor was pathologically diagnosed with grade II ependymoma. Note the several bridging vessels crossing the surface of the tumor and how to deal with it during tumor dissection.

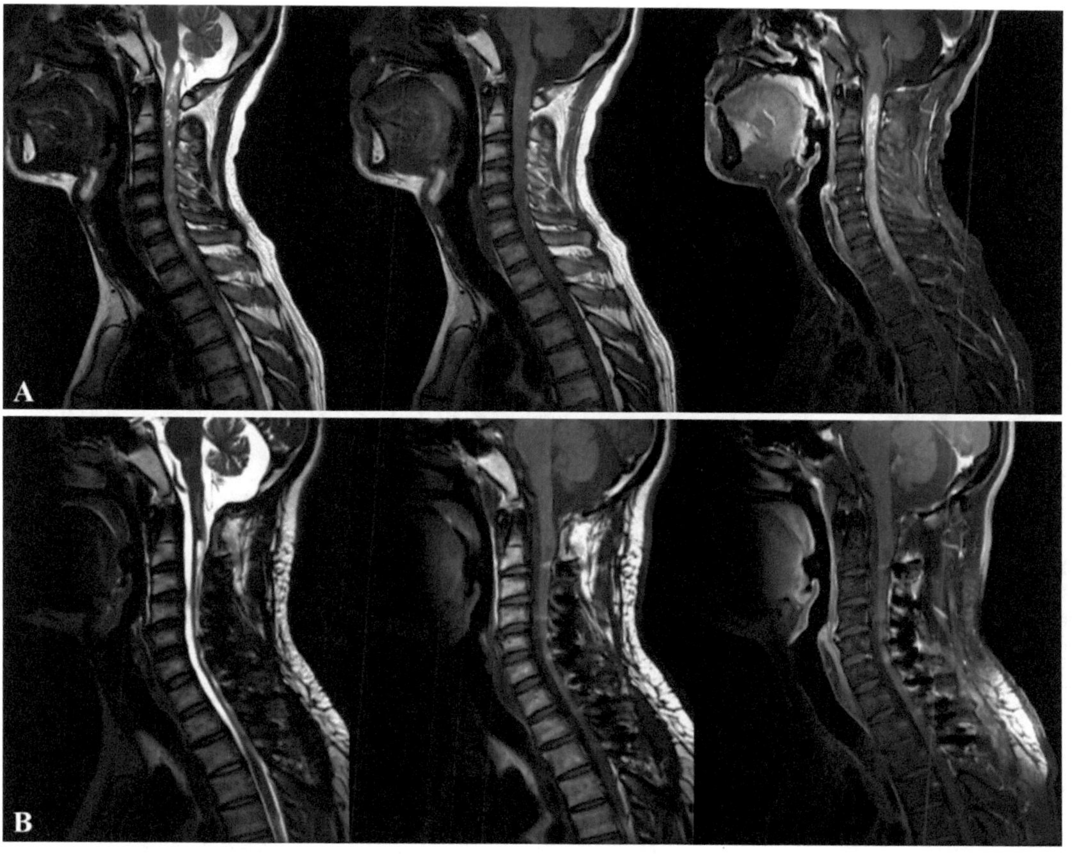

Fig. 14.3 **a** Preoperative magnetic resonance images of a 31-year-old male patient who complained of limb weakness and gait disturbance. Extensive enhancing, predominantly solid, intramedullary mass extending from C2 to T1 level is seen. Tumor-associated syrinx is accompanied at the cervicomedullary junction and upper thoracic level (T2-4). **b** There is no recurrence found in postoperative 2-year follow-up MR images

14.4.2 Case 2 (Video 2)

A 31-year-old man presented with weakness in the limbs and gait disturbance which started 1-year prior to the visit. Motor grade of his upper and lower extremities was grade IV out of V and the patient needed assistant to gait. MRI images show an extensive enhancing intramedullary mass extending through C2 to T1 level (Fig. 14.3). Tumor-associated syrinx was seen in both cranial and caudal end, and cord edema was accompanied. Having impression of ependymoma, a surgery was performed and gross total resection was achieved. Motor power improved to normal at postoperative 3 months, and he returned back to a normal life. Note how to develop dissection plane and manage adhesion between the tumor and the spinal cord.

14.4.3 Case 3 (Video 3)

A 67-year-old female patient presented with paresthesia and cold sensation which started 2 years back and progressively spreading from both legs to upper body. On presentation, the patient exhibited mild dysfunction in proprioception and fine motor of hands. MR images revealed an intramedullary mass extending from C4 to T2 with accompanied syrinx at cephalad and caudal ends (Fig. 14.4). With impression of ependymoma, the surgery was performed and

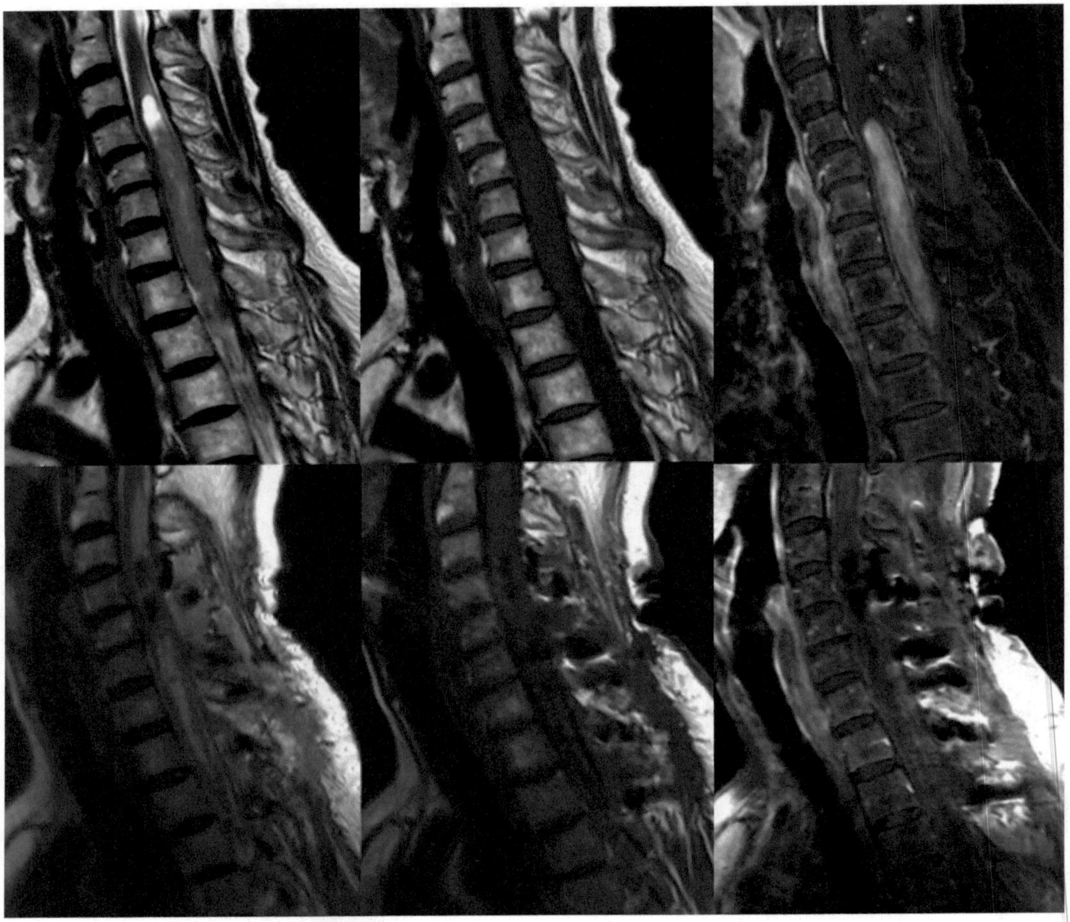

Fig. 14.4 **a** Magnetic resonance images of a 67-year-old female patient presenting with longstanding myelopathic symptoms. An 8.2 cm-sized, solid-enhancing mass with cephalo-caudal syrinx is observed at C4-T2 level. **b** Immediate postoperative MR images after achieving gross total removal

en-bloc removal was achieved. Note that getting into syrinx first and taking it is the starting point of dissection.

14.5 Conclusion

Ependymoma is often a curable disease, and surgical resection is the mainstay of treatment. Nevertheless, it is somewhat challenging to achieve a complete resection minimizing intraoperative neural damage because of its intramedullary location. Therefore, understanding its origin and anatomical relationship with surrounding tissue, and applying proper surgical techniques are imperative for the successful treatment of spinal ependymomas.

References

1. Wu J, Armstrong TS, Gilbert MR. Biology and management of ependymomas. Neuro Oncol. 2016;18:902–13.
2. Connolly ID, Ali R, Li Y, et al. Genetic and molecular distinctions in spinal ependymomas: a review. Clin Neurol Neurosurg. 2015;139:210–5.
3. Schweizer L, Sieber L, Volckmann R, et al. Molecular Classification of ependymal tumors across all CNS Compartments, histopathological grades, and age groups author contributions to the design and conduct of experiments and to the writing HHS public access. Cancer Cell. 2015;27:728–43.

4. Rushing EJ, Cooper PB, Quezado M, et al. Subependymoma revisited: clinicopathological evaluation of 83 cases. J Neurooncol. 2007;85:297–305.
5. Yuh WT, Chung CK, Park SH, et al. Spinal cord subependymoma surgery: a multi-institutional experience. J Korean Neurosurg Soc. 2018;61:233–42.
6. Taylor MD, Poppleton H, Fuller C, et al. Radial glia cells are candidate stem cells of ependymoma. Cancer Cell. 2005;8:323–35.
7. Barton VN, Donson AM, Kleinschmidt-Demasters BK, et al. Unique molecular characteristics of pediatric myxopapillary ependymoma. Brain Pathol. 2010;20:560–70.
8. Milano MT, Johnson MD, Sul J, et al. Primary spinal cord glioma: a surveillance, epidemiology, and end results database study. J Neurooncol. 2010;98:83–92.
9. Schellinger KA, Propp JM, Villano JL, et al. Descriptive epidemiology of primary spinal cord tumors. J Neurooncol. 2008;87:173–9.
10. Jung KW, Park KH, Ha J, et al. Incidence of primary spinal cord, spinal meninges, and cauda equina tumors in Korea, 2006–2010. Cancer Res Treat. 2015;47:166–72.
11. Khalid SI, Adogwa O, Kelly R, et al. Adult Spinal ependymomas: an epidemiologic study. World Neurosurg. 2018;111:e53-61.
12. McCormick PC, Stein BM. Intramedullary tumors in adults. Neurosurg Clin N Am. 1990;1:609–30.
13. Kobayashi K, Ando K, Kato F, et al. MRI characteristics of Spinal ependymoma in WHO grade II. *Spine (Phila Pa 1976)* 2018;43:E525–30.
14. Lee S, Chung CK, Kim CH, et al. with or without adjuvant radiation therapy for treatment of spinal ependymoma: a Spinal oncology research group. Neuro Oncol. 2013;15:921–9.
15. Samii M, Klekamp J. Surgical results of 100 intramedullary tumors in relation to accompanying syringomyelia. *Neurosurgery* 1994;35:865–73; discussion 873.
16. Klekamp J. Spinal ependymomas. Part 1: Intramedullary ependymomas. Neurosurg Focus 2015;39:E6.
17. Fine MJ, Kricheff II, Freed D, et al. Spinal cord ependymomas: MR imaging features. Radiology. 2014;197:655–8.
18. Cristante L, Herrmann HD. Surgical management of intramedullary spinal cord tumors: functional outcome and sources of morbidity. Neurosurgery. 1994;35:66–9.
19. Schwartz TH, McCormick PC. Intramedullary ependymomas: Clinical presentation, surgical treatment strategies and prognosis. J Neurooncol. 2000;47:211–8.
20. Epstein FJ, Farmer JP, Freed D. Adult intramedullary spinal cord ependymomas: The result of surgery in 38 patients. J Neurosurg. 1993;79:204–9.
21. Vera-Bolanos E, Aldape K, Yuan Y, et al. Clinical course and progression-free survival of adult intracranial and spinal ependymoma patients. Neuro Oncol. 2015;17:440–7.
22. Harrop JS, Ganju A, Groff M, et al. Primary Intramedullary tumors of the spinal cord. Spine *(Phila Pa 1976)* 2009;34:S69–77.
23. Oh MC, Ivan ME, Sun MZ, et al. Adjuvant radiotherapy delays recurrence following subtotal resection of spinal cord ependymomas. Neuro Oncol. 2013;15:208–15.
24. Chamberlain MC. Etoposide for recurrent spinal cord ependymoma. Neurology 2002;58:1310–1.
25. Abd-El-Barr MM, Huang KT, Moses ZB, et al. Recent advances in intradural spinal tumors. Neuro Oncol. 2018;20:729–42.
26. Morris KA, Afridi SK, Evans DG, et al. The response of spinal cord ependymomas to bevacizumab in patients with neurofibromatosis Type 2. J Neurosurg Spine. 2016;26:474–82.
27. Fakhrai N, Neophytou P, Dieckmann K, et al. Recurrent spinal ependymoma showing partial remission under Imatimib. Acta Neurochir (Wien). 2004;146:1255–8.
28. Essayed WI, Bernard A, Kalamarides M. Clinical response associated with radiographic regression of a cervicomedullary ependymoma in a NF2 patient treated by bevacizumab. J Neurooncol. 2015;125:445–6.
29. Yeboa DN, Liao K ping, Guadagnolo BA, et al. National Patterns of Care in the Management of World Health Organization Grade II and III Spinal Ependymomas. *World Neurosurg* 2019;124:e580–94.
30. Tao X, Hou Z, Hao S, et al. The clinical features and surgical outcomes of spinal cord tanycytic ependymomas: a report of 40 cases. World Neurosurg. 2017;106:60–73.
31. Keil VC, Schmitt AJ, Martin SC, et al. Optimising treatment strategies in spinal ependymoma based on 20 years of experience at a single centre. J Clin Neurosci. 2016;29:52–8.
32. Wild F, Hartmann C, Heissler HE, et al. Surgical treatment of spinal ependymomas: experience in 49 patients. World Neurosurg. 2018;111:e703–9.
33. Behmanesh B, Gessler F, Dützmann S, et al. Natural history of intramedullary spinal cord ependymoma in patients preferring nonoperative treatment. J Neurooncol. 2017;135:93–8.
34. Yanni DS, Ulkatan S, Deletis V, et al. Utility of neurophysiological monitoring using dorsal column mapping in intramedullary spinal cord surgery. J Neurosurg Spine. 2010;12:623–8.
35. Nagasawa DT, Smith ZA, Cremer N, et al. Complications associated with the treatment for spinal ependymomas. Neurosurg Focus. 2011;31:E13.
36. Jin SH, Chung CK, Kim CH, et al. Multimodal intraoperative monitoring during intramedullary spinal cord tumor surgery. Acta Neurochir (Wien). 2015;157:2149–55.
37. Sohn S, Chung CK, Kim CH. Is closed-suction drainage necessary after intradural primary spinal cord tumor surgery? Eur Spine J. 2013;22:577–83.

Dorsal Column Mapping

15

Han Gil Seo and Min-Gu Kang

Abstract

Midline myelotomy to approach an intramedullary tumor may cause dorsal column injury. Injury to the dorsal columns can result in dysfunction manifesting numbness, dysesthesias, proprioception changes, and sensory ataxia. Dorsal column mapping is a technique to identify the left and right dorsal columns, and the neurophysiological midline of the spinal cord before myelotomy during intramedullary spinal cord tumor surgeries. So far, three methods of dorsal column mapping have been introduced. They are: recording of somatosensory-evoked potentials (SEPs) on the exposed spinal cord with a miniature multielectrode, antidromic sensory nerve action potentials on the peripheral nerves, and phase-reversal SEPs on the scalp. Among them, phase-reversal technique is a fast and easy method which provide real-time feedback to identify the neurophysiologic midline of the spinal cord before myelotomy. Further study is needed to elucidate the role of this technique for prevention of dorsal column injury.

Keywords

Intraoperative neurophysiologic monitoring · Dorsal column mapping · Myelotomy · Intramedullary tumor · Phase-reversal

15.1 Introduction

Intraoperative neurophysiologic monitoring aims to prevent potential injuries which may occur during surgical procedures on the nervous system. Continuous monitoring techniques, such as motor-evoked potentials (MEPs) and somatosensory-evoked potentials (SEPs), are used to assess the functional integrity of the relevant neural structures during the procedures. On the other hand, mapping techniques are used for localization of the functional structures to avoid injuries during the resection. Dorsal column mapping is a technique to identify the left and right dorsal columns, and the neurophysiological midline of the spinal cord before myelotomy during intramedullary spinal cord tumor surgeries [1–3].

Electronic supplementary material The online version of this chapter (https://doi.org/10.1007/978-981-15-7771-0_15) contains supplementary material, which is available to authorized users.

H. G. Seo (✉) · M.-G. Kang
Department of Rehabilitation Medicine, Seoul National University Hospital, Seoul, South Korea
e-mail: hgseo80@gmail.com

M.-G Kang
e-mail: kangmingu.ryan@gmail.com

C. K. Chung (ed.), *Surgery of Spinal Cord Tumors Based on Anatomy*,
https://doi.org/10.1007/978-981-15-7771-0_15

The surgical incision of the spinal cord (i.e., myelotomy) to approach an intramedullary tumor is usually made in the dorsal median raphe because it is a neurophysiologically inactive fibrous structure. Although the dorsal median raphe can be identified anatomically between the elevated dorsal columns or by following the median dorsal sulcal vein, the anatomy may be distorted due to the tumor within the spinal cord. Misidentification of the midline of the spinal cord may lead to dorsal column injury during myelotomy.

Dorsal column dysfunction has been reported to be the most significant morbidity, which occurred more than 40% of patients, after intramedullary spinal tumor surgery [4]. The dorsal column contains the first-order afferents from the largest sensory receptors which convey sensations of fine touch, vibration, two-point discrimination, and proprioception. Injury to the dorsal columns can result in dysfunction manifesting numbness, dysesthesias, proprioception changes, and sensory ataxia. In particular, the gracile fasciculus from the lower limb and lower trunk is prone to injury during the midline myelotomy. Therefore, balance and gait dysfunction could be debilitating consequences after intramedullary spinal cord tumor surgeries.

In this chapter, we introduce the dorsal column mapping techniques to prevent dorsal column injury during myelotomy, focusing on the phase-reversal SEPs technique which is used in our institution. Interpretation, technical considerations, and clinical implications of the technique are also discussed.

15.2 Methods of Dorsal Column Mapping

So far, three methods of dorsal column mapping have been introduced.

(1) Recording of SEPs on the exposed spinal cord with a miniature multielectrode.

Kržan [5] introduced the method of recording of SEPs on the exposed dorsal cord. To record SEPs, the surgeon placed a miniature multielectrode on the midline of the dorsal spinal cord. The multielectrode consists of 8 parallel, 2 mm length Teflon-coated stainless-steel wires which are spaced 1 mm apart, embedded in a 1 cm^2 strip of silastic [5]. Each wire was used as the recording electrode, while a needle electrode was placed in nearby muscle as the reference electrode. Electrical activities were recorded by recording wires on the dorsal cord during electrical stimulation of each of the posterior tibial nerves at the medial malleolus via subdermal needles. The impedance and filter settings were 20 kΩ and 50–1700 Hz [2]. The stimulus intensity, duration, and the repetition rate were 40 mA, 0.2 ms, and 13.3 Hz, respectively [2]. After averaging two sets of 100 sweeps from the eight recording electrodes, the recording wire showing the maximal amplitude was considered to be placed on the densest fibers of the stimulated gracile fasciculus. After stimulating each side of posterior tibial nerves, the midline between the two wires of maximal amplitudes was regarded as the neurophysiological midline which was electrically inert area. Therefore, the surgeon made an incision through the line to prevent dorsal column injury.

The multielectrode could record high-quality and high-amplitude SEPs [6]. However, there are some weaknesses in this method. Above all, it needs a specially designed multielectrode which is not available in many institutions. The electrode is not easy to keep good contact with the dorsal spinal cord, especially due to pulsation artifacts. Therefore, a greater number of averages are needed. Activities in the dorsal roots and horns provoked by the higher-amplitude segmental responses might contaminate the SEPs [6]. Lastly, the variable signal-to-noise ratio can lead to amplitude fluctuation [7].

(2) Recording of antidromic sensory nerve action potentials on the peripheral nerves.

Quinones-Hinojosa et al. [1] described the method of recording of antidromic sensory nerve action potentials (SNAPs) on the peripheral nerves. Needle electrodes were placed on the medial malleoli of the patient's ankles to record the SNAPs antidromically. To stimulate the dorsal column, the surgeon used a handheld bipolar stimulator with a spacing of 2–3 mm between the anodal and cathodal tips. The filter settings were 30–300 Hz [1]. The stimulus intensity, duration, and the repetition rate were 3–8 mA, 200 μs, and 9.1 Hz [1]. A ruler with 5 mm mark was placed on the apparent anatomic midline and then five areas were stimulated in turn at 1 mm interval with the cathodal tip pointing distally. After averaging 50–100 sweeps on each point, the area showing minimal response was considered as the neurophysiological midline and selected as the incision site.

Because this method needs five points stimulation in turn with up to 100 sweeps, it is a time-consuming procedure. In addition, the surgeon should hold the stimulator still during the averaging. If the bipolar stimulator moves during the average, a new stimulation should be started. This method is technically challenging due to low amplitudes, and the action potentials can be contaminated by the compound motor action potentials (CMAPs) [7].

(3) Recording of phase-reversal SEPs on the scalp.

Simon et al. [7] introduced the method of recording of phase-reversal SEPs on the scalp. SEPs were recorded from the ipsilateral and contralateral parietal scalp area (CP3 and CP4) via scalp electrodes. To stimulate the spinal cord, the surgeon placed a minielectrode on the exposed dorsal cord perpendicular to the spine. The minielectrode consists of 8-contact strip of 2 mm stainless steel wires with 1 mm spacing. The electrical pulses were delivered via two adjacent wires. The stimulation was applied in succession from left to right. This way, the surgeon could find the neurophysiologic midline when CP3–CP4 channel showed a phase-reversal of SEPs. The stimulus intensity, duration, and repetition rate were 0.2 mA, 0.3 ms, and 3.17 Hz. The high signal-to-noise ratio could reduce the number of averages to 10 sweeps. However, there was a possibility of current spread and not only gracile fasciculus but also cuneate fasciculus could be stimulated. In addition, the minielectrode required several repositions and it was hard to sustain good contact due to the spinal cord pulsation.

Nair et al. [3] modified the phase-reversal method. CP3 and CP4 scalp recording electrodes were used the same as the previous method, but Cz–Fz channel was added to identify current spread. In place of minielectrode, the surgeon used a handheld bipolar stimulator. The stimulator was placed on the exposed dorsal cord with the prongs parallel to the cord axis and gradually repositioned from one side to the other side. The stimulus current was used from 0.3 to 0.5 mA to minimalize the current spread. The neurophysiologic midline was considered to be located in the area showing minimal amplitudes in all channels including Cz–Fz, and a phase-reversal of SEPs was observed across the area. The refined technique was thought to be a fast and reliable method which provide real-time feedback [3].

15.3 Interpretation

Recorded potentials from the scalp electrodes by stimulating the gracile fasciculus on the dorsal surface of the spinal cord are equivalent to those by stimulating the posterior tibial nerves. When stimulating the left dorsal column, initial positive and then negative peaks are usually seen in the CP3–CP4 channel (Fig. 15.1). These potentials correspond to P37 and N45 when recording the tibial nerve SEP, although the latencies are shorter when stimulating the dorsal column. The distribution of SEPs on the scalp, which is a maximum response at the vertex and a paradoxical ipsilateral extension, by stimulation of the efferent fibers from the lower extremity is known to be "paradoxical lateralization of cortical potentials." [7, 8] This phenomenon is thought to be due to the primary somatosensory region for the foot is situated on the medial surface of the contralateral postcentral gyrus in the interhemispheric fissure. Because the cortical generators are oriented transversely or horizontally to the scalp surface, the responses are best recorded in the electrodes over the ipsilateral hemisphere [8]. However, unlike the stimulation of the posterior tibial nerve, the efferent fibers from the whole

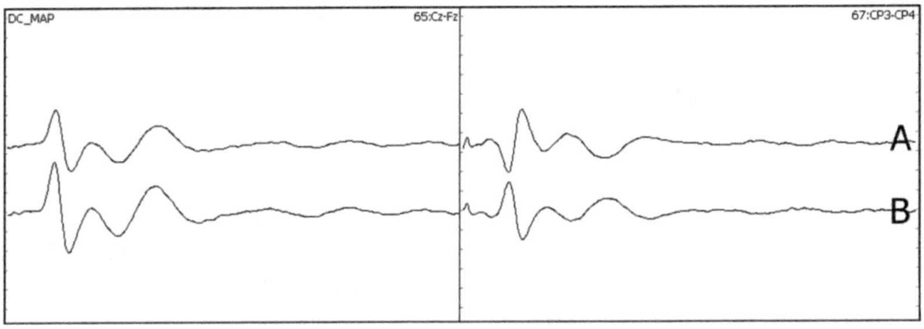

Fig. 15.1 Recorded potentials in the Cz–Fz and CP3–CP4 channels by stimulation of the left (**a**) and right (**b**) gracile fasciculi. Initial positive and subsequent negative peaks are seen in the CP3–CP4 channel when stimulating the left side, and they are reversed when stimulating the right side

lower extremity can be stimulated during the dorsal column mapping. The cortical generators of the proximal lower extremity are located superficially, not deep in the interhemispheric fissure. In some cases, only negative peaks are remarkable due to very small initial positive peaks. In our experience, the expected waveform may not appear during the mapping for a variety of reasons (Fig. 15.2).

The physiological midline of the spinal cord can be identified by a phase-reversal in the CP3–CP4 channel when the bipolar stimulator is moved across the midline. Sometimes, this mapping procedure is necessary at several different spinal cord level due to distorted anatomy by the tumor. If the bipolar stimulator is placed across the midline, both gracile fasciculi are stimulated simultaneously. In such a case, the cancellation of the polarities occurs in the CP3–CP4 channel, whereas the response remains the same or becomes larger due to summation of the same polarity potentials in the Cz–Fz channel [3]. This finding confirms that the midline is between the two electrodes of the stimulator (Fig. 15.3). If no reliable signals are recorded in both CP3–CP4 and Cz–Fz channels, the stimulation site is neurophysiologically inert region. If the location is not the dorsal median raphe, the tumor may be near the pial surface. Depending on the surgeon's preference, the incision can be made at this location without damage to the dorsal column.

15.4 Technical Considerations

Anesthetic considerations for dorsal column mapping via phase-reversal method are the same as those of SEP monitoring. Total intravenous anesthesia (TIVA) is recommended for this method because the cortical potentials are significantly affected by inhalation anesthetics. Propofol and opioids mildly suppress SEPs signals and have no significant influence on identifying changes in polarity of the evoked potentials.

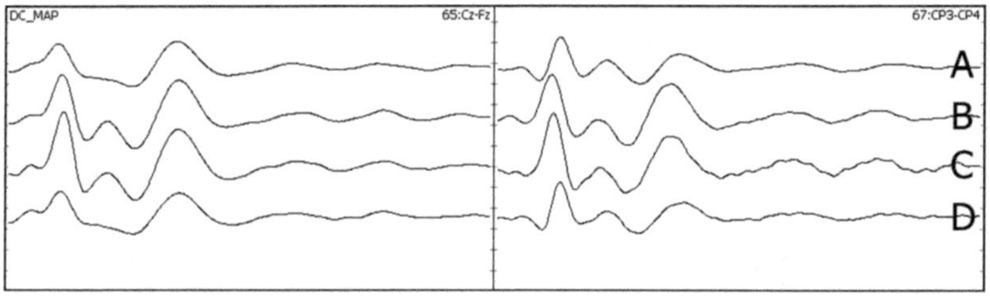

Fig. 15.2 Recorded potentials in the Cz–Fz and CP3–CP4 channels by stimulation of the left (**a**, **d**) and right (**b**, **c**) gracile fasciculi. Although small initial positive peaks are seen when stimulating the left side, only negative peaks are notable when stimulating the right side. Phase reversal is also not clear between the left and right gracile fasciculi

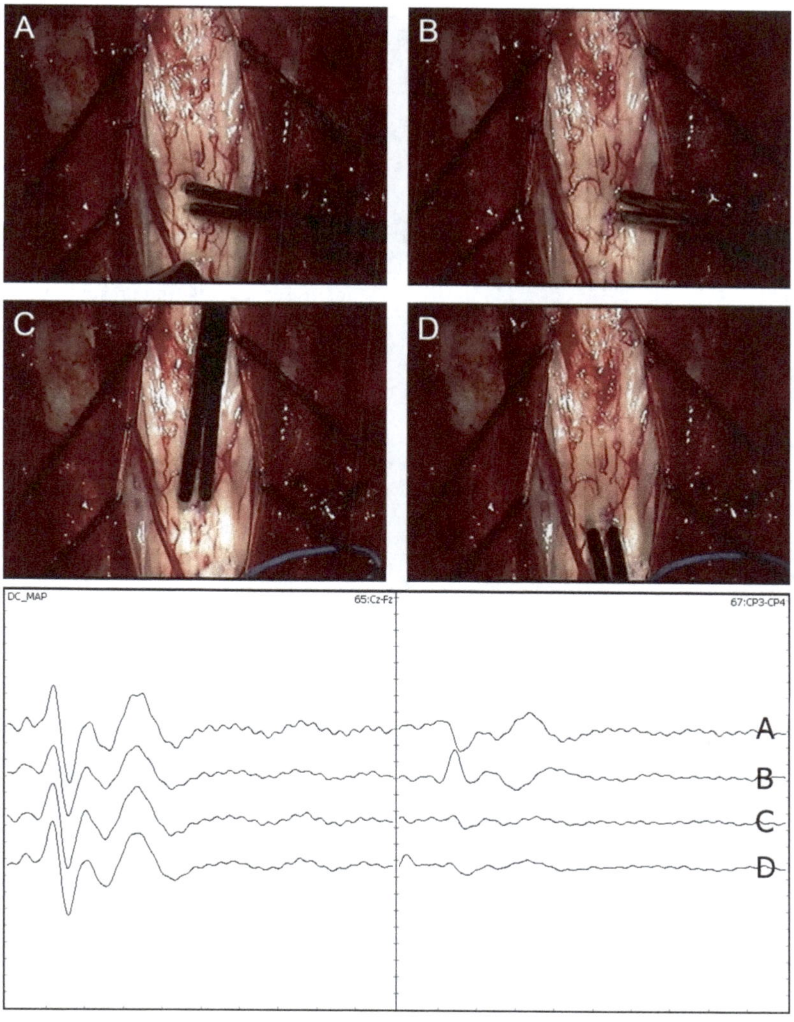

Fig. 15.3 Identification of the physiological midline by dorsal column mapping using a bipolar stimulator. In the CP3–CP4 channel, a phase-reversal is observed by stimulation of the right (**a**) and left (**b**) gracile fasciculi across the midline. When stimulating both fasciculi simultaneously using the bipolar stimulator placed across the midline, the response disappears by the cancellation of the polarities in the CP3–CP4 channel without change in the Cz–Fz channel (**c**, **d**). Therefore, the physiologic midline is located between the two electrodes

Larger number of sensory fibers are stimulated at the gracile fasciculus, more robust signals are usually obtained by this technique compared to tibial nerve SEPs. Therefore, the signal-to-noise ratio is high and a small number of averages per recorded response is necessary. An adequate response may be obtained by around 10 stimuli [7]. In a noisy environment, an average of up to 30 stimuli may be required.

15.5 Clinical Implications

Although mapping techniques provide intuitive information about the location of neural structures, the evidence of their clinical utility is hard to be established. So far, only one study, which employed recording of antidromic sensory nerve action potentials for dorsal column mapping, demonstrated significant decrease of new postoperative dorsal column dysfunction compared to the historical control (9% vs. 50%) [9]. Other studies were case reports or case series which had no controls. Nair et al. [3] reported that the phase-reversal mapping technique using a bipolar stimulator is successfully applied in 12 cases. The dorsal median raphes were localized by the mapping technique in 11 patients and no one had postoperative worsening of the dorsal column function. Yanni et al. [2] reported that dorsal column mapping by recording of SEPs on the spinal cord with a strip electrode were successful in all 10 patients. One patient showed initially worsened dorsal column function postoperatively. Kržan [5] described that reproducible spinal SEPs were obtained using a miniature multielectrode in 55 of the 65 patients without a report of postoperative outcomes.

We reviewed 39 patients who were operated for intramedullary spinal cord tumors at our hospital. Dorsal column mapping via phase-reversal method was performed in 19 out of 39 patients in which midline myelotomy was needed due to the etiology (e.g. ependymoma) of the patients. The phase-reversal was definite in 10 out of 19 patients and not clear in the other 9 patients. The rate of functional deterioration measured by Bergs Balance Scale and 10-m Walk Test was comparable between the patients with and without definite phase-reversal on dorsal column mapping. Therefore, we are still reluctant to draw the conclusion that we can confidently depend on this technique. Phase-reversal technique is a fast and easy method which provide real-time feedback to identify the neurophysiologic midline of the spinal cord before myelotomy. However, technical improvements are necessary to reduce negative mapping cases and improve the reliability of the method. In addition, further study is needed to elucidate the role of this technique for prevention of dorsal column injury during the surgery of intramedullary spinal cord tumors.

References

1. Quinones-Hinojosa A, Gulati M, Lyon R, Gupta N, Yingling C. Spinal cord mapping as an adjunct for resection of intramedullary tumors: surgical technique with case illustrations. Neurosurgery 2002;51:1199–206; discussion 206–7.
2. Yanni DS, Ulkatan S, Deletis V, Barrenechea IJ, Sen C, Perin NI. Utility of neurophysiological monitoring using dorsal column mapping in intramedullary spinal cord surgery. J Neurosurg Spine. 2010;12:623–8.
3. Nair D, Kumaraswamy VM, Braver D, Kilbride RD, Borges LF, Simon MV. Dorsal column mapping via phase reversal method: the refined technique and clinical applications. Neurosurgery 2014;74:437–46; discussion 46.
4. Manzano G, Green BA, Vanni S, Levi AD. Contemporary management of adult intramedullary spinal tumors-pathology and neurological outcomes related to surgical resection. Spinal Cord. 2008;46:540–6.
5. Kržan MJ. Intraoperative Neurophysiological Mapping of the Spinal Cord's Dorsal Columns. In: Deletis V, Shils JL, editors. Neurophysiology in neurosurgery: a modern intraoperative approach, 1st ed. Amsterdam, Boston: Academic Press;2002. pp. 153–65.
6. Deletis V, Shils J. Neurophysiology in neurosurgery: a modern intraoperative approach: Elsevier;2002.
7. Simon MV, Chiappa KH, Borges LF. Phase reversal of somatosensory evoked potentials triggered by gracilis tract stimulation: case report of a new technique for neurophysiologic dorsal column mapping. Neurosurgery. 2012;70:E783–8.
8. Cruse R, Klem G, Lesser RP, Leuders H. Paradoxical lateralization of cortical potentials evoked by stimulation of posterior tibial nerve. Arch Neurol. 1982;39:222–5.
9. Mehta AI, Mohrhaus CA, Husain AM, et al. Dorsal column mapping for intramedullary spinal cord tumor resection decreases dorsal column dysfunction. J Spinal Disord Tech. 2012;25:205–9.

Diffusion Tensor Imaging

16

Roh-Eul Yoo

Abstract

Diffusion tensor imaging (DTI) is an advanced imaging technique which enables quantification of anisotropic diffusion (i.e., restricted or preferential diffusion to one particular direction) in terms of direction and magnitude on a voxel-by-voxel basis. Serial calculation of anisotropic diffusion in neighboring voxels can provide the information on the integrity of longitudinal structures such as fiber tracts in spinal cord and therefore reflect the earlier physiological disturbance along fiber tracts prior to the development of any structural changes. Both qualitative/visual (i.e., fiber tracking techniques [tractography]) and quantitative (DTI anisotropy indices such as fractional anisotropy [FA] and apparent diffusion coefficient [ADC]) methods have been used to assess changes in anisotropic diffusion along the spinal cord. Tractography has been used for the visual assessment of the relationship between white matter tracts and spinal cord tumors and has been shown to be helpful in the differential diagnosis of intramedullary tumors. Furthermore, information on the relationship between spinal cord tumors and normal fibers from preoperative DTI tractography can further assist in surgical planning and thus help improve the surgical outcome.

Keywords

Anisotropic diffusion · Anisotropy indices · Diffusion tensor imaging (DTI) · Intramedullary tumors · Surgical planning · Tractography

16.1 Basic Concepts

(1) Diffusion

'Diffusion (or Brownian motion)' refers to a random translational moment of water molecules within body tissue, driven by inherent latent thermal energy of the molecules. Unrestricted diffusion of water molecules in all directions (as in cerebral spine fluid [CSF]) is termed 'isotropic', whereas restricted or preferential diffusion to one particular direction due to the presence of biological barriers (as in muscle fibers and axons) is termed 'anisotropic' (Fig. 16.1). Diffusion tensor imaging (DTI) is an advanced imaging technique which enables quantification of anisotropic diffusion in terms of direction and magnitude on a voxel-by-voxel

R.-E. Yoo (✉)
Department of Radiology, Seoul National University Hospital, 101 Daehak-ro, Jongno-gu, Seoul 110-744, South Korea
e-mail: roheul7@gmail.com

C. K. Chung (ed.), *Surgery of Spinal Cord Tumors Based on Anatomy*,
https://doi.org/10.1007/978-981-15-7771-0_16

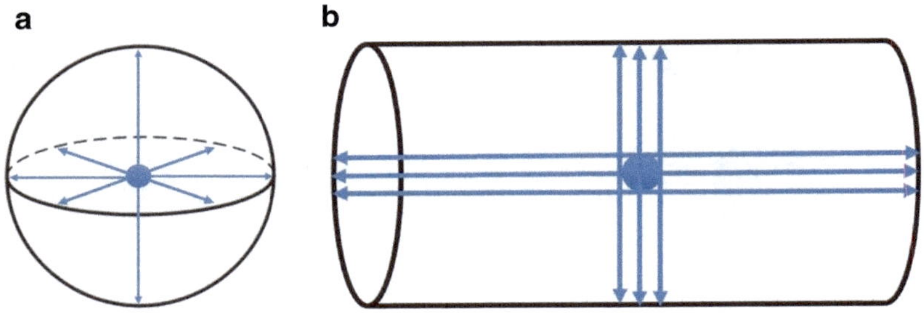

Fig. 16.1 Illustrations showing isotropic and anisotropic diffusion. Isotropic diffusion is comparable to diffusion of water molecules in a sphere (**a**) where the molecules can diffuse in all directions equally. Anisotropic diffusion is comparable to diffusion of water molecules in a cylinder (**b**) where there is a preferential diffusion of water molecules to one particular direction

basis. Serial calculation of the direction and magnitude of anisotropic diffusion in neighboring voxels can provide the information on the integrity of longitudinal structures such as fiber tracts in spinal cord. DTI may be used as an adjunct to conventional structural imaging in spinal cord, because it is thought to have the potential to reflect the earlier physiological disturbance along fiber tracts prior to the development of any structural changes. Both qualitative/visual (i.e., fiber tracking techniques [tractography]) and quantitative (DTI anisotropy indices) methods have been used to assess changes in anisotropic diffusion using DTI [1].

(2) Diffusion Tensor Tractography

Tractography provides a visual representation of the anisotropic diffusion and allows qualitative assessment of the overall diffusion status within the evaluated structure. Anisotropic diffusion in an axon, in which water molecules move preferentially in one direction over others, is compared to that in an ellipsoid (Fig. 16.2). Water molecules move along three directions (x, y, z) in an ellipsoid, represented by three eigenvectors (E1, E2, and E3), where E1 denotes the main vector along the long axis. Tractography can be derived by serially connecting the E1 vectors of adjacent voxels and color coding is often used

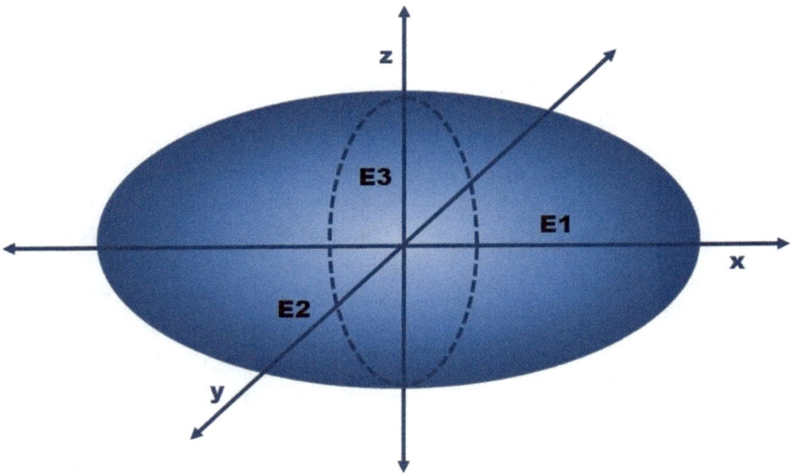

Fig. 16.2 An ellipsoid model to describe anisotropic diffusion in a neuron. The ellipsoid has three eigenvectors (E1, E2, and E3) in x, y, and z directions with E1 being the main vector along the long axis. Various diffusion tensor indices including FA and ADC can be calculated from the eigenvector values and tractography can be constructed by connecting the main eigenvector (E1)

to better represent the three different directions of diffusion—for example, red for left to right, green for anteroposterior, and blue for craniocaudal directions. In comparison to brain where multi-directionality of fibers is represented by multiple colors, tractography of spinal cords is usually shown in blue because intact fiber tracts run mainly in craniocaudal direction [1].

(3) Diffusion Anisotropy Indices
Anisotropy indices are quantitative measures for diffusion in a given voxel. Various indices indicating the direction and magnitude of diffusion can be calculated from the eigenvector values, including mean diffusivity (MD, often referred to as the apparent diffusion coefficient [ADC]), fractional anisotropy (FA), radial diffusivity (Dr), and axial diffusivity (Da). Two most popular DTI measures are FA and ADC. FA, a direction parameter, represents the fraction of the magnitude of 'anisotropic' diffusion in a voxel and its value ranges from 0 (e.g., sphere with completely isotropic diffusion) to 1 (e.g., thinnest cylinder with infinite anisotropy). High degree of anisotropy results in FA value close to 1 in intact neurons, and the FA value decreases when the diffusion becomes less restricted (more isotropic) because of the injury of axonal membrane. Apparent diffusion coefficient (ADC), a magnitude parameter, quantifies how much free diffusion of water molecules are restricted due to anatomic barriers such as local tissue microstructures (e.g., myelin sheath) within neurons. Specifically, intact neurons with well-organized nerve fibers exhibit low ADC value, whereas injured neurons with disorganized fibers demonstrate high ADC value [1].

16.2 DTI in Preoperative Evaluation of Spinal Cord Tumors

(1) Diffusion Anisotropy Indices
Among various anisotropy indices, FA is the most commonly used to reflect earlier physiological disturbance along fiber tracts. Several studies have demonstrated that FA values are significantly lower in most enhancing or non-enhancing spinal cord tumors than in normal fibers in volunteers or reference regions, which may be attributable to destruction of normal fibers by tumor infiltration. [2–12] The studies suggest that the FA map may help detect the abnormality and determine its extent in spinal cord lesions. On the other hand, quantitative ADC values have been reported to be variable in spinal cord tumors [9].

(2) DTI Fiber Tractography
Tractography has been used for the visual assessment of the relationship between white matter tracts and spinal cord tumors. [1–8, 10–18] Three major types of relationships have been previously described and used as clues for the discrimination of intramedullary ependymomas from astrocytomas as well as the diagnosis of benign spinal cord tumors: ① fibers not entering solid lesions, ② most of the tumor volume not containing fibers with only some fibers crossing tumors, and ③ most of the tumor volume containing fibers. [12] Specifically, full displacement of fibers has been regarded as an imaging characteristic of benign spinal cord tumors. [2, 4, 5, 7, 10, 12] In addition, intramedullary astrocytomas are the key differential diagnosis for ependymomas but conventional MR imaging may not suffice to differentiate the two when they lack typical features. Tractography may provide additional diagnostic clue in those cases, since spinal cord ependymomas with delicate capsules forming the interface between tumors and surrounding normal neural tissue tend to displace fibers (Fig. 16.3), whereas astrocytomas with more infiltrative growth pattern tend to encase fibers in the spinal cord (Fig. 16.4). [4, 10, 19] Nonetheless, diagnostic challenge remains, because low-grade astrocytomas, which account for the majority of astrocytomas (75%–89%), can also displace white matter tracts like ependymomas [1–3, 5, 7, 10, 12, 17, 18].

More importantly, information on the relationship between spinal cord tumors and normal fibers from preoperative DTI tractography can further assist in surgical planning [8]. First, DTI tractography may be used to determine the resectability of spinal cord tumors. Previous

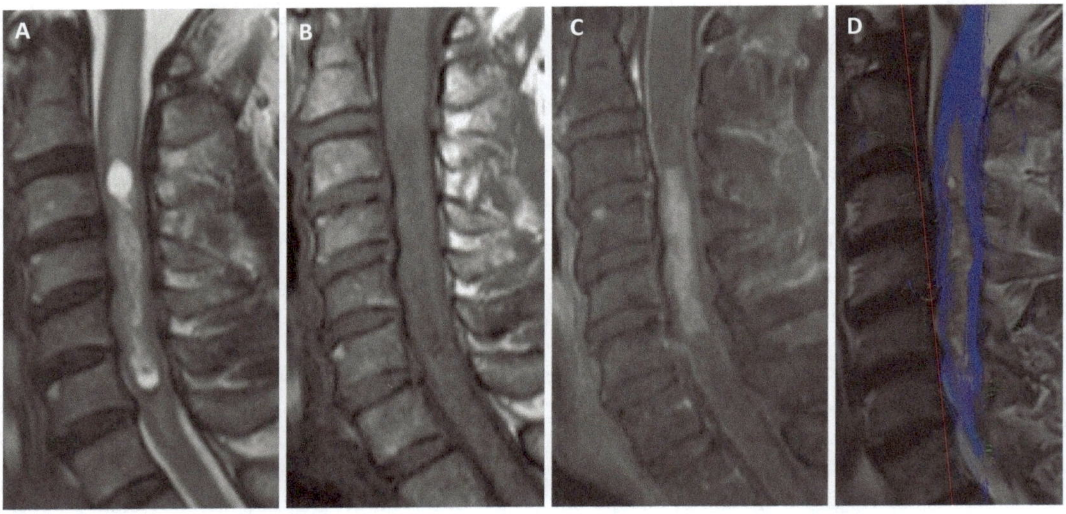

Fig. 16.3 A 66-year-old man with intramedullary ependymoma. Conventional sagittal T2-weighted (**a**), precontrast and postcontrast T1-weighted (**b** and **c**) images demonstrate an intramedullary mass at the cervical spine with an enhancing solid component and intratumoral hemorrhage. DTI tractography (**d**) well demonstrates splaying of the surrounding white matter tracts by the tumor

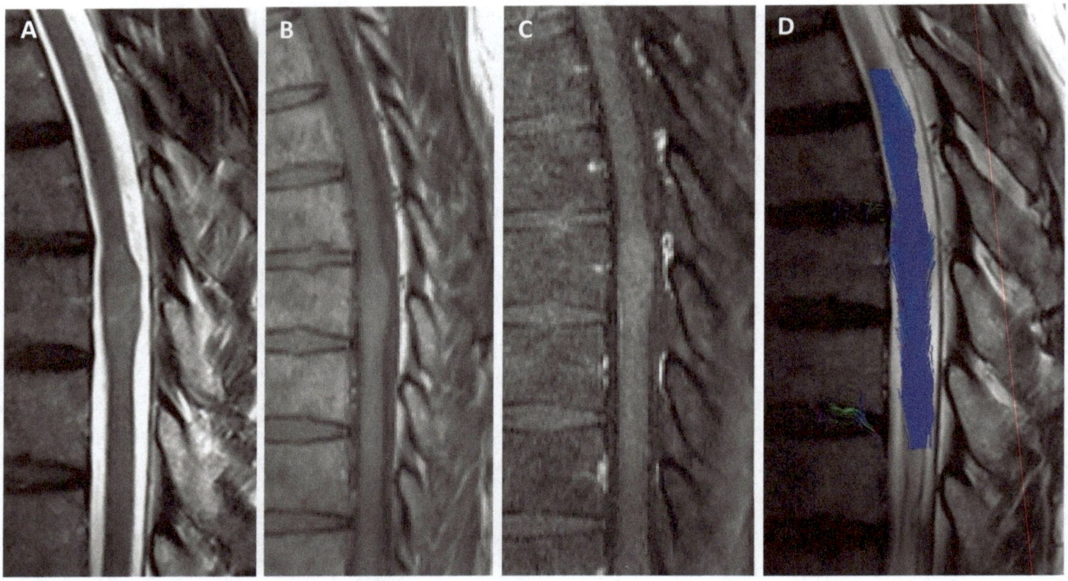

Fig. 16.4 A 60-year-old man with intramedullary astrocytoma. Conventional sagittal T2-weighted (**a**), precontrast and postcontrast T1-weighted (**b** and **c**) images depict an intramedullary mass with no definite contrast enhancement at the cervical spine. On DTI tractography (**d**), normal fibers are encased by the tumor, a finding which suggests a more infiltrative growth pattern

studies have demonstrated that the resectability determined based on the fiber course relative to the lesion show strong correlations with intraoperative and neurologic findings [11, 12]. Specifically, tumors that encase normal fibers have been considered unresectable because complete resection is likely to cause a significant neurologic deficit, whereas tumors that displace fibers have been considered resectable. Second, DTI tractography may be used to determine the optimal surgical approach that can minimize the unnecessary nerve injury and guide the surgery during neuronavigation [12]. DTI tractography-guided surgical resection is of clinical importance in that it can increase the chance of preservation of neurologic function while ensuring maximal resection of tumors, which in turn would ultimately help improve the surgical outcome [5, 7, 10].

References

1. Rajasekaran S, Kanna RM, Shetty AP. Diffusion tensor imaging of the spinal cord and its clinical applications. J Bone Joint Surg Br. 2012;94:1024–31.
2. Alkherayf F, Arab AF, Tsai E. Conus Medullaris Teratoma with utilization of fiber tractography: case report. J Neurol Surg Rep. 2015;76:e183–7.
3. Baruah D, Chandra T, Bajaj M, et al. A simplified algorithm for diagnosis of spinal cord lesions. Curr Probl Diagn Radiol. 2015;44:256–66.
4. Bloomer CW, Ackerman A, Bhatia RG. Imaging for spine tumors and new applications. Top Magn Reson Imaging. 2006;17:69–87.
5. Choudhri AF, Whitehead MT, Klimo P Jr, Montgomery BK, Boop FA. Diffusion tensor imaging to guide surgical planning in intramedullary spinal cord tumors in children. Neuroradiology. 2014;56:169–74.
6. Ducreux D, Lepeintre JF, Fillard P, Loureiro C, Tadie M, Lasjaunias P. MR diffusion tensor imaging and fiber tracking in 5 spinal cord astrocytomas. AJNR Am J Neuroradiol. 2006;27:214–6.
7. Landi A, Palmarini V, D'Elia A, et al. Magnetic resonance diffusion tensor imaging and fiber-tracking diffusion tensor tractography in the management of spinal astrocytomas. World J Clin Cases. 2016;4:1–4.
8. Liu X, Tian W, Chen H, et al. Advanced neuroimaging in the evaluation of spinal cord tumors and tumor mimics: diffusion tensor and perfusion-weighted imaging. Semin Ultrasound CT MR. 2017;38:163–75.
9. Liu X, Tian W, Kolar B, et al. Advanced MR diffusion tensor imaging and perfusion weighted imaging of intramedullary tumors and tumor like lesions in the cervicomedullary junction region and the cervical spinal cord. J Neurooncol. 2014;116:559–66.
10. Mechtler LL, Nandigam K. Spinal cord tumors: new views and future directions. Neurol Clin. 2013;31:241–68.
11. Phillips NS, Sanford RA, Helton KJ, et al. Diffusion tensor imaging of intraaxial tumors at the cervicomedullary and pontomedullary junctions. Report of two cases. J Neurosurg. 2005;103:557–62.
12. Setzer M, Murtagh RD, Murtagh FR, et al. Diffusion tensor imaging tractography in patients with intramedullary tumors: comparison with intraoperative findings and value for prediction of tumor resectability. J Neurosurg Spine. 2010;13:371–80.
13. Bosma R, Stroman PW. Diffusion tensor imaging in the human spinal cord: development, limitations, and clinical applications. Crit Rev Biomed Eng. 2012;40:1–20.
14. Ducreux D, Fillard P, Facon D, et al. Diffusion tensor magnetic resonance imaging and fiber tracking in spinal cord lesions: current and future indications. Neuroimaging Clin N Am. 2007;17:137–47.
15. Renoux J, Facon D, Fillard P, Huynh I, Lasjaunias P, Ducreux D. MR diffusion tensor imaging and fiber tracking in inflammatory diseases of the spinal cord. AJNR Am J Neuroradiol. 2006;27:1947–51.
16. Schellinger KA, Propp JM, Villano JL, McCarthy BJ. Descriptive epidemiology of primary spinal cord tumors. J Neurooncol. 2008;87:173–9.
17. Thurnher MM, Law M. Diffusion-weighted imaging, diffusion-tensor imaging, and fiber tractography of the spinal cord. Magn Reson Imaging Clin N Am. 2009;17:225–44.
18. Vargas MI, Delavelle J, Jlassi H, et al. Clinical applications of diffusion tensor tractography of the spinal cord. Neuroradiology. 2008;50:25–9.
19. Van Goethem JW, van den Hauwe L, Ozsarlak O, De Schepper AM, Parizel PM. Spinal tumors. Eur J Radiol. 2004;50:159–76.

Electrophysiological Study Including EP, EMG, NCS

17

Sung-Min Kim

Abstract

Diverse electrophysiological studies, including evoked potential, electromyography, and nerve conduction studies, are currently used in the operating room to spare the function of the spinal cord during surgery. Here, we dealt with the basic principles, advantages, and limitations of each electrophysiological study.

Keywords

Electrophysiological study · Nerve conduction study · Evoked potential · Electromyography · Nerve conduction study

17.1 Basic Principles

To understand how the electrophysiologic study can help to spare the functions of the spinal cord during surgery, it is necessary to understand the basic principles in generating the electrical potentials in the nervous system.

S.-M. Kim (✉)
Department of Neurology, Seoul National University Hospital, Seoul, South Korea
e-mail: sueh916@gmail.com

The commonly using electrophysiologic studies for intraoperative monitoring of the spinal cord include nerve conduction study, electromyography, motor evoked potential, and somatosensory evoked potentials. For any type of studies above, recording the electric signal with either the surface or needle electrodes is required to obtain the electrophysiologic signals from the designated nervous systems. In recording the electrophysiologic signals, intracellular electric potentials are transmitted through the extracellular structures. This type of transmission of electric or magnetic fields toward measuring sensors, across a distance from their source generators, is termed as volume conduction [1].

For the studies above, the volume conduction can be obtained either in the form of the near-field potentials or far-field potentials. The near-field potential can be recorded when the recording electrode is close to the source of the volume conduction. It has a higher amplitude, inversely correlated with the distance from the source to the electrode, than the far-field potential. The examples of the near-field potentials are NCS, compound muscle action potential recordings, N9 potential (recorded in the Erb's point) in SSEP, and cortically recorded potentials in SSEP (N19 or N20 for MNSEP and P37 for PTSEP). When recorded with a monopolar recording electrode, the near-field potential can produce a typical triphasic waveform

C. K. Chung (ed.), *Surgery of Spinal Cord Tumors Based on Anatomy*,
https://doi.org/10.1007/978-981-15-7771-0_17

(Fig. 17.1). In real clinical practice, it is not always possible to place electrode directly onto the nerve of interest. In this case, the electrophysiologic testing for the nervous structure should be performed using far-field potential. The exact generator of far-field potential has not been fully known, and probably multiple generators can be involved in each far-field potential. Due to its small amplitude, most of the far-field potential need to be recorded through averaging the signals that are obtained by multiple testing. The waveform P14 and N18 in the median nerve SSEP corresponds to the far-field potential.

17.2 Somatosensory Evoked Potential

The SSEP for spinal cord monitoring can usually be performed using either stimulation of the median nerve (median nerve somatosensory evoked potential, MNSEP) or the posterior tibial nerve (PTSEP). These stimulations in the peripheral nerve will travel via nervous system in an afferent way, and thereby activate the plexus (can be recorded in the Erb's point via near-field potential), nerve root, posterior column of the spinal cord, brainstem, thalamus, and finally the sensory cortex (N20 for the MNSEP and P37 for the PTSEP). For the clinical testing of SSEP for the outpatients, both the near-field potential and far-field potential are commonly adapted. However, for the intraoperative monitoring of the spinal cord, the near-field potentials that represent the volume conduction of the sensory cortex (N20 or P37) are most commonly used due to the limitation in the channel, time, etc. The name of the waveforms in SSEP was determined according to their polarity and latency. Per se, the N20 is the negative potential that is recorded after a latency of 20 ms of stimulation (Fig. 17.2). The recording of both the N20 and P37 is performed via an averaging process to have a better signal to noise ratio, especially to minimize the effect of the 60 Hz artifacts. One of the great advantages of using the SSEP for the intraoperative monitoring (IOM) is that it can produce quite constant waveforms in each testing thereby lesser inter-trial variations. The definite warning criteria for the SSEP changes during the IOM of the spinal cord can be dependent on the types of the surgery (cervical

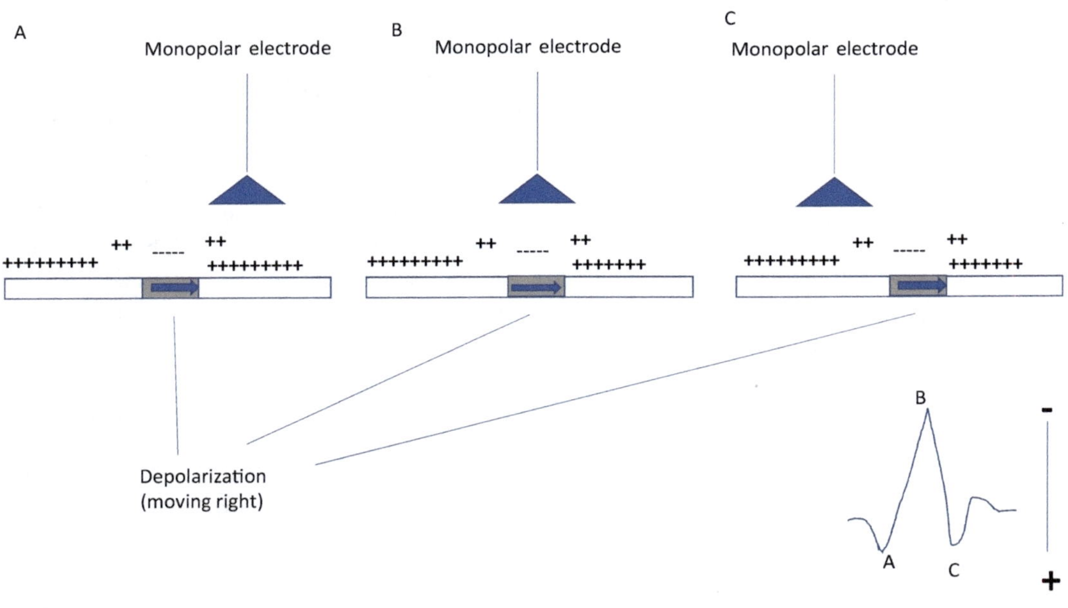

Fig. 17.1 Schematic diagram for the triphasic waveform obtained via near-field potential recording from a nerve

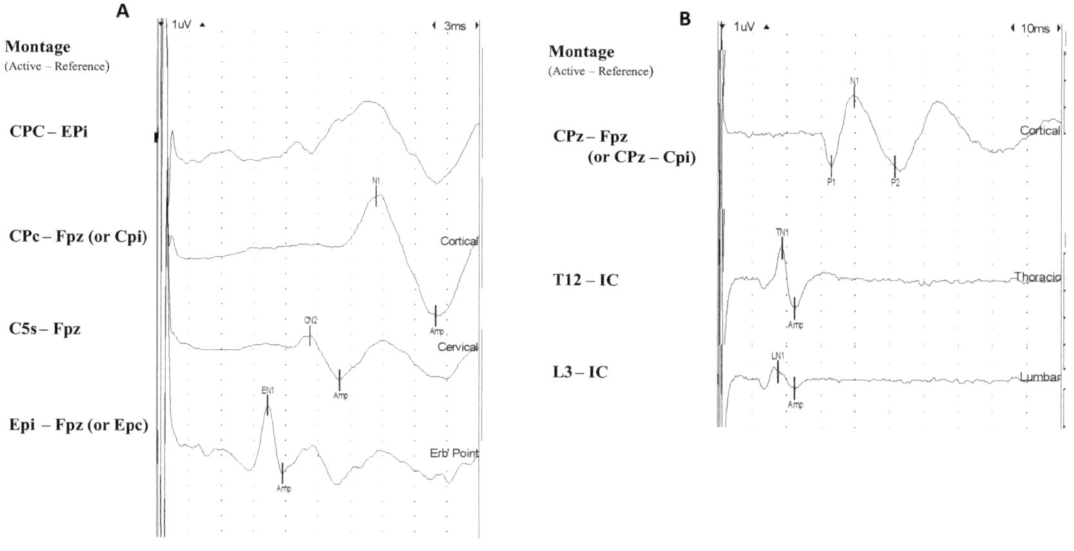

Fig. 17.2 Examples of the waveforms and montages for the somatosensory evoked potential using median nerve (**a**) and posterior tibial nerve (**b**). Abbreviations: *C5s* spinous process of 5th cervical vertebrae, *Epc* Erb's point contralateral, *EPi* Erb's point ipsilateral, *L3* spinous process of 3rd lumbar vertebrae, *T12* spinous process of 12the thoracic vertebrae. * Please refer to the 10–20 EEG system for the cephalic electrodes

spine vs thoracic spine) or the outcomes to be evaluated (predicting the presence of the immediate postoperative neural deficit versus long term outcomes). But the generally accepted warning criteria are either 10% increase in the latency of the primary SSEP cortical response (N20 or P37) or a decrease of more than 50% in cortical peak to peak amplitude, which can be indicative of a significant surgical event and thereby are criteria for intervention [2].

17.3 Motor Evoked Potentials

The motor evoked potential (MEP) is a modality that can test the function of the motor cortex and/or corticospinal tract through the stimulation of each site. It can be classified into transcranial magnetic MEP using a magnetic field and transcranial electric MEP using an electric field depending on the type of stimulation. Although transcranial magnetic MEP is mostly adapted for MEP testing in clinical practice, it requires unnecessarily large and expensive equipment, relatively small waveform, and characteristic noise. For these reasons, intraoperative MEP stimulation is currently achieved via electrical stimulation method.

Intraoperative MEP is also divided into neurogenic mixed evoked potential (MEP), D-wave, and muscle MEP, depending on the stimulus and location of the recording. Neurogenic mixed evoked potential (MEP) has been proposed as a new method to monitor the motor pathway under the influence of anesthetic agent by directly stimulating the spinal cord and recording the waveform on the peripheral nerve. It is known that the resulting waveforms reflect the antidromic conduction of the sensory pathway located in the dorsal column rather than reflecting the function of the actual motor pathway [3]. This limitation of neurogenic mixed evoke potential might cause misinterpretation of the IOM data even in case of serious damage in the motor tract [3], hence it is not commonly used as a current IOM modality during spinal surgery.

Transcranial muscle MEP is a simple and straightforward method of recording transcranial electric stimulation waveforms in the limb muscles, and currently the most widely accepted technique for MEP monitoring during surgery. However, it also has a major drawback that it has high inter-trial variability in its amplitude and shapes [4], and also its waveform can be severely reduced or damaged with just a small amount of the inhalation anesthetics/neuromuscular blockade [5]. Currently, the most commonly used anesthetic technique for the stable implementation of muscle MEP is total intravenous anesthesia (TIVA), which uses only intravenous anesthetic (mainly propofol) without using anesthetic anesthesia. The high inter-trial variability of muscle MEP cannot be fully overcome until now. Currently our center uses "presence or absence criteria" as a most reliable warning sign for the long-term neurologic deficit [6, 7] and also applies tetanic stimulation in the peripheral nerve to reduce the inter-trial variability [8].

To overcome the disadvantages of muscle MEP described above, the D-wave measurement was designed. D-wave is a method directly recording waveforms generated by stimulation of the cortex through an epidural catheter electrode placed at the distal and proximal sites of the surgical site, respectively. In contrast to muscle MEP with a very high intra-variability, D-wave has a waveform with less intra-variability. Some groups have suggested it to be one of the standard IOM modality during surgery for intramedullary spinal cord tumors [9]. However, D-wave has its own disadvantages. First, the use of an epidural electrode can potentially pose a risk for nerve damage during surgery. In addition, D-wave cannot monitor the anterior horn cell, which may be the most vulnerable structures to ischemia. Lastly, due to the amplitude of the D-wave can be highly dependent on the distance between the spinal cord and epidural electrode, some types of spinal surgery (per se, correction of the scoliosis) may not be suitable for the D-wave monitoring, where the position of the epidural electrode can change during surgery [10].

17.4 Electromyography

Needle electromyography (EMG) is a well been established tool for routine clinical evaluation of patients having disease in either motor neuron, nerve root, peripheral nerve, muscle, or sometimes neuromuscular junction. Clinical EMG testing is mainly comprised of assessing spontaneous activity in resting state and motor unit action potential after voluntary muscle contraction [11]. These basic procedures, with a minor modifications, are currently also used for intraoperative monitoring (IOM) of the spinal cord function during diverse types of spinal surgery. Two commonly used EMG monitoring technics during spinal surgery are free-running EMG and stimulated EMG.

- Free-running EMG

During free-running EMG monitoring for spinal surgery, the neurotonic discharge (tonic EMG, train activity) is the potential of interest predictive of postoperative outcomes. This neurotonic discharge can arise spontaneously in response to either the mechanical, thermal, or metabolic irritation/insults [12]. It has high frequency of 50–200 Hz and regular pattern of short bursts or long trains, which can be distinctive from motor unit action potential (MUP) activity (10–15 Hz) or fibrillation potentials (1–5 Hz) [12]. As diverse artifact from electro-cautery, wire movement, interference from anesthesia equipment as warmers and respirators, can also provoke free-running EMG signals, it is important for the IOM team to acknowledge the patterns of each waveform (Fig. 17.3). The generator for neurotonic EMG has mostly been considered to be the nerve root and the peripheral nerve; as its high frequency (up to 200 Hz) exceeds those that can arise from motor neurons [13]. Nevertheless, a recent study showed that mechanical intramedullary motor tract injury can also provoke severe EMG

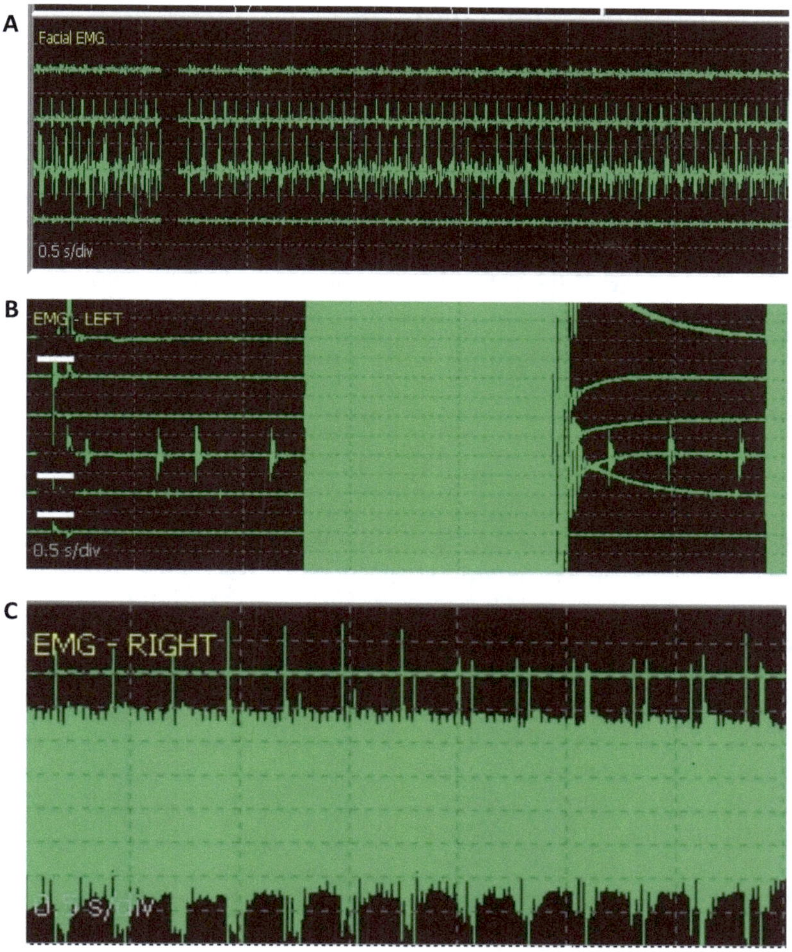

Fig. 17.3 Diverse types of EMG patterns during spontaneous EMG recording. Neurotonic discharge of high frequency during spontaneous EMG monitoring in the facial muscles (**a**). Stimulation artifact from electrocautery (**b**). Artifact in a limb that was connected with the fluid warmer via intravenous (IV) fluid line (**c**).

discharges during surgery [14]. The exact mechanism for these phenomena was not fully known, but a membrane leakage conductance and depolarization after mechanical injury to the axonal membrane has been proposed to be responsible for it [14, 15]. A previous study on patients with hereditary motor neuropathy showed that the regional treatment with curare, an antagonist of nicotinic AChRs, completely abolished the neuromyotonia of patients, which implied that neurotonic EMG can arise due to the hyperexcitability of the peripheral nerve [16]. One caveat of neuromyotonic EMG in IOM of the spinal cord is that despite its high sensitivity (up to 100%) it has a relatively poor specificity (24%) in predicting a postoperative neurologic deficit in spinal surgery [17].

– Stimulated (evoked) EMG

The stimulated EMG is fundamentally identical with the motor nerve conduction study in clinical practice. During surgery it can be used for identifying the level of the spinal root, mapping the corticospinal tract during intramedullary spinal cord tumor [18], or determining the proper screw placement [19] during spinal surgery. Nevertheless, one important issue in mapping the corticospinal tract in the spinal cord is that the compound motor action potentials of the limb muscle can also be elicited by the stimulation of the dorsal column rather than the corticospinal tract [20, 21]. A recent study proposed the method of double stimulation technique with an inter-stimuli interval of 60 ms to reliably obtain the compound motor action potential elicited from the corticospinal tract [18] that can be distinguished from those form the dorsal column.

17.5 Conclusion and Future Perspective

Diverse techniques of neurophysiologic testing can be adapted during spinal surgery to preserve the function of the spinal cord. Nevertheless, the optimal usage of these testing will be most beneficial with the proper knowledge on the basic principles. One of the major limitations of the current IOM modalities for the spinal surgery is that most of them can detect the electrophysiologic signal alterations only after the occurrence of some degree of the neural injuries. Future techniques using recording the unit potentials from small groups of cells or nerve fibers may be more beneficial in preserving the integrity of nervous system through the earlier detection of the possible neural injuries.

References

1. Rutkove SB. Introduction to volume conduction. Clinical neurophysiology primer. p. 43.
2. Available from https://cdn.ymaws.com/www.asnm.org/resource/resmgr/docs/INTRAOPERATIVE_MONITORING_US.pdf.
3. Minahan R, et al. Anterior spinal cord injury with preserved neurogenic'motor'evoked potentials. Clin Neurophysiol Off J Int Fed Clin Neurophysiol. 2001;112(8):1442.
4. Burke D, et al. Trial-to-trial variability of corticospinal volleys in human subjects. Electroencephalogr Clin Neurophysiol. 1995;97(5):231.
5. Taniguchi M, Cedzich C, Schramm J. Modification of cortical stimulation for motor evoked potentials under general anesthesia: Technical description. Neurosurgery. 1993;32(2):219.
6. Kim D-G, et al. Intraoperative motor-evoked potential disappearance versus amplitude-decrement alarm criteria during cervical spinal surgery: A long-term prognosis. J Clin Neurol (Seoul, Korea). 2017;13(1):38.
7. Jin S, et al. Multimodal intraoperative monitoring during intramedullary spinal cord tumor surgery. Acta Neurochir. 2015;157(12):2149.
8. Kim J, et al. Effect of peripheral nerve tetanic stimulation on the inter-trial variability and accuracy of transcranial motor-evoked potential in brain surgery. Clin Neurophysiol Off J Int Fed Clin Neurophysiol. 2016;127(5):2208.
9. Kothbauer K. Intraoperative neurophysiologic monitoring for intramedullary spinal-cord tumor surgery. Neurophysiol Clin/Clin Neurophysiol. 2007;37(6):407.
10. Ulkatan S, et al. Monitoring of scoliosis surgery with epidurally recorded motor evoked potentials (D wave) revealed false results. Clin Neurophysiol Off J Int Fed Clin Neurophysiol. 2006;117(9):2093.
11. Preston DC, Shapiro BE. Electromyography and neuromuscular disorders E-book: Clinical-electrophysiologic correlations (Expert Consult-Online and Print). Elsevier Health Sciences; 2012.
12. Harper C, Daube J. Facial nerve electromyography and other cranial nerve monitoring. J Clin Neurophysiol Off Publ Am Electroencephalogr Soc. 1998;15(3):206.
13. Layzer R. Neuromyotonia and myokymia.
14. Skinner S, et al. Electromyography detects mechanically-induced suprasegmental spinal motor tract injury: Review of decompression at spinal cord level. Clin Neurophysiol Off J Int Fed Clin Neurophysiol. 2009;120(4):754.
15. Galbraith J, Thibault L, Matteson D. Mechanical and electrical responses of the squid giant axon to simple elongation. J Biomech Eng. 1993;115(1):13.
16. Hahn A, et al. Neuromyotonia in hereditary motor neuropathy. J Neurol Neurosurg Psychiatry. 1991;54(3):230.
17. Gunnarsson T, et al. Real-time continuous intraoperative electromyographic and somatosensory evoked potential recordings in spinal surgery: Correlation of clinical and electrophysiologic findings in a prospective, consecutive series of 213 cases. Spine. 2004;29(6):677.
18. Deletis V, et al. Intraoperative identification of the corticospinal tract and dorsal column of the spinal cord by electrical stimulation. J Neurol Neurosurg Psychiatry. 2018;89(7):754.

19. Glassman S, et al. A prospective analysis of intraoperative electromyographic monitoring of pedicle screw placement with computed tomographic scan confirmation. Spine. 1995;20(12):1375.
20. Gandhi R, Curtis C, Cohen-Gadol A. High-resolution direct microstimulation mapping of spinal cord motor pathways during resection of an intramedullary tumor. J Neurosurg Spine. 2015;22(2):205.
21. Deletis V, et al. Letter to the Editor: Electrical activity in limb muscles after spinal cord stimulation is not specific for the corticospinal tract. J Neurosurg Spine. 2017;26(2):267.

My Surgical Experience of Spinal Cord Tumor Surgery

18

Chun Kee Chung and Dong Hwan Kim

Abstract

I've had spinal cord tumor surgery for quite some time. During about 25 years, 321 intramedullary tumors, 929 intradural extramedullary tumors, and 182 extradural tumors were operated. While I worked as a neurosurgeon, I learned a lot from patients and image like as MR. I have changed many of my practices. I used to use steroids and insert drain. However, currently, steroids are never used, and if dura is opened, no drain is added. In schwannoma, you have to meet endoneurial fluid. And spinal cord meningioma is intradural extra-arachnoidal tumor. In hemangioblastoma, it is not cauterization but dissection. In ependymoma, the tumor should be dissected from gray matter of spinal cord. The principle of cavernous malformation surgery is to open the shortest distance from the lesion. I would like to share my experience and ideas with others in this book. I've also changed and developed a lot of spinal cord tumor surgery, but I think there's still a lot to change. I hope my experiences and ideas in this book will help surgeons performing spinal cord tumor surgery.

Keywords

Surgical experience · Spinal cord tumor

C. K. Chung (✉)
Department of Neurosurgery, Seoul National University Hospital, Seoul National University College of Medicine, Seoul, Republic of Korea
e-mail: chungc@snu.ac.kr

Neuroscience Research Institute, Seoul National University Medical Research Center, Seoul, Republic of Korea

Clinical Research Institute, Seoul National University Hospital, Seoul, Republic of Korea

Department of Brain and Cognitive Sciences, Seoul National University College of Natural Sciences, Seoul, Republic of Korea

D. H. Kim
Department of Neurosurgery, Seoul National University Hospital, Seoul, Republic of Korea
e-mail: fskdh@daum.net

I have been performing a spinal cord tumor surgery since 1993 at Seoul National University Hospital. During about 25 years, 321 intramedullary tumors, 929 intradural extramedullary tumors, and 182 extradural tumors were operated. In the 90s, about 10 IM tumors and 20 IDEM tumors were operated in a year. In the last five years, an average of 27 IM tumors and 67 IDEM tumors have been removed annually. While I worked as a neurosurgeon, I have carefully considered perioperative management and control of intraoperative epidural hemorrhage and changed my practice. I was able to gain knowledge about the origin, anatomy, and tumorigenesis about several spinal cord tumor surgery. I would like to share my experience and Ideas

C. K. Chung (ed.), *Surgery of Spinal Cord Tumors Based on Anatomy*,
https://doi.org/10.1007/978-981-15-7771-0_18

with others in this book. I've also changed and developed a lot of spinal cord tumor surgery, but I think there's still a lot to change. I hope my experiences and ideas in this book will help surgeons performing spinal cord tumor surgery.

1. Value of perioperative steroids
   In perioperative period, I do not use steroids for spinal cord tumor patients. There is no evidence that steroids improve the clinical outcomes of spinal cord tumor patients, but it is much more obvious that it raises the adverse effects such as infection.
2. Laminoplasty Instead of Laminectomy

In order to access the spinal cord tumor, lamina must be opened. The more laminectomy I do, the higher probability of iatrogenic kyphosis, and we should prevent it. So I try to minimize facet injury and do only as much lateral opening as is necessary. I try to preserve the bone integrity, as far as possible, and minimize the facet joint resection. So we fix the lamina we removed back to its original position and return it to the original form. It is also helpful that lamina, which is re-secured, becomes an excellent boundary between adhesion tissues and dura when performing a re-operation.

3. How to Reduce Epidural Bleeding

First, good position is very important. I always check patient's belly when positioning patients. Reducing abdominal pressure is very important. And if you don't open arachnoid when opening dura, the epidural bleeding is reduced because it can reduce amount of CSF leakage. Dura tack-up suture reduces epidural bleeding as well because pressure is applied to the sides laterally. And when closing the dura, the knots are not tied by hands. If the knots are tied by hands, dura is pulled, which makes the epidural bleeding a lot. And, just before the dura is closed completely, the saline is injected into the dura to inflate the dural sac and apply pressure to the sides to reduce the epidural bleeding. In addition, I can also check the CSF leakage.
I don't use hemostatic agent, including gelfoam, if possible. If I have to use it, I use only surgicels. If it is bleeding from the artery, the bleeding point is precisely cauterized, and if it's bleeding from venous plexus, it is sufficiently controlled by compression with or without surgicels.

4. General Principle

A. All anatomical layers shall be opened separately until exposed from to tumor on the skin. This allows all layers to be closed when the tumor is removed and then closed again.

5. Spinal Cord Tumor

Postoperatively, The absence of a motor weakness does not mean that the patient can walk. Preservation of proprioceptive sensation is more important in predicting whether a patient can walk. When doing midline myelotomy, it is most important to minimize the damage given to the dorsal column. When I do midline myelotomy, I usually do dorsal column mapping. I always check the anatomic landmark, but I check it again with the dorsal column mapping.

B. Schwannoma

i. Epidural Schwannoma

When I first removed the epidural schwannoma, I thought that it was a tumor to go out of the dura, and I removed the entire root that included the tumor. So there was a lot of epidural bleeding. I used to control epidural bleeding by packing surgicels into the epidural space. It occurred to me that this entire epidural mass was not a tumor, but that normal root was mixed with a tumor. So my hypothesis was that since the epidural mass includes normal nerve root and tumor together, if the longitudinal incision was made in this mass and the pseudocapsule was pushed aside, only the tumor could be isolated. That is, because schwannoma originates from schwann cell, it basically comes up from only one axon. Theoretically, because several axons would come together to make one fascicle, and several fascicles would come together to make a root, only one axon with schwannoma could be removed. This led me to think about the layers. In order to expose schwannoma, root sheath must be incised. This sheath is an extension of dura. Opening this sheath is like entering an intradural space. Next, perineurium, the sheath of the fascicle is incised. This perineurium can be thought of as an extension of arachnoid membrane of spinal cord. In other words, it is like entering a subarachnoid space, CSF space. That is, you have to meet endoneurial fluid because you entered endoneurial space. Since communication exists between endoneurial fluid and subarachnoid space, the space in which schwannoma exists is the same as in CSF space, regardless of whether it is an extradural or intradural space. This thought led to the same treatment of both an intradural and extradural schwannoma. It is no longer necessary to keep the old dogma to remove the intradural tumor first when removing the intradural and extradural schwannoma. Always the extradural tumor is removed first, and when the last remaining tumor is pulled, the old concept, the intradural part, has been pulled out in most cases.

ii. Intradural Extramedullary Schwannoma

Intradural schwannoma is a classical intradural extradural tumor (IDEM). The difference between this and meningioma becomes clear whether the existing space is inside or outside the arachnoid. Schwannoma exists in intraarachnoid space and meningioma exists in extraarachnoid space. Therefore, it is necessary to open the dura and the arachnoid during surgery to expose the typical IDEM schwannoma. Once the tumor is exposed, only tumor should be dissected from several rootlets. Separation of rootlets adhering to tumor is important, especially when in cauda equina. Schwannoma is mainly from dorsal root. So in the case of non-cauda equina, it is debatable how important this dissection of peripheral rootlets is functionally, after surgery. In principle, however, all rootlets that can be dissected from the tumor as much as possible are separated. In principle, schwannoma comes from schwann cell in a single axon, so theoretically, everything else can be dissected except for a single axon that is the origin of tumor.

iii. Intramedullary Schwannoma

Intramedullary schwannoma is very rare. Usually it has an extramedullary part. Therefore, it is relatively easy to remove this intramedullary part by removing extramedullary part and entering spinal cord substance along with this plane. It should be felt that it passes through pia clearly as it enters the interior along the intramedullary part. This way, all detachable cord substance can be preserved.

C. Meningioma (IDEM)

Meningioma is a tumor that originates from the arachnoid cap cell. Therefore, as is often said, meningioma does not originate from the dura. The arachnoid cap cell, which is part of the arachnoid membrane, is the closest part to the dura, so the rest of the arachnoid membrane has nothing to do with the tumor. So this tumor is an intradural extra-arachnoidal tumor. Therefore, it is not necessary to open arachnoid membrane when meningioma is removed. The meningioma can be removed if only the dura is opened and intact arachnoid membrane and CSF space and nervous structure in it, are pushed aside. Of course, in case of ventral tumor, when it is difficult to push the arachnoid membrane aside, you can open the dorsal arachnoid membrane, enter the intra-arachnoid space then open the ventral arachnoid too, and expose the tumor. In this case, it is also easy to remove meningioma by keeping in mind that ventral arachnoid membrane defines the space in which nervous and vascular structures exist.

C. Intraparenchymal tumor

i. Hemangioblastoma

This tumor is in the intra-pial extramedullary space. Therefore, it is important to have an interface between the pia and the blood vessels. Previously, en-bloc resection was emphasized, cauterization all around the tumor should be done. As a result, the tumor does not shrink and the blood vessels rupture, so once the coagulation starts, it cannot stop. In the end, it should have been removed almost by the time the bleeding stops. So I started dissection of the tumor from the pia instead of cauterizing it with a bipolar cautery. I found that if I cauterize and cut the blood vessels that supply the tumor one by one, I could push the tumor out of the spinal cord. The dissection between the tumor and the normal spinal cord made the operation much easier. Most hemangioblastoma is supplied by blood vessels in the pia of the spinal cord. Therefore, even if only visible feeders are controlled, I can push the tumor from the spinal cord and separate from it. Almost all hemangioblastoma could be removed by approaching posteriorly. Sometimes there were tumors in the ventral location, but these were very exceptional cases. In the case of ventral location, it was not so difficult to control the feeders when the tumor was exposed through a routine midline myelotomy, and then the tumor was pushed from the spinal cord after finding the interface between the tumor and the spinal cord. Thus, preoperative angiography became less and less necessary. Also preoperative embolization didn't help much. So it was replaced by an intraoperative fluorescence angiography.

ii. Ependymoma

It is important not to damage the gray matter of the spinal cord in order to preserve the motor function of the hand during the operation of the ependymoma, especially, which occurred in the cervical enlargement.
The ependymoma and gray matter of spinal cord are difficult to distinguish. So it is better to find the ependymal layer first. I have to enter the central canal of spinal cord to find it. It is easy to find the space where cerebrospinal fluid exists. Removal of ependymoma must be done within the central canal of the spinal cord. If the surgery is performed only in the central canal of the spinal cord, the gray matter can be preserved.

iii. Myxopapillary Ependymoma

Myxopapillary ependymoma is basically a very indolent tumor. Therefore, it should be done if it can be completely removed, but if it fails to do so, it should be boldly stopped if other normal rootlets are thought to have been damaged more than expected. Therefore, the most important thing during this tumor's operation is not aggressive resection, but having the courage to stop it. In other words, a surgeon who is fully aware of the interface should boldly stop surgery if he thinks it is no longer possible to remove only the tumor. Of course, this tumor grows gradually as it progresses, and sometimes distant CSF seeding occurs. In these cases, patients may have a functional life for a considerable period of time, even if only the problematic lesions are removed and the rest are left.

iv. Subependymoma

It is very difficult to distinguish between subependymoma and ependymoma, preoperatively. However, in the case that characteristic similarity with ependymoma in surgical field of view, but difficult to separate from the spinal cord, subependymoma should be suspected.

v. Cavernous Malformation

Of course, this lesion is not a tumor. It is a kind of vascular malformation, but it grows in size each time the bleeding is repeated. Naturally, there are personal differences between patients, so it is difficult to determine which lesion will grow and which lesion will remain stationary. Therefore, for this lesion, it is most difficult to determine when it should be removed. The principle of surgery is to open the shortest distance from the lesion when approaching a lesion through the spinal cord. It is not always necessary to do midline or lateral myelotomy. If you can see lesions through the spinal cord when you open the dura and arachnoid membranes, you should open the best viewing area. I still don't know how extensive the pia has to be removed in these cases. It is relatively clear to remove hemorrhage, abnormal vasculature, and gliosis inside the pia. Surgical works only need to be done inside the gliosis. However, it is still not clear how much pia need to be removed.

Anatomical Compartment's Representative Tumor Surgery and Video

19

Young San Ko and Chun Kee Chung

Abstract

Until now, we have introduced classic example of tumors and elucidated operative strategy depending on each anatomical compartments. As mentioned at the beginning, the best benefit using the concept of anatomical compartments in surgery is that if we can confine our work in one compartment, other compartments will be beyond of our concern. In this chapter, we are going to solely focus on operative strategy for securing specific anatomical space depending on anatomical compartment of each tumor.

Keywords

Anatomical compartment · Video · And strategy

Electronic supplementary material The online version of this chapter (https://doi.org/10.1007/978-981-15-7771-0_19) contains supplementary material, which is available to authorized users.

Y. S. Ko
Department of Neurosurgery, Seoul National University Hospital, Seoul, Republic of Korea
e-mail: samkyu114@gmail.com

C. K. Chung (✉)
Department of Neurosurgery, Seoul National University Hospital, Seoul National University College of Medicine, Seoul, Republic of Korea
e-mail: chungc@snu.ac.kr

Neuroscience Research Institute, Seoul National University Medical Research Center, Seoul, Republic of Korea

Clinical Research Institute, Seoul National University Hospital, Seoul, Republic of Korea

Department of Brain and Cognitive Sciences, Seoul National University College of Natural Sciences, Seoul, Republic of Korea

19.1 Surgical Video and Demonstration of Surgical Strategy for Securing Anatomical Spaces Depending on Anatomical Compartment

19.1.1 Surgical Approach for Intradural Extra-Arachnoid Space

The intradural extra-arachnoid space is a potential one between dura and outer membrane of arachnoid. The surgical procedure depends on whether the spinal cord is pushed backward or pushed forward. When the cord is pushed forward, the dura is opened, the arachnoid is lifted (Epi-arachnoid approach) and the tumor can be removed. Find the interface between the dura and the outer layer of arachnoid membrane and secure this space is the most important point, then tumor can be easily followed through this

C. K. Chung (ed.), *Surgery of Spinal Cord Tumors Based on Anatomy*,
https://doi.org/10.1007/978-981-15-7771-0_19

interface. Once the tumor is found, peel the outer arachnoid off from the tumor using instruments such as microforcep, suction, and blunt hooks. If surgeon meets bleeding from this step of procedure, it always will happen tumor side of this interface and easily coagulate with microbipolar. Once intradural extra-arachnoid space is secured with this method, surgeon can begin to peel tumor off the dura. Damages to subarachnoid structure (particularly vascular structures) can be avoided through this approach.

On the other hand, if the cord is pushed dorsally, an epi-arachnoid approach is sometimes impossible [1]. In this case, first thing to do is find and cut dentate ligaments along the interface between the dura and the arachnoid membrane. If the outer layer of arachnoid membrane disturbs surgeon's view, open the dorsal outer layer and go into the subarachnoid space. And then, open the ventral outer layer again to approach the subdural space. In other words, the arachnoid is opened twice to enter the epi-arachnoid space (ventral epi-arachnoid) [2, 3].

Video Case

A 59-year-old female patient complained of gait disturbance. The patient also complained of leg paresthesia. Her magnetic resonance (MR) images showed that 1.7 × 1.2 × 1.1 cm sized ovoid mass at the intradural extramedullary region in the T8-9 spinal canal (Fig. 19.1). The patient underwent spinal cord tumor removal with epi-arachnoid approach. When dura was opened, the tumor was showed at epi-arachnoid space. The tumor was removed without incision of arachnoid membrane (Video 1).

A 68-year-old female patients complained of leg weakness for 3 months. She has felt tingling sense at both soles several years ago. The patient checked MR imaging, which demonstrated 1.2 × 1.1 × 1.3 cm mass at the T10 level (Fig. 19.2). Surgery for the patient was performed extra-leptomeningeal approach. After midline dura incision, the tumor was found via ventral epi-arachnoid approach. The dentate ligament was cut to make the operation field. Arachnoid membrane was dissected from the tumor and

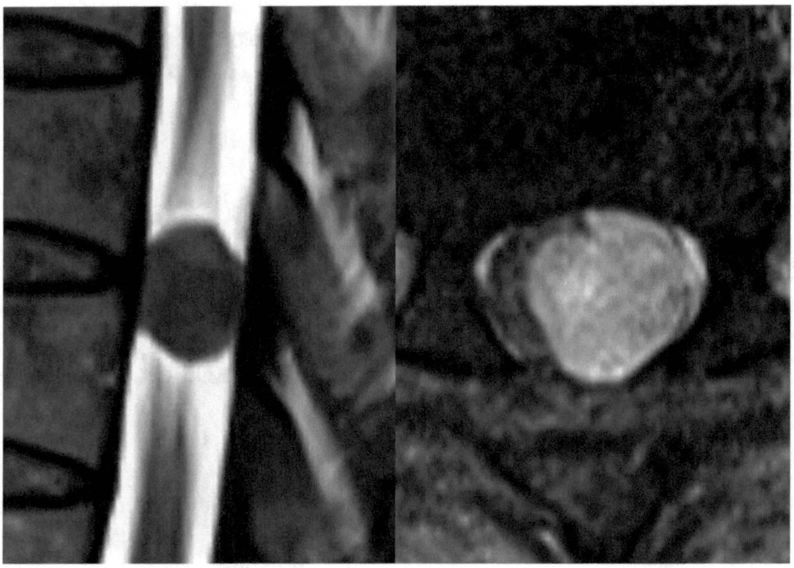

Fig. 19.1 Magnetic resonance images (MRI) of the thoracic spine revealed about 1.7 × 1.2 × 1.1 cm sized ovoid mass at left side of T8-9 intradural extramedullary region. The tumor showed homogenous enhancement. The spinal cord displaced to the right

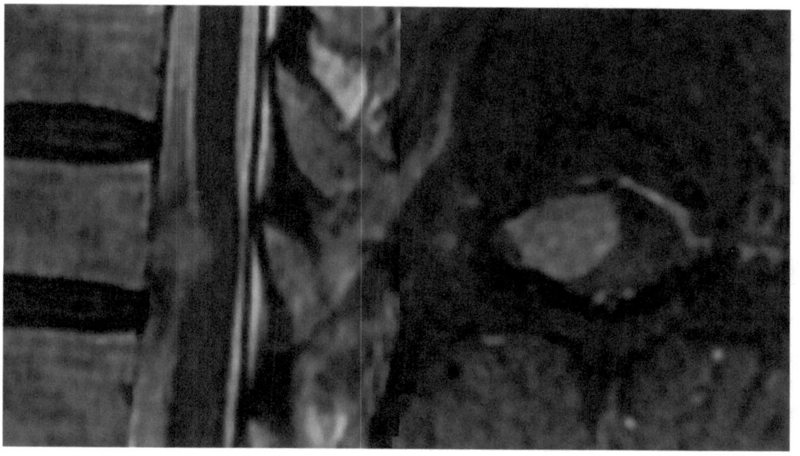

Fig. 19.2 Magnetic resonance images (MRI) of the thoracic spine revealed about 1.2 × 1.1 × 1.3 cm well enhancing mass at the right level T10. The tumor was located at intradural extramedullary region with suspicious focal dural enhancement. The spinal cord displaced to the backward

the tumor was removed piecemeal pattern. Finally, dura of the tumor origin was coagulated with curettage (Video 2).

19.1.2 Surgical Approach for Intradural Intrapial Intraependymal Space

Even though tumor located in the intradural intrapial intraparenchymal space is commonly known as intramedullary tumor, we believe its misnomer and proper name should be intrapial intraependymal tumor considering it's anatomical origin which is ependymal cell lining of the central canal of the spinal cord, when it comes to ependymoma. From this point of view, it can be said that tumor located in this space has nothing to do with parenchyma of the spinal cord itself.

The key surgical strategy is get into central canal passing through spinal cord with the shortest distance which will minimize neural damage. It is common misguided belief that dissection should be in the direction of peeling white matter from the tumor which could lead to substantial damage for gray matter [4]. The most important point is how to save this paper-thin remnant gray matter.

As previously described in previous chapters, conventional approach needs to be done before tumor exposure. Dura and arachnoid need to be opened respectively. The next step is to try best to find true midline using multiple adjuncts methods. It is known that dorsal column mapping can be useful for finding functional midline in the spinal cord. Identifying bilateral vessel is also important to find anatomical midline. Once the location of midline is identified, further step is to make midline myelotomy using ophthalmic knife. Care should be taken not to do midline myelotomy at once. Gradual, step by step myelotomy should be done at the plane between bilaterally existed vessels to reduce neural damage. The other important concept is that tumor is never located in the exact midline, but tumor is slightly one-sided as shown with lateralization of patient's symptom or imaging studies.

After myelotomy, one can find tumor easily with different gray color and consistency from spinal cord. Once tumor is exposed, the following step is to enter central canal which one can feel with gushing out of CSF. After entering into central canal, the other key point is that dissection of gray matter should be done using ependymal lining as interface between tumor and normal anatomical layer. The last point would

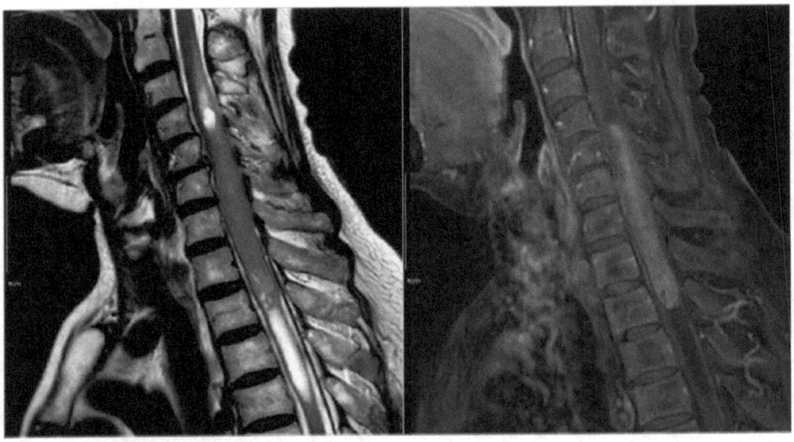

Fig. 19.3 Magnetic resonance (MR) images showed that 2 cm sized cystic enhancing mural nodule in right posterior cervicomedullary junction with prominent cord edema

like to mention is not to use cavitron ultrasonic surgical aspirator (CUSA) which will destroy layers of anatomic compartment and make the operation difficult, on the contrary to general belief [4, 5].

Video Case

A 67-year-old female patient complained of tingling sense. The patient also complained of both lower extremity weakness. Her magnetic resonance (MR) images showed that 8.2 cm sized enhancing mass at C4-T2 with cephalo-caudal syrinx formation (Fig. 19.3). The patient underwent intramedullary tumor removal. After dura opening, midline was identified with dorsal column mapping. Once myelotomy is done, tumor could be easily found and dissected after entering into central canal (Video 3).

Preoperative neurologic status of the patient. Patient couldn't carry out tandem gait (Video 4).

Postoperative neurologic status of the patient. Patient didn't show any postoperative neurological aggravation (Video 5).

19.1.3 Surgical Approach for Intradural Intraparenchymal Space

Tumor located in the intradural intraparehcymal space is true intramedullary tumor applying our concept of anatomical compartment. It can be speculated that approach to this tumor should be different from tumor located the intradural intrapial intraparenchymal space above point that their anatomical compartment is truly different. The bottom line is that there will be inevitable neural tissue damage, to minimize this damage is the key point. This can be possibly done with approaching tumor using shortest distance as possible. Depending on tumor location, myelotomy can be started in the midline or surface where closest point to the tumor. As mentioned in the ependymoma section, using CUSA makes anatomical layer non-differentiable and make the operation more difficult. The only factors we can rely on are color and consistency of tumor during the operation.

Video Case

A 30-year-old male patient complained of both extremity tingling sense. His magnetic resonance (MR) images showed that 3 cm sized enhancing mass at T11–T12 with hemosiderin cap and enhancement at the inferior portion (Fig. 19.4). The patient underwent intramedullary cord tumor removal. Since tumor was located at the midline, midline myletomy was done. Tumor could be differed from normal spinal cord with grayish color and different consistency (Video 6).

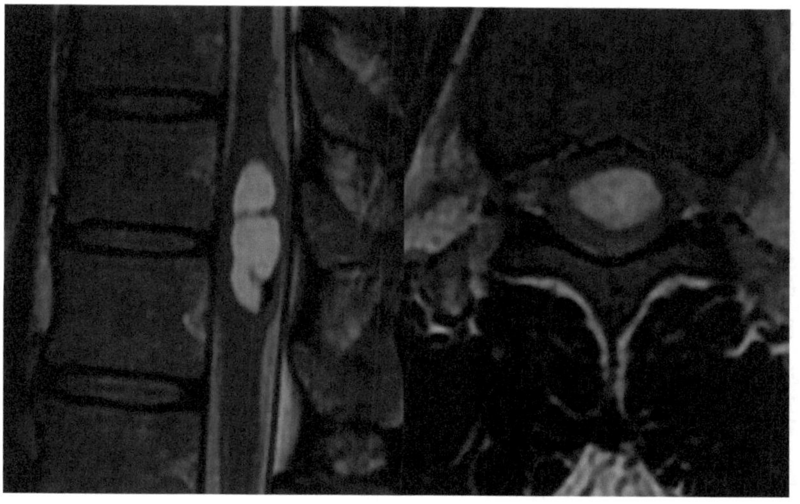

Fig. 19.4 3 cm sized enhancing mass at T11–T12 with hemosiderin cap and enhancement at the inferior portion

19.1.4 Surgical Approach for Intradural Extraparenchymal Pial Space

It is the beginning point that tumor located in the intradural extraparenchymal pial space is not true intramedullary tumor but extraparenchymal pial tumor which means tumor located at the pial surface where vascular structure exists as we know. From this point of view, it is postulated that this tumor can be dissected from spinal cord surface with different consistency of tumor from cord itself. Once one can find the interface between tumor and spinal cord, feeder is able to be separated from the cord surface. After the separation, the only thing to do is coagulate these vessels and remove the tumor [6, 7]. Classical concept of operation for tumor in this space is that one should coagulate every vascular structure that we can see under microscopic view. Our surgical strategy is slightly different from this. The most important thing is to trace tumor without loss of extraparenchymal pial space which cannot be easily differentiated after massive indiscreet coagulation.

There would be three situations for tumor in this space. First one is easier situation that tumor can be verified after dura and arachnoid opening. If surgeon can verify tumor, tumor can be peeled off from the pial surface using microsurgical instruments. Once dissection is completely done, easily identified feeder and draining vein can be coagulated in consecutive order. Other one is a difficult situation that tumor cannot be verified at the cord surface except feeders and draining veins. For this situation, the key point is to dissect every feeder and draining vein patiently from cord surface with assistance for indocyanine green angiography (ICGA) [8]. When the tumor is finally exposed, the following steps are same as previous situation. Surgeon should peel off tumor from the pial surface circumferentially, with minimize coagulation.

The other one is rare situation that purely ventrally located tumor which needs myelotomy. After myelotomy, tumor need to be verified and peeled off from the normal parenchyma. The following step is same as above situations.

Video Case

A 55-year-old female patient complained of right-hand numbness and tingling sense. Her magnetic resonance (MR) images showed that 2 cm sized cystic enhancing mural nodule in right posterior cervicomedullary junction with prominent cord edema (Fig. 19.5). The patient

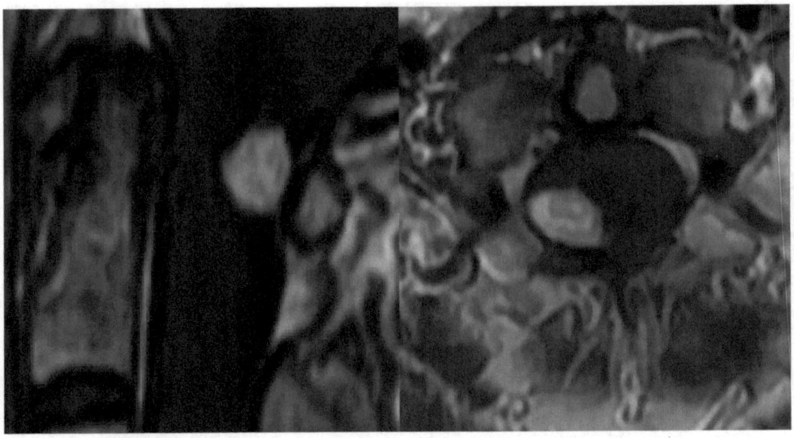

Fig. 19.5 2 cm sized cystic enhancing mural nodule in right posterior cervicomedullary junction with prominent cord edema

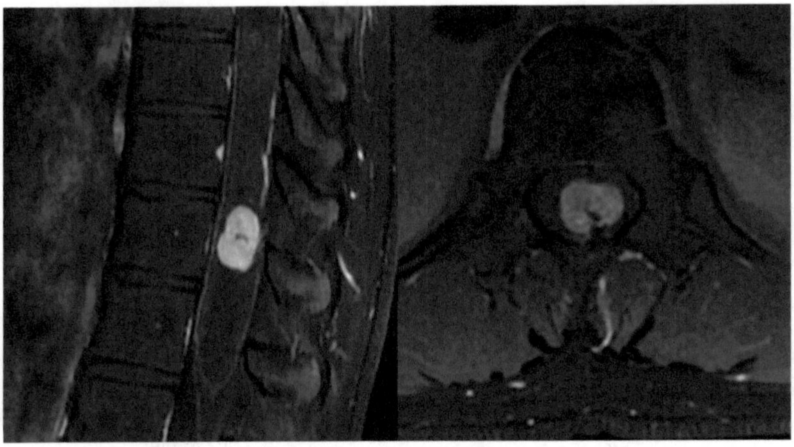

Fig. 19.6 1.4 × 1.2 × 2.2 cm sized lobulating enhancing intramedullary tumor at T12 vertebral body level with flow void at dorsal aspect of the tumor

underwent intramedullary cord tumor removal. Tumor can be easily identified after dura and arachnoid opening and could be peeled off easily from the pial surface (Video 7).

A 25-year-old male patient visited our clinic with consistent right upper extremity paresthesia for 4 months. His magnetic resonance (MR) images showed that 1.4 × 1.2 × 2.2 cm sized lobulating enhancing intramedullary tumor at T12 vertebral body level with flow void at dorsal aspect of the tumor (Fig. 19.6). Spinal angiogram showed hypervascular tumor staining through anterior spinal artery and posterior spinal artery (Video 8). The patient underwent intramedullary cord tumor removal. Tumor couldn't be easily verified in that massive vascular structure was covered whole surface of tumor. Intraoperative angiography was done with indo-cyanin green (ICG) to confirm anatomy of feeding vessels. Epi-arachnoid dissection was done firstly around main feeder, tumor can be notified underneath of main feeder. Same strategy was used for other vessels at lateral and medial location, and whole tumor could be exposed and removed at once (Video 9).

19.1.5 Surgical Approach for Extradural Intra-epineurial Intra-perineurial Space

To understand the concept of anatomical compartments in intra-epineurial and intra-perinuerial space, the starting point is to have speculation that endoneurium of peripheral nervous system (PNS) is extension of pia mater at central nervous system (CNS), perineurium is extension of arachnoid mater, and epineurium is extension of dura mater.

When approach to this space, we can apply same strategy as we do tumors in intradural extramedullary space such as schwannoma. As described in previous chapters, tumor in intradural extramedullary space is located under arachnoid space and we can only approach it after arachnoid opening. To access and remove tumor located in this space, epineurium and perineurium should be opened using same concept above.

When the most outside tumor capsule is exposed, this capsule is epineurium and opened after verification of no functional neural tissue underneath. The next capsule is epineurium and also opened the same technique as we do for perineurium. Now one can already know that we are in this space with existence of clear fluid as CSF existence in subarachnoid space. Tumor can be easily dissected from the other fascicle and outer capsule using circumferential dissection with instrument and cottonoid without any damage to endoneurium of other nerve fascicle. En-bloc removal can be usually achieved after dissection.

Video Case

A 39-year-old female known neurofibromatosis type 2 patient complained of left axillary pain for several months. Her magnetic resonance (MR) images showed that 5.1 × 4.5 cm sized encapsulated T2 hyperintense mass at left axillary area, abutting left brachial plexus (Fig. 19.7). The patient underwent extradural tumor removal. Axillary approach was done with help of thoracic surgeon. Tumor could be identified after dissection of pectoralis minor and teres minor muscle with prominent capsule.

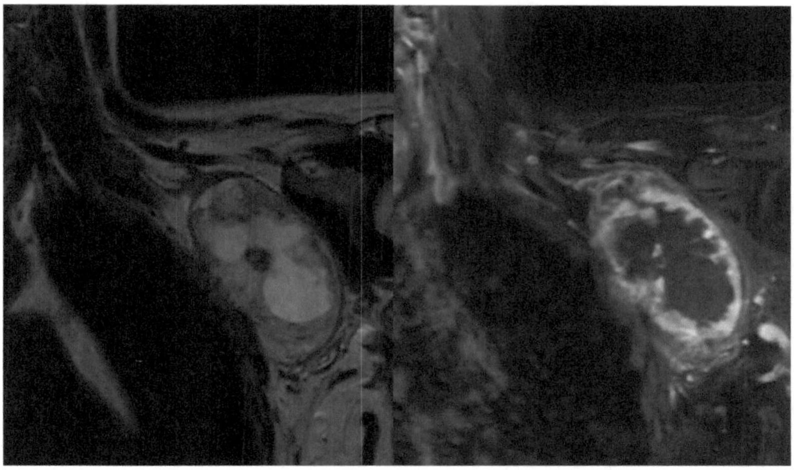

Fig. 19.7 1 × 4.5 cm sized encapsulated T2 hyperintense mass at left axillary area, abutting left brachial plexus with peripheral enhancement and cystic change

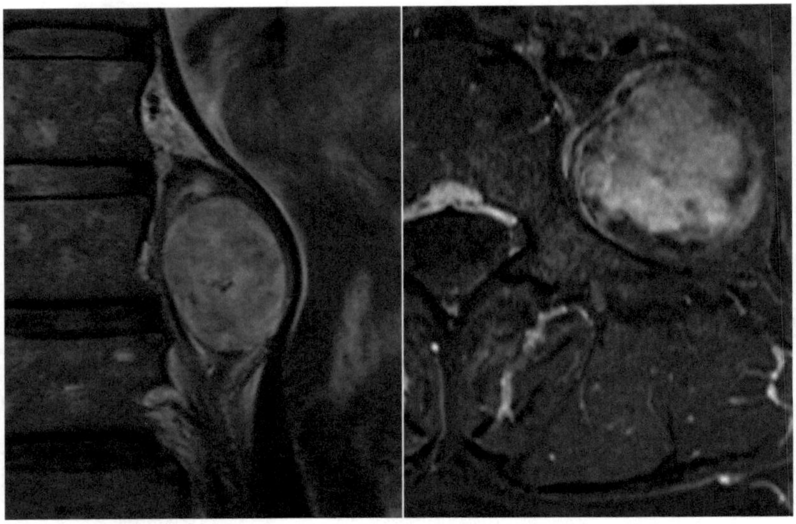

Fig. 19.8 3.7 × 3.2 × 5 cm sized T2 hyperintense, enhancing fusiform mass in the left paraspinal area extending from the L2 and L3 neural foramen to the left psoas muscle

After the opening of epineurium (most outside capsule) and perineurium (next underneath capsule), tumor can be easily dissected from the capsule and removed (Video 10).

A 48-year-old female patient visited clinic due to radiating pain from left back to thigh for a year. Her magnetic resonance (MR) images showed that 3.7 × 3.2 × 5 cm sized T2 hyperintense, enhancing fusiform mass in the left paraspinal area (Fig. 19.8). The patient underwent lateral retroperitoneal approach with tumor removal. Tumor capsule could be identified after dissection of psoas muscle. After verifying no functional neural tissue underneath of tumor capsule, epineurium (most outside capsule) and perineurium (next underneath capsule) was sequentially opened, tumor can be easily dissected and removed (Video 11).

19.2 Conclusion

Tumors located in the intradural extra-arachnoid space, intrapial intraependymal space, intraparenchymal space, extraparenchymal pial space, and extradural intra-epineurial intra-perineurial space can be safely removed with the concept of anatomical compartment.

References

1. Sohn S, Chung CK. Conventional posterior approach without far lateral approach for ventral foramen magnum meningiomas. J Korean Neurosurg Soc. 2013;54:373–8.
2. Kim CH, Chung CK. Surgical outcome of a posterior approach for large ventral intradural extramedullary spinal cord tumors. Spine (Phila Pa 1976). 2011;36:E531–7.
3. Yoon SH, Chung CK, Jahng TA. Surgical outcome of spinal canal meningiomas. J Korean Neurosurg Soc. 2007;42:300–4.
4. Kucia E, Bambakidis N, Chang S, Spetzler R. Surgical technique and outcomes in the treatment of spinal cord ependymomas, Part 1: Intramedullary ependymomas. Neurosurgery. 2010;68:57–63; discussion 63.
5. Sciubba DM, Liang D, Kothbauer KF, Noggle JC, Jallo GI. The evolution of intramedullary spinal cord tumor surgery. Neurosurgery. 2009;65:84–91; discussion 91–82.
6. Pojskic M, Arnautovic KI. Microsurgical resection of spinal cord hemangioblastoma: 2-Dimensional operative video. Oper Neurosurg (Hagerstown). 2018;15:E88–9.

7. Joaquim AF, Ghizoni E, dos Santos MJ, Valadares MG, da Silva FS, Tedeschi H. Intramedullary hemangioblastomas: Surgical results in 16 patients. Neurosurg Focus. 2015;39:E18.
8. Suero Molina E, Stummer W. Where and when to cut? Fluorescein guidance for brain stem and spinal cord tumor surgery-technical note. Oper Neurosurg (Hagerstown). 2018;15:325–31.

Results of Representative Tumor Surgery of Each Anatomical Compartment

20

Hyeseon Kim and Chung Kee Chung

Abstract

The extent of tumor resection and nature of tumor appear to determine the surgical outcomes of the spinal cord tumors. Surgical techniques and perioperative management of spinal cord tumors have evolved over time, improving the outcomes of patients in general. In this chapter, we review surgical and clinical outcomes of different types of spinal tumors based on our experience.

Keywords

Spinal cord tumor · Surgery · Treatment · Outcome

20.1 Intradural Tumors

20.1.1 Intrapial Tumors

20.1.1.1 Astrocytoma

Kim et al. reviewed a total of 30 operations performed on 28 patients (male 19, female 9) for spinal astrocytoma between April 1978 and June 1999 [1, 2]. Gross total resection (GTR) was achieved only in 3 patients with low grade astrocytomas. Subtotal or partial resection was seen in 21 patients and biopsy was done in 6. One patient underwent biopsy and syringosubarachnoid shunt simultaneously, and another patient received syringosubarachnoid shunt only.

Postoperatively, one patient achieved better functional outcome with improved Nurick grade. The grades remained the same in 21 patients, but 4 of them, who had low grade astrocytomas, reported to have improved sensory or motor symptoms. The neurological status and Nurick grade deteriorated in 6 patients.

The mean observation period was 6.5 months (range 0.5–184 months), 11 patients died during

H. Kim
Department of Neurosurgery, Seoul National University Hospital, Seoul, South Korea
e-mail: hskim29@gmail.com

C. K. Chung (✉)
Department of Neurosurgery, Seoul National University Hospital, Seoul National University College of Medicine, Seoul, Republic of Korea
e-mail: chungc@snu.ac.kr

Neuroscience Research Institute, Seoul National University Medical Research Center, Seoul, Republic of Korea

Clinical Research Institute, Seoul National University Hospital, Seoul, Republic of Korea

Department of Brain and Cognitive Sciences, Seoul National University College of Natural Sciences, Seoul, Republic of Korea

C. K. Chung (ed.), *Surgery of Spinal Cord Tumors Based on Anatomy*,
https://doi.org/10.1007/978-981-15-7771-0_20

this period. The survival rates were significantly different according to the histological grades. For low grade astrocytoma ($n = 18$), the cumulative survival was 62.3% after 8.5 years, whereas the higher grade astrocytomas ($n = 10$) showed a poorer outcome with the survival of 19.1% after 11 months ($p = 0.00117$).

Postoperative complications included neurological deterioration in 6 patients and CSF leakage in 1 patient. No death was reported within 2 months of surgery.

We looked at the more recent patient pool, which included a total of 11 patients who underwent surgery and had histologically proven spinal cord astrocytoma between 2012 and 2015. There were 3 men and 8 women. Of the 11 patients, 3 had diffuse astrocytoma, 5 anaplastic astrocytoma, 2 pilocytic astrocytoma and 1 glioblastoma. GTR of the tumor was achieved in one patient, whereas partial or subtotal resection was done in 6 and biopsy only in 4. The mean follow-up period was 32.7 months (range 0.7–72 months). Preoperative and postoperative neurological status was assessed using the Modified McCormick scale (MMS). No patient died during the period but neurological deterioration was reported in 6 patients. One patient improved functional status postoperatively and 4 patients remained stationary. The grade of astrocytoma did not have correlation with the final neurological status of patients ($p = 0.196$).

Postoperative complication was observed in one patient with anaplastic astrocytoma. The patient underwent a revision surgery due to wound dehiscence.

These two studies, which were performed a decade apart, revealed no significant changes in the extent of tumor resection and postoperative outcomes over time. Authors believed that both features completely depend on the characteristics of astrocytoma.

20.1.1.2 Ependymoma [3]

Eight-eight patients (male 60, female 28) who had been diagnosed with ependymoma between January 1989 and December 2009 were reviewed. Surgery was done once in 84 patients, twice in 2 patients, and three times in 2 patients. Overall, GTR of tumor was achieved in 82 patients, subtotal resection (STR) in 15 patients, and partial removal in 1 patient. Postoperatively, 6 of the 88 patients reported to have improved neurological status, whereas 46 patients remained unchanged and 36 deteriorated; paralyzes and/or bladder/bowel dysfunction in 14, proprioceptive deficits in 20, dysesthesia and/or paresthesia in 11.

In terms of postoperative complication, 3 patients experienced postoperative CSF leakage and all of them were treated with a revision surgery and/or lumbar drainage. Seven patients developed wound problems and 3 developed postoperative kyphosis.

Of the 88 patients, 20 underwent postoperative radiotherapy and one received chemotherapy due to diffuse meningeal seeding. Even with adjuvant therapies, 15 patients presented with recurrent or progressive disease during the median follow-up period of 7.29 months. The postsurgical mortality rate within two months was 0%. However, 2 patients with anaplastic ependymoma died 12 and 22 months after surgery, respectively.

Also, we retrospectively reviewed the more recent patient data between December 2011 and January 2017 (Table 20.1). A total of 41 patients (30 patients with ependymoma and 11 patients with myxopapillary ependymoma (ME)) were identified. Anaplastic ependymoma was not seen during this period. Surgery was performed once only in all patients and GTR of tumor was possible in the majority of patients: only 1 patient with ependymoma and two with ME underwent subtotal resection of tumor. The two patients with ME received adjuvant radiotherapy: one had leptomeningeal seeding of ME on initial presentation and the other received subtotal resection of tumor due to the tumor inseparable from the cauda equina. The mean follow-up duration was 3.4 year and recurrence or progression of tumor have not been reported.

Postoperatively, MMS score improved in 14 patients: 7 in ependymoma and 7 in ME. On the other hand, symptoms or neurological status worsened postoperatively in 11 patients (10 in ependymoma and 1 in ME); 7 complained of worsening motor weakness, 3 sensory change,

Table 20.1 Comparison of outcomes of patients with ependymoma (unpublished data)

Parameter	No. of patients (1989–2009)			No. of patients (2011–2017)		
	Ependymoma ($n=64$)	Myxopapillary ($n=24$)	Total ($n=88$)	Ependymoma ($n=30$)	Myxopapillary ($n=11$)	Total ($n=41$)
Type of surgery						
GTR	52	20	72	29	10	39
STR	11	4	15	1	1	2
Partial	1	0	1	0	0	0
Adjuvant therapy						
Radiotherapy	13	7	20	0	2	2
Chemotherapy	1	0	1	0	0	0
Complication						
Motor weakness	6	0	6	6	1	7
Bladder/bowel	3	5	8	1	0	1
Sensory change	N/A	N/A	N/A	3	0	3
CSF leakage	2	1	3	0	0	0
Wound problem	5	2	7	0	0	0
Postop kyphosis	3	0	3	1	0	1

1 urinary symptom, and 1 postoperative kyphosis. No one experienced CSF leakage or wound problem.

These two studies, also performed a decade apart, showed improvements in the extent of tumor resection and postoperative patient outcome over time (Table 20.1). Understanding that ependymoma is intra-ependymomal in origin has made a great contribution to the change.

(Unpublished data).

20.1.2 Pial-Extrapial

20.1.2.1 Hemangioblastoma [4]

The surgical outcome of hemangioblastoma has been discussed in the chapter 9. Please refer to the chapter.

20.1.3 Sub-Arachnoidal

20.1.3.1 Schwannoma

From March 2010 to December 2014, a total of 87 patients underwent operation and had pathologically proven intradural schwannomas. Of the 87 cases, intradural extramedullary (IDEM) type was the most frequently encountered entity ($n=64$), followed by dumbbell shaped in 21, and invasive in 2.

Surgery was performed once in 78 patients, twice in 5 and three or more times in 4. Overall, GTR was achieved in 79 patients, NTR in 2 and STR in 6. Postoperatively, 84 of the 87 patients (96.6%) reported to have symptoms improved or unchanged. Three patients experienced worsened symptoms postoperatively, but one of them recovered to their preoperative status, whereas the other two did not.

Complications included vertebral artery injury, CSF leakage, infection and neurological deterioration.

Vertebral artery (VA) injury was seen in 2 patients; both of them had dumbbell-shaped schwannoma. VA was sutured in one patient and the other underwent trapping of VA as it was not a dominant VA. Both of them recovered without neurological sequelae.

CSF leakage was seen in one patient leading to the formation of pseudomeningocele. This patient later presented with discharge and required further surgeries. One patient reported to have deteriorated motor power postoperatively.

Compared to the above-mentioned schwannomas, intramedullary schwannomas are very rare. Only 9 cases (male 4, female 6) were seen between 1995 and 2010 and they accounted for 2.7% of all spinal cord schwannomas [5]. They all underwent surgery: GTR was achieved in 8 and STR in 2. In those with STR, the magnetic resonance imaging (MRI) showed no interval change in the residual tumors during their 45- and 55-month follow-up. Overall, the Japanese Orthopedic Association (JOA) score significantly improved ($p < 0.01$) postoperatively. However, 4 patients had remaining motor deficits and 2 had remaining sensory disturbance.

(Unpublished data).

20.1.4 Extra-Arachnoidal

20.1.4.1 Meningioma

A total of 38 patients (male 7, female 31) were reviewed with spinal canal meningioma [6]. Thirty-four cases were located in intradural space, 2 in epidural and 2 in intradural and extradural space. All underwent microsurgical resection: GTR in 32 and STR in 6. Using the Simpson grading, 10 achieved Gr I resection, Grade II in 17, Gr III in 4, and Gr 6 in 4. The extent of resection was not clear for one patient as he underwent surgery at other hospitals.

During the average follow-up of 73 months, no radiological evidence of tumor recurrence was seen in patients with Simpson Gr I, II, or III resection. Six recurrence cases were observed; 5 patients with Gr IV resection and one with an unknown extent of resection. Five recurrence cases underwent one additional surgery and one case proven to be malignant meningioma underwent two additional surgeries.

No immediate postoperative death occurred but two patients died of progression of malignant meningioma. Two cases of postoperative CSF leakage were reported and the other two had worsened neurological status after the surgery.

Kim et al. performed a retrospective review in 20 patients who had Simpson grade II removal of spinal meningiomas [7]. They reviewed the final neurological status and tumor recurrence rates of patients and compared them to those of patients with Simpson grade I removal of meningiomas. No neurological deterioration was observed in patients with Simpson grade II removal and only one patient had a recurrent tumor 92 months postoperatively. These results lead the authors to suggest that Simpson grade II removal may be an alternative option to Simpson grade I removal if the risk of complications is likely to be high with Simpson grade I removal.

20.2 Dural Tumors

20.2.1 Solitary Fibrous Tumor/Hemangiopericytoma

Due to its rarity, only 6 cases of primary solitary fibrous tumor/hemangiopericytoma have been seen at our institute between 2010 and 2017. Five patients had grade II tumors and 1 had grade III tumor. Overall, GTR was achieved in 4 cases and STR in 2. Those 2 patients with STR both showed regrowth of tumor in 58 months and 6 months, respectively. The patient with anaplastic solitary fibrous tumor underwent the first surgery at other hospitals and the immediate postoperative MRI scan showed no evidence of residual tumor. However, lower extremity pain occurred 65 months after the initial operation and the follow-up MRI showed an IDEM tumor at a different spinal level. The pathological examination confirmed a diagnosis of anaplastic solitary fibrous tumor and the patient received adjuvant radiotherapy. 2.5 year postoperatively, the patient remained asymptomatic with no evidence of recurrence in the follow-up MRIs.

(Unpublished data).

20.3 Extradural Tumors

20.3.1 Schwannoma

Schwannomas originating outside the dural sac can mimic the symptoms of IDEM or dumbbell-shaped schwannoma. From March 2010 to December 2014, 4 foraminal schwannomas and 5 paraspinal schwannomas were seen. The main presenting symptoms of the patients were pain and sensory change, which were the same as the symptoms of patients with IDEM or dumbbell shaped. Surgical removal was attempted in all cases but only one foraminal case and 3 paraspinal cases were resected completely. Three foraminal schwannomas achieved STR and 2 paraspinal schwannomas had STR and NTR, each of 9 extradural schwannoma patients, symptoms improved or remained unchanged in 8. Only one patient reported worsened symptoms postoperatively but they returned back to the preoperative status. One complication was seen: A patient with paraspinal schwannoma had VA tear intraoperatively and the VA was sutured. The patient made a full recovery without neurological deficits.

(Unpublished data).

20.3.2 Neurofibroma

Between 2012 and 2017, 11 patients with spinal neurofibroma were identified. Three of them had previously diagnosed neurofibromatosis type I (NF1) and one had neurofibromatosis type 2 (NF2). One patient was suspected to have NF1 but the clinical information was incomplete. The rest of them did not have NF1 or NF2. All but one had dumbbell-shaped tumor. The patient with NF2 had multiple IDEM tumors in the lumbar region. Initially, schwannomas were suspected but the pathological examination revealed that they were neurofibromas.

They all underwent surgery. GTR was achieved in 8 patients, STR in 3. Neurological status improved or remained stationary in 8. Three patients reported deterioration of their symptoms: two patients had reduced motor power and one reported worsening pain. Reoperation was performed in one patient due to postoperative CSF leakage.

Tumor recurrence was seen in one patient but the patient was treated conservatively as she remained symptom free. In patients with STR of tumors, the lesions remained unchanged in the follow-up MRIs.

(Unpublished data).

References

1. Kim MS, Chung CK, Kim HJ, Kim SS, Choe G, Chi JG. Long term results of adult spinal cord astrocytoma. J Korean Nuerosurg Soc 2002;35:234–40.
2. Kim MS, Chung CK, Choe GY, Kim IH, Kim HJ. Intramedullary spinal cord astrocytoma in adults: postoperative outcome. J Neurooncol. 2001;52(1):85–94.
3. Lee SH, Chung CK, Kim CH, Yoon SH, Hyun SJ, et al. Long-term outcomes of surgical resection with or without adjuvant radiation therapy for treatment of spinal ependymoma: a retrospective multicenter study by the Korea Spinal Oncology Research Group. Neuro Oncol. 2013;15(7):921–9.
4. Lee DK, Choe WJ, Chung CK, Kim HJ. Spinal cord hemangioblastoma: surgical strategy and clinical outcome. J Neuroonco 3003;61:27–34.
5. Lee SE, Chung CK, Kim HJ. Intramedullary schwannomas: long-term outcomes of ten operated cases. J Neuroonco. 2013;113:75–81.
6. Yoon SH, Chung CK, Jahng TA. Surgical outcome of spinal canal meningioma. J Korean Nuerosurg Soc. 2007;42:300–4.
7. Kim CH, Chung CK, Lee SH, Jahng TA, Hyun SJ, et al. Long-term recurrence rates after the removal of spinal meningiomas in relations to Simpson grades.

The Future Direction to Improve the Outcome of Surgery for Spinal Cord Tumors

21

Chun Kee Chung

Abstract

At present, the concept of compartmentalization is helpful in surgery for spinal cord tumors. However, in near future, the following advancements could further improve the outcome, including optics for better visualizing the tumor, physiological tools for better delineation of the individual tracts, genomic input for understanding tumorigenesis of spinal cord tumors, and finally better understanding of the natural history.

Keywords

Optics · Physiology · Tumorigenesis · Natural history

C. K. Chung (✉)
Department of Neurosurgery, Seoul National University Hospital, Seoul National University College of Medicine, Seoul, Republic of Korea
e-mail: chungc@snu.ac.kr

Neuroscience Research Institute, Seoul National University Medical Research Center, Seoul, Republic of Korea

Clinical Research Institute, Seoul National University Hospital, Seoul, Republic of Korea

Department of Brain and Cognitive Sciences, Seoul National University College of Natural Sciences, Seoul, Republic of Korea

This book emphasizes the concept of compartment in surgery for spinal cord tumors. With the current technologies at hand, the addition and application of the concept of compartmentalization is definitely helpful to improve the outcome of surgery for spinal cord tumors. However, still we have limitations which need to be improved.

When a certain spinal cord tumor developed and is confined to one compartment, we neurosurgeons could remove that tumor without incurring any more damage to the neighboring structures at least theoretically. In that sense, surgery of the spinal cord tumor is not any more a kind of wait and see surgery. We could expect its outcome with a reasonable accuracy.

However, we still have a formidable limitation in the tumor which does not abide by the compartment. Representative is the malignant tumors, although it is not limited to malignant tumors. One of the examples is neurofibromas, particularly plexiform type, since it follows the nerves, but does not grow in a globoid form. It has a tendency to extend through the normal nerve fibers. Hence, although we could remove the neurofibromas, there always remains a possibility that a tumor remnant would be left behind. The most important difference between the systemic tumors and spinal cord tumors is that spinal cord is indispensable. If we resect a portion of the normal spinal cord with its appendages, there is always a consequence. Only in a small portion of tumors without evident

C. K. Chung (ed.), *Surgery of Spinal Cord Tumors Based on Anatomy*,
https://doi.org/10.1007/978-981-15-7771-0_21

compartmentalization, we could achieve marginal resection if the involved part is dispensable such as dura or nerve roots. Here we could proceed the surgery with results expected and acceptable by patients if we discuss the following risk preoperatively.

The whole chapters of this book emphasize the concept of compartment. Up until the present moment, our surgery heavily relies upon the operative microscope which provides us an excellent illumination and magnification. However, the future would lie on the technologies which may replace or compete with operative microscope. Most promising technology in the horizon is the endo- or exoscopy with high resolution (at least over 4 K resolution) and 3D. However, even with the popularity of endo- or exoscopy, there would remain a room for a conventional microscopy, which still could provide a much higher resolution, enabling the most dexterous surgery possible, particularly for the surgery using fine anatomy of compartment. However, the technology providing the visualization of fiber tracts could change the whole game, since the outcome of surgery of spinal cord tumors is dependent upon how we could save the normal tracts and remove the tumor only. Hence, the need for such technology is immense. I have an opinion that the current development of optics could fill the gap. Firstly I am looking for the optical computed tomography as the candidate. It has a potential to change our practice as it changed the ophthalmology. Also confocal microscope or two-photon microscope are looming in the horizon. However, those tools providing higher magnification beyond the human visuomotor capacity has their own constraint, which delimit their application to the clinical theater.

Aforementioned comment is from an anatomical perspective. From the physiological perspective, I wholeheartedly feel that the current mapping technology is at its infancy. There is a lack of mapping tracts in the spinal cord, although we are using several evoked potential and electromyography monitoring. Dorsal column mapping should be the starting point of such an endeavor. Combined with anatomical imaging such as birefringence imaging, in near future we are going to map almost all tracts we are aware of and determinant for the functional outcome postoperative.

For malignant IM cord tumors, surgery has a limited value, since it could not change the outcome as we expect it should. To improve its outcome, we need to understand its biology. Usually they do not abide by the compartment. They are not pushing the normal structure, but invading the normal structures with intermixing. Hence, we are not certain whether we remove the tumor only and save the normal structure. Also since the spinal cord is indispensable in our lives, we could not resect the spinal cord with tumors. The traditional concept of marginal resection is not applicable to the spinal cord surgery. Now it becomes consensus that in low grade gliomas in the brain, the extent of resection is critical for the survival. The more we resect, the better the outcome. To achieve that goal, we should devise a better tool to visualize the normal structure mixed with tumors. Here I stress that visualizing the normal structure should be more emphasized than visualizing tumors.

As far as we know, the spinal cord resembles neural tube most than any other central nervous structures. The malignant tumor in the spinal cord would represent the whole spectrum of central nervous tumors. However, there are dearth of genetic studies in the spinal cord tumors. In the following years, I would expect there would be a plethora of genomic data from the spinal cord tumors. Also once we understand the tumorigenesis and its biological behavior, we may have a better tools to hinder its devastating effect. I presume that the trial from the spinal cord tumors would easily translate to the whole central nervous tumors, since the spinal cord is the prototype of whole central nervous structures. Particularly I am interested in molecular changes in tumor cell of origin and geno-phenotyping. Once we achieve some success in the spinal cord tumors, then we are in a sense prepared to address the brainstem tumors, which is in a worse shape than spinal cord tumors in terms of treatment. The translation from the spinal cord tumors to brainstem tumors makes more sense than that from brain tumors to brainstem tumors, since as I wrote above understanding the prototype here spinal cord tumors is much easier than understanding the end product here brain tumors.

To make a real advance in malignant spinal cord tumors, we need a better systemic treatment modality. We have failed to devise a systemic treatment even in tumors with well-known genetic background, including neurofibromatosis, von Hippel-Lindau disease, and multiple CNS cavernous angiomas. In the near future, I expect we would have a better systemic treatment modalities for these entities.

Last but not least, we have to have a better understanding for the natural history of spinal cord tumors. We have the issue of incidental tumors with advancement and popularity of imaging studies. However, pure lack of understanding of natural history makes us feel uneasy for whether to proceed to surgery, when to have a surgery, how to follow-up, (and) what the risk–benefit would be, etc.

To wit, I expect the future treatment of spinal cord tumors will be changed with advancement of optics for better visualizing the tumor, physiological tools for better delineation of the individual tracts, genomic input for understanding tumorigenesis of spinal cord tumors, which is a prototype of all central nervous tumors, and finally with better understanding of the natural history, which enables us to make better professional opinion.

I hope the next edition of this book could incorporate the advancement which I have mentioned above.

Index

C. K. Chung (ed.), *Surgery of Spinal Cord Tumors Based on Anatomy*,
https://doi.org/10.1007/978-981-15-7771-0